PREVENTIVE CARDIOLOGY

SECOND EDITION

CONTEMPORARY CARDIOLOGY

CHRISTOPHER P. CANNON, MD
SERIES EDITOR-IN-CHIEF
ANNEMARIE M. ARMANI, MD
EXECUTIVE EDITOR

PREVENTIVE CARDIOLOGY

Insights Into the Prevention and Treatment of Cardiovascular Disease

Second Edition

Edited by

JOANNE MICALE FOODY, MD

Section of Cardiovascular Medicine, Department of Internal Medicine, Yale University School of Medicine, New Haven, CT

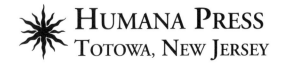

HUMANA PRESS
TOTOWA, NEW JERSEY

© 2006 Humana Press Inc.
999 Riverview Drive, Suite 208
Totowa, New Jersey 07512

www.humanapress.com

Production Editor: Melissa Caravella

Cover design by Patricia F. Cleary

Cover Illustration: From Fig. 2 in Chapter 1, "The Unstable Plaque: *Implications and Opportunities for Prevention,*" by JoAnne Micale Foody and Steven E. Nissen.

For additional copies, pricing for bulk purchases, and/or information about other Humana titles, contact Humana at the above address or at any of the following numbers: Tel.: 973-256-1699; Fax: 973-256-8341, E-mail: orders@humanapr.com; or visit our Website: www.humanapress.com

This publication is printed on acid-free paper. ∞
ANSI Z39.48-1984 (American National Standards Institute) Permanence of Paper for Printed Library Materials.

Printed in the United States of America. 10 9 8 7 6 5 4 3 2 1

eIBSN 1-59745-096-0

Library of Congress Cataloging-in-Publication Data

Preventive cardiology : insights into the prevention and treatment of
    cardiovascular disease / edited by JoAnne Micale Foody. -- 2nd ed.
       p. ; cm. -- (Contemporary cardiology)
    Includes bibliographical references and index.
    ISBN 1-58829-521-4 (alk. paper)
    1. Coronary heart disease--Prevention. 2. Coronary heart disease
--Risk factors. 3. Coronary heart disease--Pathophysiology. I. Foody,
JoAnne Micale. II. Series: Contemporary cardiology (Totowa, N.J. :
Unnumbered)
    [DNLM: 1. Coronary Arteriosclerosis--therapy. 2. Coronary Arterio-
sclerosis--prevention & control. 3. Coronary Arteriosclerosis--physio-
pathology. 4. Risk Factors. WG 300 P9457 2006]
RC685.C6P675 2006
616.1'23--dc22

2005033068

PREFACE

Preventive cardiology is a fast moving field that places emphasis on the prevention and treatment of coronary disease. *Preventive Cardiology: Insights Into the Prevention and Treatment of Cardiovascular Disease, Second Edition* is intended for clinical cardiologists, internists, primary care providers, and allied health care professionals who wish to extend their knowledge and expertise in the rapidly expanding field of preventive cardiology. It is the mission of this book to provide clinicians with the understanding and tools necessary to implement prevention in their daily practices.

Recent changes in the delivery of health care in the United States and abroad, in conjunction with new scientific evidence supporting the role of preventive strategies in the maintenance of cardiovascular health, have focused new attention and efforts on the field of cardiovascular disease prevention. The field of cardiology is thus making a gradual transition from the technology-driven, intervention-oriented perspective of the last several decades to a new, preventive, molecular-based perspective. As fresh evidence amasses that preventive measures produce a considerable decrease in the incidence of both primary and secondary cardiac events and mortality, there is growing, widespread acknowledgment that health care providers from all arenas must initiate preventive strategies in the management and care of their patients.

Preventive Cardiology: Insights Into the Prevention and Treatment of Cardiovascular Disease, Second Edition hopes to provide clinicians with both the knowledge and expertise to incorporate preventive strategies into their everyday practices. It will not only provide practical information for the management of patients at risk for cardiovascular disease, but also offer an overview of the new paradigms in the pathophysiology of coronary artery disease (CAD). The first part of the book focuses on the atherosclerotic process, the important central role of the endothelium in the maintenance of cardiovascular health, and the role of inflammation in CAD. This section provides a novel current perspective on important emerging concepts in the pathophysiology of coronary atherosclerosis.

The second part focuses on traditional cardiovascular risk factors and provides insights into gender-specific aspects of CAD risk. These insights offer thorough, concise reviews of the various risk factors with preventive strategies outlined for the clinician. The final part of the book provides an overview of approaches for the identification of patients at risk for CAD events and reviews of stress testing in patients with CAD and the important role of antiplatelets in coronary disease. Finally, given the imperatives of cost-containment and health care resource allocation, a chapter on pharmacoeconomics of preventive strategies is included. The goal of *Preventive Cardiology: Insights Into the Prevention and Treatment of Cardiovascular Disease, Second Edition* is to provide an overview of the exciting opportunities to prevent the progression, and in some instances to regress the process, of coronary atherosclerosis and incorporate these strategies into the daily practice of clinical medicine.

JoAnne Micale Foody, MD

CONTENTS

PART III STRATEGIES FOR PREVENTION

CONTRIBUTORS

GORDON G. BLACKBURN, PhD • *Department of Cardiology, Cardiac Health Improvement and Rehabilitation Program, The Cleveland Clinic Foundation, Cleveland, OH*

ROBYN BERGMAN BUCHSBAUM, MHS, CHES • *Formerly Affiliated with The Heart Center, The Cleveland Clinic Foundation, Cleveland, OH*

JEFFREY CRAIG BUCHSBAUM, MD, PhD • *Department of Radiation Oncology and Department of Pediatrics, Milton S. Hershey Medical Center, Penn State University College of Medicine, Hershey, PA*

MATTHEW M. BURG, PhD • *Section of Cardiovascular Medicine, Yale University School of Medicine, New Haven CT*

CHRISTOPHER R. COLE, MD • *Colorado Cardiac Alliance Research Institute, Colorado Springs Cardiologists, Colorado Springs, CO*

RON COREY, PhD, MBA, RPH • *Department of Economic Strategies, Pharmacia Corporation, Peapack, NJ*

JOANNE MICALE FOODY, MD • *Section of Cardiovascular Medicine, Department of Internal Medicine, Yale University School of Medicine, New Haven, CT*

JOSEPH P. FROLKIS, MD, PhD, FACP • *Department of Preventive Medicine, New Milford Hospital, New Milford, CT*

MARGARITA R. GARCES, MD • *Department of Rheumatology, University of Miami, Miami, FL*

BRENDON L. GRAEBER, MD • *Section of Cardiovascular Medicine, Yale University School of Medicine, New Haven, CT*

BYRON J. HOOGWERF, MD • *Section of Preventive Cardiology, Department of Cardiology, Department of Endocrinology, Diabetes & Metabolism, The Cleveland Clinic Foundation, Cleveland, OH*

MICHAEL A. LAUER, MD • *Division of Cardiology, William Beaumont Hospital, Royal Oak, MI*

MICHAEL S. LAUER, MD • *Section of Cardiology, Cleveland Clinic Foundation, Cleveland, OH*

ERIC H. LIEBERMAN, MD • *Director of Research Department, South Florida Heart Institute, Delray Beach, FL*

FRANCISCO LOPEZ-JIMENEZ, MD, MSc • *Department of Cardiology, Mayo Clinic, Rochester, MN*

ANDREW I. MACKINNON, MD • *Department of Cardiology, Wilford Hall Medical Center, Lackland Air Force Base, San Antonio, TX*

WILLIAM F. MCGHAN, PharmD, PhD • *Graduate Program in Pharmacy Administration, University of the Sciences, Philadelphia, PA*

SCOTT A. MOORE, MD • *Department of Cardiology, Wilford Hall Medical Center, Lackland Air Force Base, San Antonio, TX*

KRISTINE NAPIER, RD, MPH • *Registered Chef and Dietician, Madison, WI*

STEVEN E. NISSEN, MD • *Section of Cardiology, Cleveland Clinic Foundation, Cleveland, OH*

MELANIE OATES, PhD, MBA, RN • *Philadelphia College of Pharmacy, University of the Sciences, Philadelphia, PA*

JOHN F. SETARO, MD • *Section of Cardiovascular Medicine, Yale University School of Medicine, New Haven, CT*

RAHMAN SHAH, MD • *Section of Cardiovascular Medicine, Yale University School of Medicine, New Haven, CT*

GREGORY M. SINGER, MD • *Section of Cardiovascular Medicine, Yale University School of Medicine, New Haven, CT*

AARON SOUFER • *Yale University School of Medicine, New Haven, CT*

ROBERT S. SOUFER, MD • *Section of Cardiovascular Medicine, Yale University School of Medicine, New Haven, CT*

STEVEN R. STEINHUBL, MD • *Division of Cardiovascular Medicine, University of Kentucky, Lexington, KY*

I NEW PARADIGMS IN THE PATHOPHYSIOLOGY OF CORONARY ARTERY DISEASE

1

The Unstable Plaque
Implications and Opportunities for Prevention

JoAnne Micale Foody, MD *and Steven E. Nissen,* MD

CONTENTS

INTRODUCTION

During this past decade, clinical trials have added to our understanding of the pathophysiology and prevention of coronary atherosclerosis. Evidence is accumulating that cholesterol lowering has immediate consequences that may favorably affect the coronary atheroma and subsequent coronary events. Intravascular ultrasound (IVUS) provides a new modality by which to better understand the atheroma.

CORONARY HEART DISEASE: AN OVERVIEW

In the United States, approx 14 million adults have a current diagnosis of coronary heart disease (CHD) *(1)*. One-third of the 1.5 million individuals who experience myocardial infarctions each year will die. The estimates of the financial costs (i.e., treatment and lost wages) that are associated with CHD in Americans range between $50 billion and $100 billion per year *(1,2)*. Although the incidence of death from CHD has decreased in the United States, the total number of deaths from CHD has recently begun to increase

From: *Contemporary Cardiology: Preventive Cardiology:*
Insights Into the Prevention and Treatment of Cardiovascular Disease, Second Edition
Edited by: J. M. Foody © Humana Press Inc., Totowa, NJ

after a previous steady decline. Most likely, this is the result of the increased number of middle-aged and elderly people in the population. Clearly, primary and secondary CHD prevention measures that are more effective are required. CHD prevention in the future will be the result of the ground-breaking research that has been conducted during the past 25 yr. For example, in the 1970s, data from the Framingham Epidemiological Study demonstrated that increases in serum cholesterol levels in the general population were associated with an increased risk of death from CHD *(3–5)*. In 1988, the National Cholesterol Education Program (NCEP) identified elevated low-density lipoprotein cholesterol (LDL-C) as a primary risk factor for CHD *(6)*. In the 1993 NCEP Adult Treatment Panel II Report, this conclusion was further strengthened by the addition of aggressive dietary and drug therapy recommendations for patients with known CHD *(2)*. In 1995, Gould and associates reported meta-analysis data on 35 randomized clinical trials that lasted longer than 2 yr and were designed to reduce serum cholesterol levels *(7)*. They concluded that for every 10 percentage points of cholesterol lowering, CHD mortality was reduced by 13% ($p < 0.002$) and total mortality by 10% ($p < 0.03$). According to the most recently reported US National Health and Nutrition Examination Survey III, an estimated 5.5 million Americans with CHD should be treated with lipid-lowering medications under the NCEP guidelines *(8)*. Presently, less than one-third of those CHD patients who require lipid-lowering medications actually receive treatment, and only a small proportion of those who do receive treatment achieve NCEP target levels *(1)*. In controlled clinical trials, hydroxymethylglutaryl (HMG)-coenzyme A (CoA) reductase inhibitors have been shown to lower total and LDL-C levels; decrease CHD-related morbidity and mortality in patients with CHD; and slow progression of, and, in some cases, cause regression of coronary atherosclerosis *(1,7,9,10)*.

During the past decade, new scientific evidence strongly supporting the role of preventive interventions in the maintenance of health has focused much needed attention and efforts on cardiovascular prevention. New trials of lipid lowering have added to our understanding of the pathophysiology and prevention of coronary atherosclerosis *(11–19)*. As this new evidence is amassing, there is widespread acknowledgment that lipid lowering with statins should be a mainstay of treatment for the patient with chronic coronary artery disease (CAD). IVUS is a new imaging study that provides the opportunity to more directly view the atheroma and study its response to risk-factor modification.

PATHOGENESIS OF CAD

Classic theory on the pathogenesis of acute coronary syndromes taught that the atherosclerotic process led to plaque formation and subsequent coronary artery luminal narrowing (Fig. 1). At some point, these lesions developed an overlying platelet-containing thrombus that acutely diminished coronary perfusion and resulted in an acute coronary syndrome. A new paradigm for acute coronary syndromes has emerged. New data suggest that most acute coronary syndromes involve coronary artery segments that do not have high-grade anatomic stenoses documented by recent coronary angiograms *(20)*. Moreover, it seems that less stenotic lesions, characterized by thin fibrous caps, large concentrations of soft lipid accumulations, large numbers of monocytes and macrophages, and depletion of smooth muscle cells, cause the majority of acute events (Fig. 2). These "vulnerable plaques" seem highly prone to rupture, thereby allowing blood to come in contact with highly thrombogenic substances found in the lipid plaque *(20–22)*. Reduction of cholesterol may not only decrease the lipid content of the plaque, but can

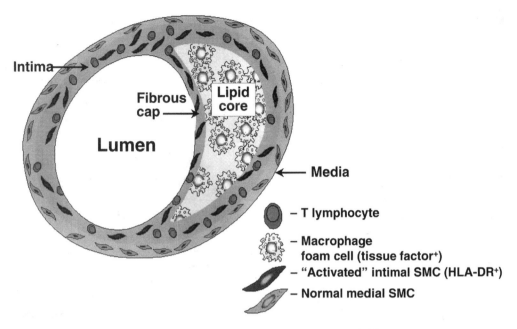

Fibrous cap

Lipid core

Intima

Lumen

Media

– T lymphocyte

– Macrophage
foam cell (tissue factor⁺)

– "Activated" intimal SMC (HLA-DR⁺)

– Normal medial SMC

Fig. 1. Unstable plaque. (Adapted from ref. *20.*)

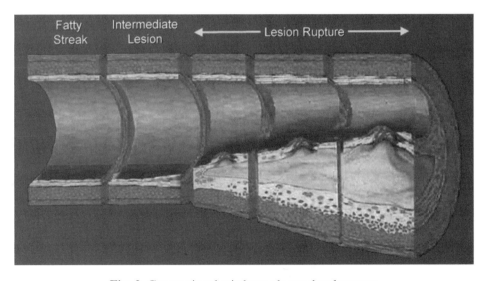

Fatty Streak

Intermediate Lesion

Lesion Rupture

Fig. 2. Conventional wisdom: plaque development.

also reduce the accumulation of monocytes and macrophages, thereby helping to transform these "vulnerable" into less active or "quiescent" plaques *(19,21,22)* (Fig. 3).

This proposed mechanism of plaque stabilization may help to explain why numerous clinical trials using lipid-lowering regimens in patients with CHD have shown that reductions in rates of coronary events and mortality are far greater than would be expected from the results of lesion regression analysis performed using quantitative coronary angiography (QCA) *(4,13,20,23)*. For example, in the Familial Atherosclerosis Treatment Study,

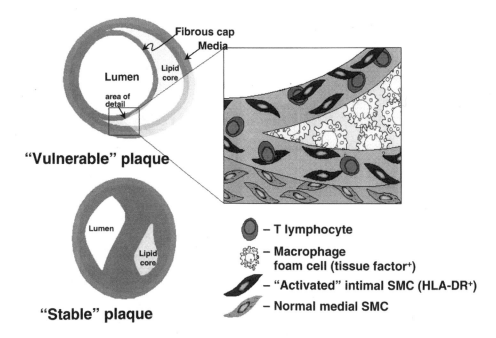

Fig. 3. Unstable vs stable plaque; characteristics of plaques prone to rupture. (Adapted from ref. *20*.)

intensive lipid-lowering therapy improved stenosis severity by less than 2%, and only 12% of lesions showed regression *(24)*. Although the decrease in minimum diameter of the coronary artery was only a fraction of a millimeter, the risk of coronary events decreased by more than 70%. These types of data strongly suggest that the beneficial effects of lipid-lowering therapy on atherosclerotic plaques are complex and dependent on multiple synergistic processes.

CORONARY ARTERY REMODELING IN ATHEROSCLEROSIS

The phenomenon known as "coronary artery remodeling" was first described by Glagov and coworkers *(25)* (Fig. 4). This process results in outward displacement of the external vessel wall in segments with atherosclerosis *(25–28)*. In the early stages of coronary disease, this adventitial enlargement prevents the atheroma from encroaching on the lumen ("positive remodeling"), thereby, concealing the presence of a lesion on contrast angiography. According to pathology studies, lumen reduction may not occur until the plaque occupies more than 40% of the total vessel cross-sectional area *(25)*. Although such lesions do not restrict blood flow, observational studies demonstrate that minimal, nonobstructive angiographic lesions represent an important substrate for acute coronary syndromes *(29)*. It has recently been suggested that coronary lumen reduction can occur either by plaque accumulation that has exceeded the capacity of the adventitia to expand (i.e., exhaustion of "remodeling" potential) or by failure of the adventitia to expand in the presence of a small or moderate plaque burden (i.e., "negative remodeling") *(30–32)*.

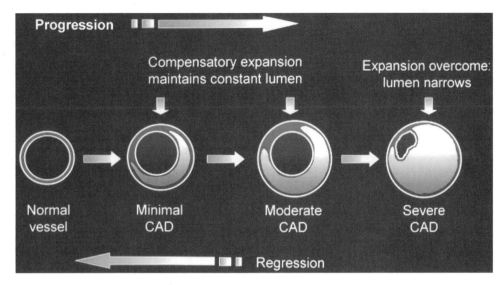

Fig. 4. Glagov's coronary remodeling hypothesis. (Adapted from ref. *25*.)

QUANTITATIVE ANALYSIS OF CORONARY ATHEROSCLEROSIS: THE LIMITS OF OUR CURRENT GOLD STANDARD FOR CHARACTERIZING CAD

The quantification of progression, regression, or development of new coronary athero-sclerotic lesions has traditionally been determined by QCA *(33,34)*. However, coronary angiography provides information regarding the atherosclerotic plaque only when the luminal dimensions of the coronary artery are substantially reduced (Fig. 5). Therefore, subtle changes in atheroma are not detectable. Several multicenter, randomized lipid-lowering trials using both angiographic criteria and clinical assessments have shown improvement in luminal caliber of only 1 to 3%. Yet these same studies demonstrated a 25 to 75% reduction in acute events, including myocardial infarction *(3,35–37)*.

Comparisons of angiography and postmortem specimens have documented that angiog-raphy significantly underestimates the extent of atherosclerosis as compared with postmor-tem histological examination *(38–41)*. Several inherent properties in the methodology can explain the inaccuracy and large observer variability of coronary angiography. An-giography is a two-dimensional imaging modality, depicting complex coronary cross-sectional anatomy as a planar silhouette of the contrast-filled arterial lumen. However, necropsy and IVUS studies demonstrate that coronary lesions are often highly complex, exhibiting markedly distorted or eccentric shapes. Accordingly, arbitrary viewing angles may misrepresent the true extent of luminal narrowing. Although orthogonal angiograms should accurately reflect the severity of many complex lesions, optimal imaging angles are frequently unobtainable because the vessel is obscured by side branches, disease at a bifurcation, or foreshortening *(35)*.

The method most commonly used to assess the severity of angiographic lesions uses visual or computer measurements to determine the percentage of stenosis. This approach compares the luminal diameter within the lesion with the caliber of an adjacent, uninvolved "normal" reference segment. However, necropsy and epicardial echocardiographic exami-

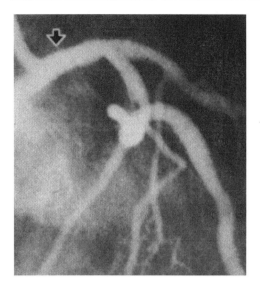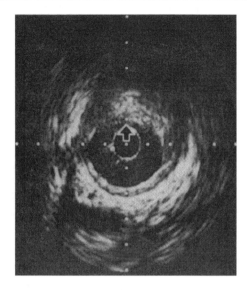

Fig. 5. Angiographically inapparent atheroma. (Figure courtesy of Dr. Steven Nissen.)

nations have demonstrated that coronary atherosclerosis is often diffuse, involving long segments of the diseased vessel *(39–42)*. In many patients, no truly normal segment exists, preventing accurate calculation of diameter reduction *(41,43)*. In the presence of diffuse vessel involvement, determination of percent diameter stenosis will predictably underestimate true disease severity. Diffuse, concentric, and symmetrical coronary disease can affect the entire length of the vessel, resulting in an angiographic appearance of a small artery with minimal luminal irregularities. The limits of this diagnostic modality may be the reason why many of the clinical trials of lipid lowering that used coronary angiography as the endpoint, although having significant reductions in clinical events, were remarkably negative in relation to angiographic findings.

IVUS IMAGING OF CORONARY ARTERIES: A NOVEL VIEW OF THE PLAQUE AND ARTERY WALL

Until recently, atherosclerotic coronary lesions could not be visualized directly by any available imaging modality. Detection of CAD has relied on indirect methods that either evaluate the vessel lumen (angiography) or unmask the ischemic effect of coronary obstructions (nuclear or stress echocardiography). However, both methods are insensitive to the early, minimally obstructive coronary atherosclerosis, the precursor to acute coronary syndromes.

During the last decade, an alternative imaging system, IVUS, has become available and is providing a radically different way to view vascular anatomy *(44–51)*. The incremental value of coronary ultrasound originates from:

1. The cross-sectional, tomographic perspective of the images.
2. The ability to image atheroma directly.

Whereas contrast angiography depicts the complex cross-sectional anatomy of a coronary artery as a planar silhouette, ultrasound permits direct visual examination of the vessel wall, allowing the precise measurement of atheroma size, distribution, and com-

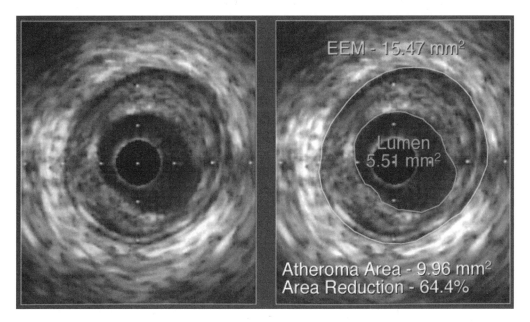

Fig. 6. Standard IVUS atheroma measurements: boundaries. (Figure courtesy of Dr. Steven Nissen.)

position. The tomographic orientation of ultrasound enables 360° visualization of the vessel wall, rather than a two-dimensional projection of the lumen. Direct planimetry can now be performed on a cross-sectional image, which, unlike contrast angiography, is not dependent on the projection angle. Unlike angiographic stenosis sizing, which requires careful calibration of the analysis system to correct for radiographic magnification, ultrasound imaging systems overlay an internal electronic distance scale on the image. Because the velocity of sound in soft tissues is almost constant, ultrasound measurements are accurate and do not require special calibration methods *(52)* (Fig. 6).

In general, normal contrast coronary angiograms are present in 10–15% of patients undergoing angiography for suspected CAD *(53)*. However, using IVUS, Erbel and colleagues have observed that atherosclerotic changes are present in 48% of patients with suspected CAD and a normal coronary angiogram *(53)*. Alfonso and coworkers have demonstrated that, in patients undergoing coronary angioplasty, 80% of the angiographically normal proximal coronary segments have atheroma *(54)*. Typically, these plaques often had a semilunar shape and did not disrupt the luminal contour. Often, atherosclerotic changes in coronary arteries are detected angiographically only when the plaque occupies more than 40% of the potential vessel lumen *(55)*. Therefore, using IVUS, it is not surprising that the "lesion count" is often 10-fold greater than by contrast angiography. As originally noted by Glagov et al., adventitial remodeling blunts changes in luminal size during progression of atherosclerosis *(25,56–59)*. IVUS can show increases or decreases in the atheroma area despite changes in the adventitial size *(27,28,55,57–59)*. In addition, IVUS can increase our understanding of "positive" vs "negative" remodeling on the natural history of CAD. As a result, one can expect that an in vivo study of coronary atherosclerosis progression and/or regression can be best shown by serial IVUS examinations *(78)*. Additionally, IVUS should permit evaluation of atheroma regression or progression using a smaller sample size than would be necessary using either contrast angiography or clinical events.

LIPID LOWERING AND REGRESSION: THE LIMITS OF ANGIOGRAPHIC TRIALS

A number of small trials have evaluated the effect of aggressive lipid lowering on actual vessel blockage. These so-called regression trials assessed the degree of atherosclerotic progression and regression by either ultrasonography of the carotid arteries or, more often, by coronary angiography (18,19). Two important observations were made from these trials. First, although lesion regression was uncommon, the rate of lesion progression was often slowed appreciably. Second, the modest degree of change in vascular endpoints has been disproportionate to the substantial reductions in clinical events observed in some regression trials. These observations suggest that mechanisms beyond change in lumen size may account for impressive clinical benefits. Several factors may mediate the risk for plaque rupture, including the functional state of the vascular endothelium and the morphological and biochemical makeup of the atherosclerotic plaque.

The small changes in luminal narrowing observed with lowering total cholesterol are unlikely to be the principal mechanism by which lipid lowering achieves a reduction in clinical events and revascularization rates. Endothelium-dependent vasomotor function and the cellular characteristics of plaques that seem to be intimately related to rupture and thrombosis are factors that might explain the clinical success after correcting the dyslipidemias.

Regression Growth Evaluation Statin Study

The Regression Growth Evaluation Statin Study (REGRESS) (18) treated 885 hypercholesterolemic men with either pravastatin or a placebo for 2 yr. The 778 (88%) patients had a final angiogram adequate for QCA. Patients had moderate hypercholesterolemia at entry (total cholesterol, 155–310 mg/dL). The mean segment diameter worsened by 0.10 mm in the placebo group and worsened by 0.06 mm in the pravastatin group, which represents a significant ($p = 0.02$) reduction in the rate of progression. The median minimum obstruction diameter decreased 0.09 in the placebo group vs 0.03 mm in the pravastatin group ($p = 0.001$). Patients in the lowest quartile of LDL-C (85–147 mg/dL) had the greatest reduction in progression of atherosclerotic disease. At the end of the follow-up period, 89% of the pravastatin patients and 81% of the placebo patients were without new cardiovascular events. There was a 57% reduction in the need for percutaneous transluminal coronary angioplasty (PTCA) in the pravastatin-treated group ($p < 0.001$). From REGRESS, it may be concluded that, in symptomatic men with significant CHD and normal-to-moderately elevated serum cholesterol, small but significant changes by QCA were noted. There was less progression of coronary atherosclerosis and fewer new cardiovascular events in the group treated with pravastatin than in the placebo group.

Pravastatin Limitation of Atherosclerosis in the Coronary Arteries

The Pravastatin Limitation of Atherosclerosis in the Coronary Arteries study was conducted in 480 male patients with CHD documented by coronary angiography (19). These patients, with LDL-C levels between 130 and 190 mg/dL (mean LDL-C = 164 mg/dL), were treated with either pravastatin or placebo for 3 yr. Pravastatin decreased total cholesterol by 19% and LDL-C by 28% ($p \leq 0.001$ vs placebo for both). Pravastatin reduced progression of atherosclerosis by 40% for minimal vessel diameter ($p = 0.04$), particularly in lesions with less than 50% stenosis at baseline. There were fewer new lesions in patients assigned pravastatin compared with placebo ($p < 0.03$).

Although no significant differences were evident for change in mean vessel diameter and percent vessel diameter stenosis between the pravastatin and placebo groups, a striking 60% reduction in risk of myocardial infarction was noted during active treatment ($p < 0.05$), with the benefit beginning to emerge after 1 yr. Thus, in patients with CHD and mild-to-moderate cholesterol elevations, pravastatin reduces progression of coronary atherosclerosis and myocardial infarction. These effects were most marked in mild lesions (<50% diameter stenosis at baseline) and in preventing new lesion formation.

CLINICAL TRIALS OF LIPID LOWERING WITH HMG-CoA REDUCTASE INHIBITORS

Conclusive evidence from rigorous, large-scale, randomized clinical trials, such as the Scandinavian Simvastatin Survival Study (4S) *(11–14)*, the Cholesterol and Recurrent Events (CARE) *(16,17)* and the West of Scotland Coronary Prevention Study (WOSCOPS) *(15)* has further strengthened the position of lipid-lowering strategies in clinical medicine (Fig. 7; Table 1).

The landmark 4S *(11–14)* randomized 4444 patients with CHD to either simvastatin (20–40 mg/d) or placebo. Significantly, therapy with simvastatin resulted in a 35% reduction in LDL-C, a 25% reduction in total cholesterol, a 42% reduction in CHD mortality, a 34% reduction in the risk of coronary events, a 37% reduction in the requirement of coronary bypass grafting or PTCA, a 30% reduction in cerebrovascular events, and, finally, an impressive 30% reduction in the risk of total mortality. Coronary event reduction was seen across all baseline LDL-C levels. The impact of simvastatin on CHD, which was evident after 1 yr of therapy, was significant at 1.5 yr and increased steadily thereafter. These results translate into a 16% reduction in CHD mortality and a 12% reduction in total mortality for each 10% reduction in levels in total cholesterol. The 4S study was the first major secondary prevention study to show a reduction in total mortality and major coronary events in CHD patients receiving lipid-lowering therapy.

WOSCOPS *(15)* was a primary prevention trial of 6595 men, with an age range of 45 to 64 yr and no history of myocardial infarction, randomized to either pravastatin (40 mg/d) or placebo. At entry, participants had moderate hypercholesterolemia (mean total cholesterol, 272 mg/dL; and mean LDL-C, 192 mg/dL). In this study, participants receiving pravastatin had 20% lower total cholesterol and 26% lower LDL-C, a 33% lower risk of death from CHD, a 31% reduction in the risk for the combined primary endpoint of definite nonfatal myocardial infarction and CHD death. A risk reduction of 22% was noted for total mortality ($p = 0.051$), as was a 32% risk reduction for death from all cardiovascular causes ($p = 0.033$). In this population, there was a reduction of 37% in the rate of coronary revascularization procedures ($p = 0.009$). WOSCOPS was the first major study to use an HMG-CoA reductase inhibitor in primary prevention and to demonstrate the clinical benefit of lipid lowering for CHD in this population.

The CARE trial *(16,17)* was a 5-yr study of treatment with pravastatin (40 mg/d) or placebo in 4159 patients with myocardial infarction. At entry, total cholesterol levels were less than 240 mg/dL and LDL-C levels were between 115 and 174 mg/dL (mean, 139 mg/dL), representing a moderate risk population. Compared with placebo, pravastatin resulted in a 30% reduction in LDL-C (from 139 mg/dL to 97 mg/dL), a 24% reduction in the primary endpoint of fatal coronary event or a nonfatal myocardial infarction ($p = 0.003$), and a 20% reduction in CHD mortality. There was also a 26% reduction in the requirement of coronary bypass grafting ($p = 0.005$) and a 23% reduction in the need for

Primary Prevention	Secondary Prevention
WOSCOPS	4S
AFCAPS/TexCAPS	CARE LIPID

LDL-c

Fig. 7. Lipid-lowering trials.

Table 1
Major Primary and Secondary Prevention Trials, Endpoints, and Risk Reduction

Study	Intervention	Endpoint	Risk reduction (%)
Primary prevention trials			
WOSCOPS	Pravastatin	Fatal CAD/nonfatal MI	31
		Total mortality	22
AFCAPS/TEXCAPS	Mevacor	Fatal CAD/nonfatal MI	36

Study	Intervention	Endpoint	Event rate/5 yr (%)		Risk reduction (%)
Secondary prevention trials					
4S	Simvastatin	Total mortality	11.5	8.2	30
		Fatal CAD/nonfatal MI	28.0	19.0	44
CARE	Pravastin	Fatal CAD/nonfatal MI	13.2	10.2	24
LIPID	Pravastatin	CAD mortality	n/a	n/a	34

PTCA ($p = 0.01$). Of note, there was a 31% reduction in cerebrovascular events ($p = 0.03$). No significant differences in overall mortality or mortality from noncardiovascular causes was found. The reduction in coronary events was greater in patients with higher baseline LDL-C levels. The benefits of pravastatin are first measurable 12 to 18 mo after initiation of therapy. The CARE trial extended the benefit of cholesterol-lowering therapy with an HMG-CoA reductase inhibitor to the majority of patients with CHD who have "average" cholesterol levels.

LDL Lowering and Revascularization

The Atorvastatin Versus Revascularization Treatment (AVERT) *(61)* study provides intriguing data on the role of lipid lowering in the management of patients with mild coronary atherosclerosis. It is known that lipid lowering has been effective in the reduction of percutaneous revascularization rates. In the 4S trial, PTCA was reduced by 37% with aggressive lipid lowering ($p = 0.00001$). Studies of PTCA vs standard therapy, including the Angioplasty Compared to Medicine trial, the Multicentre Anti-Atheroma study, and the Randomized Intervention Treatment of Angina 2 study, have failed to demonstrate a significant reduction in coronary events. Therefore, it was hypothesized that, in a population with mild-to-moderate CAD under consideration for coronary

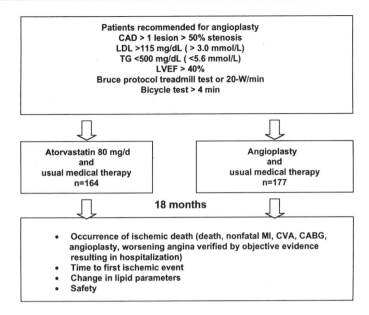

Fig. 8. The AVERT trial: Study design and inclusion criteria. (From ref. *61*.)

revascularization via PTCA, aggressive lipid lowering would provide a significant reduction in clinical events and improved outcomes.

The AVERT trial randomized 341 patients with CAD (one lesion of at least 50% stenosis), LDL-C level greater than 115 mg/dL, left ventricular ejection fraction greater than 40% either to PTCA plus standard care or to medical management and aggressive lipid lowering with 80 mg/dL atorvastatin. Patients with left main CAD or its equivalent of three-vessel CAD were excluded (Fig. 8).

The AVERT trial showed a trend toward improved outcomes with medical therapy and aggressive lipid lowering compared with PTCA plus standard medical care. There was a 13% ischemic event rate in those receiving atorvastatin vs a 21% ischemic event rate in those randomized to PTCA. This represented a 36% reduction in events in the group treated with high-dose atorvastatin, although this did not represent a statistically significant difference ($p = 0.048$) (Fig. 9). In general, high-dose atorvastatin was well tolerated, with only a 2.4% incidence of aspartate aminotransferase or alanine aminotransferase abnormalities (more than three times normal). The AVERT trial was a small, underpowered trial with a short follow-up time. It represents a highly selected population that may not have clinical relevance. It does however, serve as an interesting hypothesis-generating trial that adds insights into the role of lipid lowering in patients undergoing revascularization and points to the potential therapeutic benefits in this subset of patients.

Response of the Atheroma to Lipid Lowering

Given the limits of coronary angiography and the striking disparity between angiographic findings and clinical events noted in the regression trials, it is intriguing to consider the potential role of this new modality to image the atheroma. It is hypothesized that plaque composition and atheroma remodeling may constitute the beneficial effects of lipid lowering. As a two-dimensional image of the coronary lumen, angiography

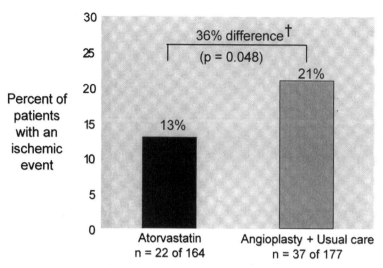

Fig. 9. The AVERT trial: reduction in clinical events. (From ref. *61*.)

cannot provide a view of these changes. IVUS may provide a more powerful tool for understanding these intra-arterial changes. With this in mind, the Reversal of Atherosclerosis with Aggressive Lipid Lowering (REVERSAL) *(62)* study was designed to provide insight into the response of the atheroma to lipid lowering.

The REVERSAL study was a multicenter, double-blind, comparative, parallel trial involving 654 patients. Of these patients, 502 had evaluable IVUS examinations at baseline and after 18 mo of treatment. Patients were randomly assigned to receive a moderate lipid-lowering regimen consisting of 40 mg of pravastatin or an intensive lipid-lowering regimen consisting of 80 mg of atorvastatin. The primary outcome was the percentage change in atheroma volume (follow-up value minus baseline value). In this study, baseline LDL-C level (mean, 150.2 mg/dL [3.89 mmol/L] in both treatment groups) was reduced to 110 mg/dL (2.85 mmol/L) in the pravastatin group and to 79 mg/dL (2.05 mmol/L) in the atorvastatin group ($p < 0.001$). C-reactive protein decreased by 5.2% with pravastatin and by 36.4% with atorvastatin ($p < 0.001$). The primary endpoint (percentage change in atheroma volume) showed a significantly lower progression rate in the atorvastatin (intensive) group ($p = 0.02$). Similar differences between groups were observed for secondary efficacy parameters, including change in total atheroma volume ($p = 0.02$), change in percentage atheroma volume ($p < 0.001$), and change in atheroma volume in the most severely diseased 10-mm vessel subsegment ($p < 0.01$). For the primary endpoint, progression of coronary atherosclerosis occurred in the pravastatin group (2.7%; 95% confidence interval, 0.2% to 4.7%; $p = 0.001$) compared with baseline. Progression did not occur in the atorvastatin group (–0.4%; 95% confidence interval –2.4% to 1.5%; $p = 0.98$) compared with baseline. Thus, the REVERSAL study demonstrates that, for patients with CHD, intensive lipid-lowering treatment with atorvastatin reduced progression of coronary atherosclerosis compared with pravastatin. Compared with baseline values, patients treated with atorvastatin had no change in atheroma burden, whereas patients treated with pravastatin showed progression of coronary atherosclerosis.

CONCLUSION

During the past decade, clinical trials have added to our understanding of the pathophysiology and prevention of coronary atherosclerosis. Evidence is accumulating that cholesterol lowering has immediate consequences that may favorably affect the coronary atheroma and subsequent coronary events. IVUS provides and important new tool for understanding these intra-arterial changes and suggests mechanisms by which plaque may be modified and result in reduced progression of disease.

REFERENCES

1. Eisenberg DA. Cholesterol lowering in the management of coronary artery disease: the clinical implications of recent trials. Am J Med 1998;104(2A):2S–5S.
2. Expert Panel on Detection, Evaluation, and Treatment of High Blood Cholesterol in Adults. Summary of the second report of the national cholesterol education program (NCEP) expert panel on detection, evaluation, and treatment of high blood cholesterol in adults (Adult Treatment Panel II). JAMA 1993;269:3015–3023.
3. Kannel WB. The Framingham Study: an epidemiological investigation of cardiovascular disease, Section 30. Some characteristics related to the incidence of cardiovascular disease and death: the Framingham Study. 18-year follow-up. Department of Health, Education and Welfare, Washington, DC, Publication No. (NIH) 74-599, 1974.
4. Kannel WB. Range of serum cholesterol values in the population developing coronary artery disease. Am J Cardiol 1995;76:69C–77C.
5. Kannel WB, Castelli WP, Gordon T, et al. Lipoprotein cholesterol in the prediction of atherosclerotic disease: new perspectives based on the Framingham Heart Study. Ann Int Med 1979;90:85–91.
6. Report of the National Cholesterol Education Program on detection, evaluation, and treatment of high blood cholesterol in adults. Arch Int Med 1988;148:36–39.
7. Gould AL, Rossouw JE, Santanello NC, et al. Cholesterol reduction yields clinical benefit: a new look at old data. Circulation 1995;91:2274–2282.
8. Sempos CT, Cleeman JI, Carrol MD, et al. Prevalence of high blood cholesterol among US adults. An update based on guidelines from the second report of the National Cholesterol Education Program Adult Treatment Panel. JAMA 1993;269:3009–3014.
9. Hunninghake DB. Therapeutic efficacy of the lipid-lowering armamentarium: the clinical benefits of aggressive lipid-lowering therapy. Am J Cardiol 1998;104(2A):9S–13S.
10. Holme I. Cholesterol reduction and its impact on coronary artery disease and total mortality. Am J Cardiol 1995;76:10C–17C.
11. Scandinavian Simvastatin Survival Study Group. Randomized trial of cholesterol lowering in 4444 patients with coronary heart disease: the Scandinavian Simvastatin Survival Study (4S). Lancet 1994;334:1383–1389.
12. Bertolini S, Bon GB, Campbell LM, et al. Efficacy and safety of atorvastatin compared to pravastatin in patients with hypercholesterolemia. Atherosclerosis 1997;130:191–197.
13. Tonkin AM. Management of the long-term intervention with pravastatin in ischaemic disease (LIPID) study after the Scandinavian simvastatin survival study (4S). Am J Cardiol 1995;76:107C–112C.
14. Gotto AM Jr. Risk factor modification: rationale for management of dyslipidemia. Am J Cardiol 1998;104(2A):6S–8S.
15. Sheperd J, Cobbe SM, Ford I, et al. for the West of Scotland Coronary Prevention Study Group. Prevention of coronary heart disease with pravastatin in men with hypercholesterolemia. N Engl J Med 1996;335:1001–1009.
16. Pfeffer MA, Sacks FM, Lemuel A, et al. Cholesterol and recurrent events: a secondary prevention trial for normolipidemic patients. Am J Cardiol 1995;76:98C–106C.
17. Sacks FM, Pfeffer MA, Moye LA, et al. The effect of pravastatin on coronary events after myocardial infarction in patients with average cholesterol levels. N Engl J Med 1996;335:1001–1009.
18. Jukema JW, Bruschke AV, van Boven AJ, et al. Coronary artery disease/myocardial infarction: effects of lipid lowering by pravastatin on progression and regression of coronary artery disease in symptomatic men with normal to moderately elevated serum cholesterol levels: The Regression Growth Evaluation Statin Study (REGRESS). Circulation 1995;91:2528–2540.

19. Pitt B, Mancini GB, Ellis SG, et al. Pravastatin limitation of atherosclerosis in the coronary arteries (PLAC I): reduction in atherosclerosis progression and clinical events. J Am Coll Cardiol 1995;26:1133–1139.
20. Libby P, Schoenbeck U, Mach F. Current concepts in cardiovascular pathology: the role of LDL cholesterol in plaque rupture and stabilization. Am J Med 1998;104(2A):14S–18S.
21. Tzivoni D, Klein J. Improvement of myocardial ischemia by lipid lowering drugs. Eur Heart J 1998;19:230–234.
22. Massy ZA, Keane WF, Kasiske BL, et al. Inhibition of the mevalonate pathway: benefits beyond cholesterol reduction? Lancet 1996;347:102–103.
23. Rossouw JE. Lipid-lowering interventions in angiographic trials. Am J Cardiol 1995;76:86C–92C.
24. Brown BG. Regression of coronary artery disease as a result of intensive lipid-lowering therapy in men with high levels of apolipoprotein B. N Engl J Med 1990;323:1289–1298.
25. Glagov S, Weisenberg E, Zarins CK. Compensatory enlargement of human coronary arteries. N Engl J Med 1987;316:1371–1375.
26. Zarins CK, Weisenberg E, Kolettis G. Differential enlargement of artery segments in response to enlarging atherosclerotic plaques. J Vasc Surg 1988;7:386–394.
27. Weissman NJ, Mendelsohn FO, Palacios IF, et al. Development of coronary compensatory enlargement in vivo: sequential assessments with intravascular ultrasound. Am Heart J 1995;130:1283–1285.
28. Berglund H, Luo H, Nishioka T, et al. Highly localized arterial remodeling in patients with coronary atherosclerosis: an intravascular ultrasound study. Circulation 1997;96:1470–1476.
29. Little WC, Constaantinescu M, Applegate RJ, et al. Can arteriography predict the site of a subsequent myocardial infarction in patients with mild-to-moderate coronary artery disease? Circulation 1988;78:1157–1166.
30. Pasterkamp G, Wensing PJ, Post MJ, et al. Paradoxical arterial wall shrinkage may contribute to luminal narrowing of human atherosclerotic femoral arteries. Circulation 1995;91:1444–1449.
31. Mintz GS, Kent KM, Pichard AD, et al. Contribution of inadequate arterial remodeling to the development of focal coronary artery stenoses: an intravascular ultrasound study. Circulation 1997;95:1791–1798.
32. Vavuranakis M, Stefanadis C, Toutouzas K, et al. Impaired compensatory coronary artery enlargement in atherosclerosis contributes to the development of coronary artery stenosis in diabetic patients: an in vivo intravascular ultrasound study. Eur Heart J 1997;18:1090–1094.
33. Kane JP, Malloy MJ, Ports TA, et al. Regression of coronary atherosclerosis during treatment of familial hypercholesterolemia with combined drug regimens. JAMA 1990;264:3007–3012.
34. Brown G, Albers JJ, Fisher LD, et al. Regression of coronary artery disease as a result of intensive lipid-lowering therapy in men with high levels of apolipoprotein B. N Engl J Med 1990;323:1289–1298.
35. Topol E, Nissen SE. Our preoccupation with coronary luminology: the dissociation between clinical and angiographic findings in ischemic heart disease. Circulation 1995;92:2333–2342.
36. Brown BG, Zhao XQ, Sacco DE, et al. Arteriographic view of treatment to achieve regression of coronary atherosclerosis and to prevent plaque disruption and clinical cardiovascular events. Br Heart J 1993;69:S48–S53.
37. Scandinavian Simvastatin Survival Study Group. Randomized trial of cholesterol lowering in 4444 patients with coronary heart disease: the Scandinavian Simvastatin Survival Study. Lancet 1994;344:1383–1389.
38. Eusterman JH. Atherosclerotic disease of the coronary arteries. A pathologic–radiologic correlative study. Circulation 1962;26:1288–1295.
39. Arnett EN, Isner JM, Redwood DR, et al. Coronary artery narrowing in coronary heart disease: comparison of cineangiographic and necropsy findings. Ann Intern Med 1979;91:350–356.
40. Freudenberg H, Lichtlen PR. The normal wall segment in coronary stenoses—a postmortal study. Z Kardiol 1981;70:863–869.
41. Roberts WC. Quantitation of coronary arterial narrowing at necropsy in sudden coronary death. Am J Cardiol 1979;44:39–44.
42. McPherson DD, Hiratzka LF, Lamberth WC, et al. Delineation of the extent of coronary atherosclerosis by high-frequency epicardial echocardiography. N Engl J Med 1987;316:304–309.
43. Blankenhorn DH, Curry PJ. The accuracy of angiography and ultrasound imaging for atherosclerosis measurement: a review. Arch Pathol Lab Med 1982;106:483–490.
44. Nishimura RA, Edwards WD, Warnes CA, et al. Intravascular ultrasound imaging: in vitro validation and pathologic correlation. J Am Coll Cardiol 1990;16:145–154.
45. Fitzgerald PJ, Ports TA, Yock PG. Contribution of localized calcium deposits to dissection after angioplasty in vivo assessed by intravascular ultrasound imaging. Circulation 1992;86:74–70.

46. Siegel RJ, Chae JS, Maurer G, et al. Histopathologic correlation of the layered intravascular ultrasound appearance of normal adult human muscular arteries. Am Heart J 1993;126:872–878.
47. Hodgson JM, Reddy KG, Suneja R, et al. Intracoronary ultrasound imaging: correlation of plaque morphology with angiography, clinical syndrome and procedural results in patients undergoing coronary angioplasty. J Am Coll Cardiol 1993;21:35–44.
48. Hausmann D, Lundkvist AJ, Friedrich G, et al. Lumen and plaque shape in atherosclerotic coronary arteries assessed by in vivo intracoronary ultrasound. Am J Cardiol 1994;74:857–863.
49. Tuzcu EM, Hobbs, RE, Rincon G, et al. Occult and frequent transmission of atherosclerotic coronary disease with cardiac transplantation—insights from intravascular ultrasound. Circulation 1995;91:1706–1713.
50. Weissman NJ, Palacios IF, Weyman AE. Dynamic expansion of the coronary arteries: implications for intravascular ultrasound measurements. Am Heart J 1995;130:46–51.
51. Takagi T, Yoshida K, Akasaka T, et al. Intravascular ultrasound analysis of reduction in progression of coronary narrowing by treatment with pravastatin. Am J Cardiol 1997;79:1673–1676.
52. De Mario C. Clinical application and image interpretation in intracoronary ultrasound. Eur Heart J 1998;19:207–229.
53. Erbel R, Ge J, Bockisch A, et al. Value of intracoronary ultrasound and Doppler in the differentiation of angiographically normal coronary arteries: a prospective study in patients with angina pectoris. Eur Heart J 1996;17:880–889.
54. Alfonso F, Macaya C, Goicolea J, et al. Intravascular ultrasound imaging of angiographically normal coronary segments in patients with coronary artery disease. Am Heart J 1994;127:536–544.
55. Hausmann D, Johnson JA, Sudhir K, et al. Angiographically silent atherosclerosis detected by intravascular ultrasound in patients with familial hypercholesterolemia and familial combined hyperlipidemia: correlation with high density lipoproteins. J Am Coll Cardiol 1996;27:1562–1570.
56. Ge J, Erbel R, Zamorano J, et al. Coronary artery remodeling in atherosclerotic disease: an intravascular ultrasonic study in vivo. Coron Artery Dis 1993;4:981–986.
57. Hermiller JB, Tenaglia AN, Kisslo KB, et al. In vivo validation of compensatory enlargement of atherosclerotic coronary arteries. Am J Cardiol 1993;71:665–668.
58. Losordo DW, Rosenfield K, Kaufman J, et al. Focal compensatory enlargement of human arteries in response to progressive atherosclerosis. Circulation 1994;89:2570–2577.
59. Gerber TC, Erbel R, Gorge G, et al. Extent of atherosclerosis and remodeling of the left main coronary artery determined by intravascular ultrasound. Am J Cardiol 1993;73:666–671.
60. Tuzcu EM, De Franco AC, Goormastic M, et al. Dichotomous pattern of coronary atherosclerosis 1 to 9 years after transplantation: insights from systematic intravascular ultrasound imaging. J Am Coll Cardiol 1996;27:839–846.
61. Pitt B, Waters D, Brown WV, et al. for the Atorvastatin Vs. Revascularization Treatment Investigators. Aggressive lipid-lowering therapy compared with angioplasty in stable coronary artery disease. N Engl J Med 1999;341:70–76.
62. Nissen SE, Tuzcu EM, Schoenhagen P, et al. Effect of intensive compared with moderate lipid lowering therapy on progression of coronary atherosclerosis: a randomized controlled trial. JAMA 2004;291:1071–1080.

2 Endothelial Function and Insights for Prevention

Eric H. Lieberman, MD, *Margarita R. Garces,* MD, *and Francisco Lopez-Jimenez,* MD, MSc

CONTENTS

INTRODUCTION

When William Harvey described the circulatory system in 1628, it was believed that the endothelium was an inert organ whose mere function was to line the arteries. Extensive research, however, has demonstrated that the endothelium is one of the most sophisticated organs in the system, playing a substantial role in the homeostasis of the circulatory system *(1)*. The endothelium serves as one of the largest paracrine organs in the body by playing a pivotal role in the regulation of such important tasks as vascular growth, vascular tone, and hemostasis. Additionally, the endothelium maintains the balance between opposing states: vasodilation vs vasoconstriction, growth promotion vs inhibition, antithrombosis vs fibrinolysis, antioxidation vs oxidation, and anti-inflammation vs proinflammation.

SUBSTANCES PRODUCED BY THE ENDOTHELIUM

In the early 1980s, Furchgott and Zawadski observed that vascular rings with intact endothelium exhibited vasodilation in response to acetylcholine. In contrast, when the vascular rings were denuded of endothelium, administration of acetylcholine resulted in vasoconstriction *(2)*. They concluded that the endothelium produced a substance capable of causing vasodilation, endothelium-derived relaxing factor (EDRF) *(3)*. It was subsequently shown that EDRF is nitric oxide (NO) or a substance capable of delivering NO.

From: *Contemporary Cardiology: Preventive Cardiology:*
Insights Into the Prevention and Treatment of Cardiovascular Disease, Second Edition
Edited by: J. M. Foody © Humana Press Inc., Totowa, NJ

NO is synthesized in the endothelium by the NO synthase (NOS), which catalyzes the reduction of L-arginine to produce NO and citruline. There are three isoforms of NOS: neuronal NOS, cytokine-inducible NOS, and endothelial NOS *(4,5)*. Activation of neuronal NOS and endothelial NOS depends on the intracellular concentrations of calcium ions, reduced nicotinamide adenine dinucleotide phosphate, and tetrahydrobiopterin. The inducible NOS is an inducible enzyme present in neutrophils and macrophages that is activated by bacterial endotoxin and cytokines, and that contains calmodulin and is not activated by calcium *(6)*.

NO relaxes the vascular smooth muscle cells by the stimulation of soluble guanylate cyclase, a cytosolic enzyme, and the formation of cyclic guanosine monophosphate, which is associated with the inhibition of the contractile apparatus. In normally functioning endothelium, low levels of NO are released constantly to keep the blood vessel dilated. Physical and humoral stimuli modulate the release of NO. Shear stress, pulsatile stretching of the vessel wall, and low partial pressure of oxygen seem to be the major physiological factors for NO release in the normal endothelium *(7)*. Several studies showed that increases in flow stimulate the release of NO and prostacyclin from the endothelial cells of the arteries. Endogenous substances that can stimulate the release of NO include catecholamines, vasopressin, bradykinin, and histamine, as well as serotonin, adenosine diphosphate, and thrombin *(8)*.

Platelet aggregation and platelet adhesion are inhibited in vitro by NO. The activation of platelets, with its release of adenosine diphosphate, serotonin, and thrombin, leads to a massive production of NO, which activates soluble guanylate cyclase, elevates cyclic guanosine monophosphate in the platelets, and reduces cytosolic-free calcium, resulting in vascular smooth-muscle relaxation. Platelet adhesion is also inhibited on the endothelium surface as a result of the release of NO in the vessel lumen *(9)*. Secretion of the granules of the platelets can be inhibited by NO. Gries et al. suggested that NO-dependent inhibition of platelet aggregation might be caused by a decrease in fibrinogen binding to the platelet glycoprotein IIb/IIIa *(10)*.

The endothelium has also been implicated in the regulation of smooth-muscle cell proliferation through the complimentary release of growth promoters and growth inhibitors. The growth promoters include angiotensin II, endothelin, fibroblast growth factor, and platelet-derived growth factor. The growth inhibitors include NO and endothelium-derived heparinoids, the former acting as a short-term inhibitor of growth, and the latter exerting a prolonged control of growth *(11)*.

Prostacyclin and thromboxane A2 are prostaglandins derived from arachidonic acid through catalysis by cyclooxygenase *(12)*. Prostacyclin is formed primarily in endothelial cells in response to shear stress, hypoxia, and other mediators of NO production. Prostacyclin causes relaxation of the vascular smooth muscle by activating adenylate cyclase and increasing the production of cyclic adenosine monophosphate. However, the contribution of prostacyclin to vasodilation is negligible when compared with NO. In addition to its vasomotor properties, prostacyclin is released by the normal endothelium to inhibit the activation and aggregation of platelets.

Thromboxane A2 is a potent platelet aggregator formed by the action of the enzyme thromboxane A2 synthase on cyclic endoperoxides. It is primarily produced in the platelets, although smaller quantities are synthesized in macrophages, lungs, kidneys, and heart. Thus, the balance between the production of thromboxane A2 and the production of prostacyclin by the endothelial cell is the primary factor in the regulation of hemostasis.

Bradykinin, a vasoactive kinin liberated through the action of kallikrein on kininogen, is a potent endothelium-dependent vasodilator, produced by endothelial cells in response to flow. It is also a potent stimulator of NO, prostacyclin, tissue plasminogen activator (t-PA), and endothelium-derived hyperpolarizing factor (EDHF) release *(13)*.

EDHF causes vasodilation by hyperpolarizing vascular smooth muscle through the stimulation of efflux through potassium ion channels *(14)*. In large arteries, both NO and EDHF contribute to endothelium-dependent vasodilation. Although NO predominates in normal circumstances, in these arteries, EDHF can mediate nearly normal, endothelium-dependent vasodilation if the release of NO is impaired.

Endothelin, the most potent vasoconstrictor known, was first isolated by Yanagisawa et al. *(15)* from porcine aortic endothelial cells. It is produced by endothelial cells in response to stimulation by thrombin, transforming growth factor-β, interleukin-1, epinephrine, angiotensin II, arginine vasopressin, calcium ionophores, and phorbol ester. Endothelin production is regulated by three inhibitory mechanisms: cyclic guanosine monophosphate-dependent inhibition, cyclic adenosine monophosphate-dependent inhibition, and an inhibitory factor produced by vascular smooth muscle. Intravascular administration of endothelin produces vasoconstriction through the endothelin A receptors located in the smooth-muscle cells. It also produces transient vasodilation because of the release of NO and prostacyclin via endothelin B receptors in the endothelial cells *(16)*. Numerous studies suggest that endothelin is a potent stimulator of endothelium hyperplasia and vascular hypertrophy. It has been shown that endothelin mediates the synthesis of collagen type I in vascular smooth-muscle cells *(17)*.

The angiotensin-converting enzyme (ACE) is found in the endothelial cell membrane. There, it converts angiotensin I to angiotensin II and degrades bradykinin. Angiotensin II is not only a strong vasoconstrictor, but also a mediator of smooth muscle growth and an enhancer of superoxide formation. In addition, angiotensin II has been found to enhance endothelin gene expression in animal endothelial cells *(18)*.

t-PA factor, a protease inhibitor that converts plasminogen to plasmin, is synthesized and released by the endothelial cell. Production of t-PA is directly related to stress, bradykinin, cytokines, and thrombin. This substance is inhibited by plasminogen activator inhibitor-1, an important modulator of fibrinolysis. A normal endothelium exhibits a delicate balance between t-PA factor and plasminogen activator inhibitor-1, in which the presence of excess plasminogen activator inhibitor-1 may lead to increased thrombosis.

von Willebrand factor (vWF) is the main cofactor in the adhesion of platelets to the endothelium. It also stabilizes and binds coagulation factor VIII in plasma. vWF is produced and stored as granules in the endothelial cell and its release is regulated by histamine, vasopressin, adrenaline phorbol esters, fibrin, and vascular endothelial growth factor *(19)*. Increased plasma levels of vWF have been associated with endothelial dysfunction *(20)*. Thrombomodulin, a protein composed of 556 amino acids, is expressed in the endothelial cells and can be regulated by the exposure of the endothelium to interleukins, hypoxia, and endotoxins. Thrombomodulin binds to thrombin and forms a complex, changing the conformation of thrombin, impeding the activation of platelets, the activation of Factor V, and the cleavage of fibrinogen.

CLINICAL MEASUREMENTS OF ENDOTHELIAL DYSFUNCTION

Ludmer and colleagues *(21)* first demonstrated that endothelial function could be assessed in vivo in the human coronary circulation. Graded concentrations of acetylcho-

line were infused directly into the coronary arteries. It was found that patients with angiographically smooth coronary arteries dilated in response to acetylcholine; however, arteries that had angiographic evidence of atherosclerosis had paradoxical vasoconstriction to acetylcholine. Additional research has shown that endothelial function can also be assessed using physiological stimuli such as increase in flow or in response to pacing. Patients with atherosclerotic coronary arteries have impaired flow-mediated dilation. Additional studies have demonstrated that atherosclerotic coronary arteries demonstrate paradoxical vasoconstriction in response to increases in heart rate induced by cardiac pacing. Administering NOS inhibitors, such as monomethyl-L-argine, can eliminate the vasodilator response to acetylcholine *(22)*.

Recently, a noninvasive technique has been used to assess flow-mediated vasodilation in the brachial artery using high-resolution ultrasound. Various studies validated and reproduced this technique *(23)*. The technique involves locating the brachial artery above the antecubital fossa and obtaining a baseline measurement using a linear phased array transducer attached to an ultrasound machine. After a baseline measurement is taken, a blood pressure cuff is placed in the forearm and is inflated to suprasystolic pressures, leading to transient ischemia of the arm. The resultant ischemia results in marked vasodilation of the resistance vessels. After release of the blood pressure cuff, there is a marked increased in flow through the brachial artery. The increase in flow results in the release of NO from the brachial artery and subsequent vasodilation. Endothelial function can be assessed by the degree of vasodilation that occurs in response to this increase in flow. There is good correlation between the endothelial responses of the coronary arteries tested with acetylcholine and the brachial artery tested using the noninvasive technique *(24)*.

FACTORS ASSOCIATED WITH ENDOTHELIAL DYSFUNCTION

Endothelial dysfunction can appear before the development of overt atherosclerosis. Furthermore, endothelial dysfunction is a diffuse and generalized process occurring in all vascular beds. The degree of endothelial dysfunction has been shown to correlate with the total number of traditional risk factors for coronary artery disease (CAD). Endothelial dysfunction generally precedes the development of clinical atherosclerosis and may be an early marker of the atherosclerotic process *(25)*.

Estrogen

Premenopausal women have a much lower incidence of CAD than age-matched men. However, this difference disappears after women become menopausal. Ovarian hormones, especially estradiol, have been suggested to mediate the gender-related difference in atherogenesis *(26)*. In animal experiments, replacement of estrogen in ovariectomized monkeys has been reported to reduce the severity of coronary atherosclerosis produced by a high-cholesterol diet. Furthermore, endothelium-dependent vasodilation varies during the menstrual cycle, and endogenous estradiol has been suggested to be responsible for that variation *(27)*. Ovariectomized monkeys have impaired endothelial-dependent vasodilation compared with ovariectomized monkeys receiving estrogen-replacement therapy. A number of investigators have shown that estrogen can acutely improve endothelial response in postmenopausal women. In addition, administration of estrogen during a period of weeks to months has also been shown to improve endothelial-dependent vasodilation *(28)*.

Smoking

Cigarette smoking is the most important modifiable risk factor for CAD and cardiovascular diseases in general. Smoking has been associated to impaired endothelial function, with a detrimental effect beginning from a young age *(29)*. Although the effect of cigarette smoking is dose-dependent and is directly related to pack-years, its consequences can be seen in as little as 1 h after smoking one cigarette *(30)*. Furthermore, passive smoking has also been linked to impairment in flow-mediated vasodilation *(31)*. It has been recently demonstrated that cigar smoke can also significantly impair endothelium-dependent vasodilation *(32)*. Smoking also potentiates the impact of other risk factors on endothelial dysfunction *(33)*.

The specific component of smoking that is responsible of the endothelial injury has not been defined. However, it is likely that the damage is the consequence of an interaction among several factors, such as carbon monoxide, nicotine, and tar, among others. Smokers have a higher level of oxidative stress, enhanced monocyte and platelet adherence to endothelial cells, and a lower level of plasma high-density lipoprotein cholesterol. Smoking may also increase nuclear damage to endothelial cells *(34,35)*.

Hyperlipidemia

A high cholesterol level is a widely known risk factor for CAD. Evidence from epidemiological and experimental studies support the hypothesis that high cholesterol levels induce vascular disease. Hypercholesterolemia impairs endothelial function of both the large conduit vessels and the smaller resistance vessels. The development of endothelial dysfunction precedes the development of overt atherosclerosis *(36)*. In coronary circulation, the degree of endothelial dysfunction correlates with total serum cholesterol levels *(37)*.

The mechanisms by which hypercholesterolemia impairs endothelial function is multifactorial. In general, the possible mechanisms include reduced synthesis of EDRF, impaired release of EDRF, or increased destruction of EDRF *(38–42)*. Oxidized low-density lipoprotein (LDL) has been shown to induce the expression of endothelial adhesion molecules, such as vascular cell adhesion molecule (VCAM)-1 and P-selectine, and enhance the production of endothelial production of chemokines. In addition, oxidized LDL particles induce monocyte recruitment and macrophage formation with the subsequent production of cytokines and growth factors *(43)*. Hypercholesterolemia also reduces the bioavailability of endothelium-derived NO, probably via reduced availability of L-arginine, the precursor of NO. It has been shown that abnormal vascular response in patients with hypercholesterolemia could be corrected by intravenous administration of L-arginine *(44,45)*. Other mechanisms by which hypercholesterolemia impairs endothelial function are by reducing the expression of endothelial NOS and also inactivating NO via superoxide anions or oxidized lipoproteins *(46)*. Years before the macroscopic features of atherosclerosis appear, hyperlipidemia causes abnormal conductance and resistance of the vessels.

Hypercholesterolemia induces endothelial dysfunction many years before clinical manifestations of CAD are present. A study showed that children with familiar hypercholesterolemia have endothelial dysfunction early in life when compared with healthy controls *(47)*. A study in young adults showed that subjects in the upper quartile of normal cholesterol level had much worse endothelium-dependent vasodilation than patients in the lowest quartile of cholesterol level *(48)*.

Early studies of the beneficial effect of lipid-lowering therapy on endothelial function had a clinical confirmation of effectiveness few months later *(49)*. Anderson showed that a medical regimen with lovastatin combined with antioxidant therapy reduced cholesterol levels and improved endothelial-dependent vasomotor responses to acetylcholine after 1 yr of treatment *(50)*. Similarly, Treasure and colleagues showed improved endothelium-mediated vasodilator response to acetylcholine after a mean of only 5.5 mo of therapy with lovastatin administered to hypercholesterolemic patients *(51)*. Furthermore, full restoration of endothelial functions *(52)* was shown in patients with hypercholesterolemia receiving fluvastatin for 1 yr. Simultaneously, clinical trials showed that statins reduced the risk of total and cardiovascular death, as well as the incidence of coronary events after several years of treatment. This fact emphasizes the reliability of endothelial dysfunction assessment for early identification of potentially beneficial interventions to prevent the development and progress of atherosclerosis.

Hypertension

Hypertension is a well-known risk factor for CAD. Endothelial dysfunction occurs because of high blood pressure, probably mediated by reduction of NO, a phenomenon that has been demonstrated in most forms of experimental hypertension models. Hypertension decreases the release or activity of NO. In addition to endothelial dysfunction, hypertension is also associated with vascular remodeling that leads to medial hypertrophy of the vessels. It is likely that the increase in smooth muscle mass may increase the degree of vasoconstriction in response to neurohormones, accentuating systemic vascular resistance and perpetuating hypertension. Whether the reduction in systemic blood pressure correlates with improvement in endothelial function is still controversial *(53–55)*. It is likely that experimental models of hypertension oversimplify a very complex vascular and metabolic disorder such as hypertension. A clinical trial showed that after 6 mo of treatment with quinapril, hypertensive patients improved their endothelium-mediated coronary vasodilation when compared with patients receiving placebo. It has been suggested that the beneficial effect of ACE-I on patients with a history of CAD may not be limited to inhibition of ACE but also to improvement in endothelial function.

Diabetes Mellitus

Cardiovascular disease is highly prevalent in patients with diabetes mellitus. Endothelial function is abnormal in experimental models of diabetes and also in patients with the diabetes mellitus *(56,57)*. The principal mediator of injury in diabetics may be hyperglycemia *(58)*. In an experimental model with rings of isolated rabbit aorta, abnormal relaxation to acetylcholine is induced after exposure to high concentrations of glucose in vitro. The glucose-induced endothelial dysfunction occurs because of several factors. Hyperglycemia increases the synthesis of sorbitol, which acts as an osmolyte, resulting in cell swelling and damage. Furthermore, endothelial dysfunction induced by hyperglycemia may be also associated with an increased release of prostanoids, such as thromboxane A2 and prostaglandin F2α.

The impairment of endothelial function in diabetic patients may be also related to abnormal intracellular signaling mechanisms, inducing the release of vasoactive mediators by the endothelial cell. Protein kinase C activation via phorbol esters induces an impaired endothelium-dependent relaxation, similar to the one seen in patients with diabetes. Other mechanisms through which hyperglycemia may induce endothelial dys-

function include an increased production of oxygen-derived free radicals, a decreased Na-K-ATPase activity level, and the presence of advanced glycosylation end products, which has been shown to inhibit NO in vitro.

Other Risk Factors

Age is an independent risk factor for the development of CAD. The effect of age is not only dependent on a longer exposure time to other directly harmful factors, but also through degeneration and aging of endothelial cells *(59,60)*. The estimated life-span of a human endothelial cell is approx 30 yr, after which the cell is replaced by regenerated endothelium. These regenerated cells tend to lose their capacity to release NO in response to platelet aggregation and thrombin.

Homocysteine is an amino acid formed during metabolism of methionine. Hyperhomocysteinemia is an independent risk factor for atherosclerosis and thrombosis. A graded response has also been demonstrated between homocysteine plasma level and the risk for CAD. The atherogenic propensity associated with hyperhomocysteinemia may be partially explained by its deleterious effect on endothelial function. Endothelium-dependent vasodilation of the brachial artery in patients with a mean homocysteine level of 35 mol/L was 40% lower than the dilation seen in patients with average homocysteine level *(61)*. Whether normalization of the plasma homocysteine level is followed by improvement in endothelial function or by a risk reduction for cardiovascular events is yet to be defined. Several ongoing clinical trials will help to clarify this issue.

Epidemiological evidence suggests that diets high in fruits and vegetables are associated with a reduced risk for atherosclerosis. One of the many potential mechanisms by which vitamin-enriched diets improve cardiovascular outcomes is restoring endothelial function. Vitamins are antioxidants: therefore, they have a protective effect against free radicals derived from reactive oxygen species. Administration of antioxidants, including vitamins C and E, has shown to improve endothelium-dependent vasodilation in humans *(62,63)*. Because folic acid decreases homocysteine levels, it may possibly reduce the risk of coronary events. Furthermore, vitamins may prevent LDL cholesterol oxidation, thereby producing an anti-atherogenic effect. Additionally, a high-fat diet can impair endothelial function acutely *(64)*, and the impairment can be prevented with concurrent intake of vitamin C.

CLINICAL APPLICATIONS OF ASSESSMENT OF ENDOTHELIAL DYSFUNCTION

Assessment of endothelial function is primarily limited to research studies. Endothelial function testing is useful in assessing the response to risk modification in a number of studies. The usefulness of endothelial function testing in the clinical arena remains unclear. However, it is likely that, in the near future, assessment of endothelial function will be a useful marker in determining the risk for cardiovascular clinical events and as a measurement of efficacy of medical interventions intended to reduce the cardiovascular risk.

REFERENCES

1. Luscher TF, Rubanyi GM, Masaki T, Vane JR, Vanhoutte PM. Endothelial control of vascular tone and growth. Circulation 1993;87(Suppl V):VI–V2.

2. Furchgott RF. The discovery of endothelium-dependent relaxation. Circulation 1993;87(Suppl V):V3–V8.
3. Furchgott RF, Zawadrki JV. The obligatory role of endothelial cells in the relaxation of arterial smooth muscle by acetylcholine. Nature 1980;288:373–376.
4. Vanhoutte PM, Perrault LP, Vilaine JP. Endothelial dysfunction and vascular disease. In: Rubanyi GM, Dzau VJ, eds. The Endothelium in Clinical Practice. Source and Target of Novel Therapies. Marcel Dekker, New York, 1997, pp. 265–289.
5. Parkinson IF, Phillips GB. Nitric oxide synthases: enzymology and mechanism-based inhibitors. In: Rubanyi GM, Dzau VJ, eds. The Endothelium in Clinical Practice. Source and Target of Novel Therapies. Marcel Dekker, New York, 1997, pp. 95–123.
6. Ikeda U, Shimada K. Nitric oxide and cardiac failure. Clin Cardiol 1997;20:837–841.
7. Busse R, Mulsch A, Fleming I, Hecker M. Mechanisms of nitric oxide release from the vascular endothelium. Circulation 1993;87(Suppl V):V18–V25.
8. Pohl U, Holte J, Busse R, Bassenge E. Crucial role of endothelium in the vasodilator response to increase to increase flow in vivo. Hypertension 1986;8:37–44.
9. Vanhoutte PM, Shimokawa H. Endothelium-derived relaxing factor and coronary vasospasm. Circulation 1989;80:1–9.
10. Gries A, Bode C, Peter K, et al. Inhaled nitric oxide inhibits platelet aggregation, P-selectin expression, and fibrinogen in vitro and in vivo. Circulation 1998;97:1481–1487.
11. Scoft-Burden T, Vanhoutte PM. The endothelium as a regulator of vascular smooth muscle proliferation. Circulation 1993;87(Suppl V):V51–V55.
12. Mehta JL, Yang BC. Prostacyclin and thromboxane: role in ischemic heart disease. In: Rubanyi GM, Dzau VJ, eds. The Endothelium in Clinical Practice. Source and Target of Novel Therapies. Marcel Dekker, New York, 1997, pp. 45–69.
13. Groves P, Kurz S, Hanjorg J, Drexler H. Role of endogenous bradykinin in human coronary vasomotor control. Circulation 1995;92:3424–3430.
14. Campbell WE, Gebredmedhin D, Pratt PF, Harder DR. Identification of oxyeicosatrienoic acids as endothelium-derived hyperpolarizing. Circ Res 1996;78:415–423.
15. Yanagisawa M, Kurihara H, Kimura S, et al. A novel potent vasoconstrictor peptide produced by vascular endothelial cells. Nature 1988;332:411–415.
16. Masaki T. Overview: reduced sensitivity of vascular response to endothelin. Circulation 1993;87(Suppl V):V33–V35.
17. Stewart D. Impact of endothelin-1 on vascular structure and function. A symposium: endothelial function and cardiovascular disease: potential mechanisms and interventions. Am J Cardiol 1998;82:14S–15S.
18. Luscher TF, Boulanger CM, Yang Z, Noll G, Dohi Y. Interactions between endothelium-derived relaxing and contracting factors in health and cardiovascular disease. Circulation 1993;87(Suppl V):V36–V44.
19. Kalafatis M, Egan J, Maim K. Coagulation factors. In: Rubanyi GM, Dzau VJ, eds. The Endothelium in Clinical Practice. Source and Target of Novel Therapies. Marcel Dekker, New York, 1997, pp. 245–264.
20. Dormandy J, Belcher G. Clinical use of prostacyclin. In: Rubanyi GM, Dzau VJ, eds. The Endothelium in Clinical Practice. Source and Target of Novel Therapies. Marcel Dekker, New York, 1997, pp. 71–94.
21. Ludmer FL, Selwyn AP, Shook TL, et al. Paradoxical vasoconstriction induced by acetylcholine in atherosclerotic coronary arteries. N Engl J Med 1986;315:1046–1051.
22. Lefroy DC, Crake T, Uren NG, et al. Effect of inhibition of NO synthesis on epicardial coronary artery caliber and coronary flow in humans. Circulation 1993;88:43–54.
23. Uehata A, Lieberman EH, Gerhard MD, et al. Noninvasive assessment of endothelium-dependent flow mediated dilation of the brachial artery. Vasc Med 1997;2:87–92.
24. Anderson TJ, Uehata A, Gerhard MD, et al. Close relation of endothelial function in the human coronary and peripheral circulations. J Am Coll Cardiol 1995;26:1235–1241.
25. Anderson TJ, Gerhard MD, Meredith IT, et al. Systemic nature of endothelial dysfunction in atherosclerosis. Am J Cardiol 1995;75:71B–74B.
26. Celerimajer DS, Sorensen K, Spiegelhalter DJ, et al. Aging is associated with endothelial dysfunction in healthy men years before the age-related decline in women. J Am Coll Cardiol 1994;24:471–476.
27. Hashimoto M, Akishita M, Eto M, et al. Modulation of endothelium-dependent flow-mediated dilatation of the brachial artery by sex and menstrual cycle. Circulation 1995;92:3431–3435.
28. Lieberman EH, Gerhard M, Uehata A, et al. Estrogen improves endothelium dependent flow-mediated vasodilation in post menopausal women. Ann Intern Med 1994;121:936–941.
29. Panza JA, Casino PR, Kiloyne CM, Quyyumi AA. Role of endothelium-derived nitric oxide in the abnormal endothelium-dependent vascular relaxation of patients with essential hypertension. Circulation 1993;87:1468–1474.

30. Celermajer DS, Sorensen KE, Georgakopoulos D, et al. Cigarette smoking is associated 20 with dose-related and potentially reversible impairment of endothelium-dependent dilation in healthy young adults. Circulation 1993;88:2149–2155.
31. Celermajer DS, Adams MR, Clarkson P, et al. Passive smoking and impaired endothelium-dependent arterial dilation in healthy young adults. N Engl J Med 1996;334:150–154.
32. Santo-Tomas M, Lopez-Jimenez F, Aldrich HR, et al. Debunking the yuppie habit: cigars and endothelial function. J Am Coll Cardiol 1999;33:232A.
33. Heitzer T, Yla-Herttuala S, Luoma J, et al. Cigarette smoking potentiates endothelial dysfunction of fore-arm resistance vessels in patients with hypercholesterolemia. Role of oxidized LDL. Circulation 1996;93:1346–1353.
34. Griendling KK, Alexander RW. Oxidative stress and cardiovascular disease. Circulation 1997;96:3264–3265.
35. Reilly M, Delanty N, Lawson JA, Fitzgerald GA. Modulation of oxidant stress in vivo in chronic cigarette smokers. Circulation 1996;94:19–25.
36. Creager MA, Cooke JP, Mendelsohn ME, et al. Impaired vasodilation of forearm resistance vessels in hypercholesterolemic humans. J Clin Invest 1990;86:228–234.
37. Zeiher AM, Drexler H, Saurbier B, et al. Correlation of endothelial dysfunction in coronary microcirculation of hypercholesterolemic patients by L-arginine. Lancet 1991;338:1546–1550.
38. Verbeuren TJ, Jordaens FH, Zonnckeyn LL, et al. Effect of hypercholesterolemia on vascular reactivity in the rabbit. Circ Res 1986;58:552–564.
39. Cohen RA, Zitnay KM, Haudenschild CC, et al. Loss of selective endothelial cell vasoactive functions caused by hypercholesterolemia in pig coronary arteries. Circ Res 1988;63:903–910.
40. Shimokawa H, Vanhoutte RM. Impaired endothelium-dependent relaxation to aggregating platelets and related vasoactive substances in porcine coronary arteries in hypercholesterolemia and atherosclerosis. Circ Res 1989;64:900–914.
41. Galle J, Mulsch A, Busse R, et al. Effects of native and oxidized low density lipoproteins on formation and inactivation of EDRF. Arterioscler Thromb 1991;11:198–203.
42. Tagawa H, Tomoike H, Nakamura M. Putative mechanisms of the impairment of endothelium-dependent relaxation of the aorta with atheromatous plaque in heritable hyperlipidemic rabbits. Circ Res 1991;68:330–337.
43. Steinberg D. Oxidative modification of LDL and atherogenesis. Circulation 1997;95:1062–1071.
44. Cooke JP, Dzau VJ, Creager MA. Endothelial dysfunction in hypercholesterolemia is corrected by l-arginine. Basic Res Cardiol 1991;86(Suppl 2):173–181.
45. Creager MA, Gallagher SJ, Girerd XJ, et al. L-arginine improves endothelium dependent vasodilation in hypercholesterolemic humans. J Clin Invest 1992;90(4):1248–1253.
46. Casino PR, Kilcoyne CM, Quyyumi AA, et al. The role of nitric oxide in endothelium-dependent vasodilation of hypercholesterolemic patients. Circulation 1993;88:2541–2547.
47. Sorensen KE, Celermajer DS, Georgakopoulos D, et al. Impairment of endothelium-dependent dilation is an early event in children with familiar hypercholesterolimia and is related to the lipoprotein (a) level. J Clin Invest 1994;93:50–55.
48. Steinberg PR, Bayazeed B, Hook G, et al. Endothelial dysfunction is associated with cholesterol levels in the high normal range in humans. Circulation 1997;96:3287–3293.
49. Leung WH, Lau CP, Wong CK. Beneficial effect of cholesterol-lowering therapy on coronary endothelium-dependent relaxation in hypercholesterolemic patients. Lancet 1993;341:1496–1500.
50. Anderson TJ, Meredith IT, Yeung AC, et al. The effect of cholesterol lowering and antioxidant therapy on endothelium in patients with coronary artery disease. N Engl J Med 1994;332:488–493.
51. Treasure CB, Klein JL, Weintraub WS, et al. Beneficial effects of cholesterol lowering therapy on the coronary endothelium in patients with coronary artery disease. N Engl J Med 1994;332:481–487.
52. Schmieder RE, Schobel HP. Is endothelial dysfunction reversible? Am J Cardiol 1995;76(2):117A–121A.
53. Berkenboom F, Langer I, Carpentier Y, Grosfils K, Fontaine J. Ramipril prevents endothelial dysfunction induced by oxidized low-density lipoproteins. Hypertension 1997;30:371–376.
54. Creager MA, Roddy MA. Effect of captopril and enalapril on endothelial function in hypertensive patients. Hypertension 1994;24:499–505.
55. Schlaifer JD, Wargovich TJ, O'Neill B, et al. Effects of quinapril on coronary blood flow in coronary artery disease patients with endothelial dysfunction. J Am Coll Cardiol 1997;80:1594–1597.
56. Johnstone MT, Creager SJ, Scales KM, et al. Impaired endothelium-dependent vasodilation in patients with insulin-dependent diabetes mellitus. Circulation 1993;88:2510–2516.

57. Williams SB, Cusco JA, Roddy MA, et al. Impaired nitric oxide-mediated vasodilation in patients with non-insulin-dependent diabetes mellitus. J Am Coll Cardiol 1996;27:567–574.

58. Cosentino F, Hishikawa K, Katusic ZS, Luscher TF. High glucose increases nitric oxide synthase expression and superoxide anion generation in human aortic endothelial cells. Circulation 1997;96:25–28.

59. Zeiher AM, Drexler H, Saurbier B, Just H. Endothelium mediated coronary blood flow modulation in humans: effects of age, atherosclerosis, hypercholesterolemia, and hypertension. J Clin Invest 1993;92:652–662.

60. Barton M, Cosentino F, Brandes RP, et al. Anatomical heterogeneity of vascular aging: role of nitric oxide and endothelin. Hypertension 1997;30:817–824.

61. Woo KS, Chook F, Lolin YI, et al. Hyperhomocystein(e)imia is a risk factor for arterial endothelial dysfunction in humans. Circulation 1997;96:2542–2544.

62. Levine GN, Frei B, Koulouris SN, et al. Ascorbic acid reverses endothelial vasomotor dysfunction in patients with coronary artery disease. Circulation 1996;93:1107–1113.

63. Ting HH, Timimi FK, Boles KS, et al. Vitamin C improves endothelium-dependent vasodilation in patients with non-insulin-dependent diabetes mellitus. J Clin Invest 1996;97:22–28.

64. Vogel RA, Correti MC, Plotnick GD. Effect of a single high-fat meal on endothelial function in healthy subjects. Am J Cardiol 1997;79:350–354.

3

Inflammation and Infection in Coronary Artery Disease

Michael A. Lauer, MD

CONTENTS

INTRODUCTION

It has recently been recognized that atherosclerosis in all stages of development and progression—from the fatty streak to the ruptured plaque causing a myocardial infarction (MI)—is a specialized inflammatory response. The central role of inflammation in atherosclerosis is underscored by the last two papers authored by the late Russell Ross, whose pioneering research and writing shaped much of our understanding of the pathology during the last 30 yr. Both of these reviews asserted unequivocally that "atherosclerosis is an inflammatory disease" *(1,2)*.

Although the understanding of atherosclerosis as an inflammatory disease at the pathological and molecular biology levels has been well-described and accepted, the development of animals models of atherosclerosis by inducing chronic inflammation is at a more formative stage. Numerous observational studies delineating clinical markers of inflammation and the relationship of inflammation to the development and progression of atherosclerosis have recently been reported, although widespread acceptance and verification of these studies are ongoing. There is recent evidence that chronic infection with viral agents or bacteria, such as *Chlamydia pneumoniae*, may contribute to the progression of atherosclerosis. Several small trials of antibiotic therapy reducing cardiovascular events have prompted larger-scale trials. Clinical trials of treatments targeted at specific mediators in the inflammatory process as a means of interrupting the atherosclerotic process are in the formative stages.

From: *Contemporary Cardiology: Preventive Cardiology:*
Insights Into the Prevention and Treatment of Cardiovascular Disease, Second Edition
Edited by: J. M. Foody © Humana Press Inc., Totowa, NJ

This chapter briefly reviews the pathobiology of the atherosclerosis development and progression, emphasizing the inflammatory nature of this disease. Second, the role of markers of inflammation in detecting early or progressive atherosclerotic disease and potentially guiding therapy or detection of a vulnerable plaque is discussed. Finally, the evidence for infectious agents as risk factors and possible etiological agents of atherosclerosis is presented, along with a review of the current trials exploring antibiotic therapy as possible treatment and prevention of atherosclerosis. The data reviewed in this chapter are not likely to dramatically modify the current management of patients; instead, the data present a modified approach to the understanding of atherosclerosis that should provide a revised framework to consider new and revised therapies in the coming years.

ATHEROSCLEROSIS IS AN INFLAMMATORY DISEASE

Early Lesions

The fatty streak is the earliest identifiable lesion of atherosclerosis, appearing early in childhood (3). The fatty streak is a purely inflammatory lesion (4). The process begins when monocyte-derived macrophages and T-lymphocytes, in response to a variety of insults to the vascular endothelium, in the form of free radicals caused by cigarette smoking, hypertension, modified lipoproteins, glycosylation products of diabetes, or elevated homocysteine, enter the arterial wall (1). The inflammatory response to these various inciting factors is generalized stereotypical response (Fig. 1) (5). The first step in this inflammatory response to injury is an upregulation of intracellular adhesion molecules, such as vascular cell adhesion molecule-1, intracellular adhesion molecule-1, and E-selectin (6–9). These adhesion molecules, along with chemoattractants secreted by the endothelium, such as monocyte chemoattract protein (2), macrophage colony-stimulating factor, and interleukins (ILs), begin a parade of monocyte-derived macrophages and T lymphocytes into the arterial wall (10). With the uptake of oxidized (ox) low-density lipoproteins (LDL), these macrophages become foam cells, and the collection of inflammatory cells is recognizable as a fatty streak (11).

Intermediate Lesions

As the monocyte-derived macrophages and T-lymphocytes accumulate in the arterial wall, they secrete a variety of proinflammatory cytokines, such as IL-1, IL-6, and tumor necrosis factor (TNF)-α, which further upregulate the adhesion molecules as well as promote the uptake of ox-LDL (12). These cytokines, along with growth factors, such as platelet-derived growth factor and fibroblast growth factor, stimulate the proliferation of smooth muscle cells that form layers between the expanding pool of macrophages and foam cells to form the intermediate plaque (13). Another product of the macrophages is a group of elastases, collagenases, and proteinases known collectively as the matrix metalloproteinases. Several of these degrading enzymes are present in developing atheroma, especially those associated with aneurysmal disease. It may be that these enzymes are responsible for the degradation of the arterial wall, allowing outward expansion of the developing atheroma without impinging on the lumen until a relatively late stage (14–21).

Complex Lesions and Plaque Rupture

As the atherosclerotic plaque continues to develop, a thin fibrous cap consisting largely of collagen develops, overlying a mixture of monocytes, extracellular matrix and lipid,

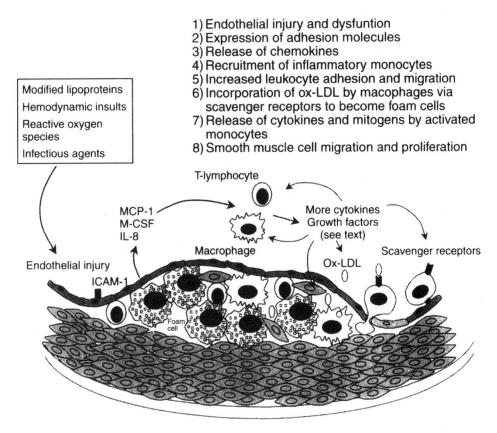

1) Endothelial injury and dysfuntion
2) Expression of adhesion molecules
3) Release of chemokines
4) Recruitment of inflammatory monocytes
5) Increased leukocyte adhesion and migration
6) Incorporation of ox-LDL by macophages via
   scavenger receptors to become foam cells
7) Release of cytokines and mitogens by activated
   monocytes
8) Smooth muscle cell migration and proliferation

Modified lipoproteins
Hemodynamic insults
Reactive oxygen species
Infectious agents

T-lymphocyte

MCP-1
M-CSF
IL-8

More cytokines
Growth factors
(see text)

Macrophage

Ox-LDL

Scavenger receptors

Endothelial injury
ICAM-1

Foam cell

Fig. 1. Inflammation and formation of fatty streak. (Adapted from ref. *5*.)

smooth muscles cells, and areas of necrosis *(22)*. Thus, the fibrous cap can erode or rupture. Such ruptures most frequently occur at the shoulder region at the edge of a plaque, where the fibrous cap is often thin and shear stresses are at a maximum because of local geometry and the Law of LaPlace *(23,24)*. Macrophages and other inflammatory cells accumulate at these shoulder regions, and, with the release of matrix metalloproteinases, contribute to erosion and rupture of the vulnerable, thin, fibrous cap *(10,14,25,26)*. With exposure of the bloodstream to the underlying lipid core, which is highly thrombogenic, this small erosion or rupture can lead to mural thrombosis and MI.

MARKERS OF INFLAMMATION IN ATHEROSCLEROSIS

Elevated C-Reactive Protein as a Risk Factor for Cardiovascular Events

C-reactive protein (CRP) is a protein produced solely in the liver under the influence of IL-6 and other inflammatory cytokines. It is named for its affinity for the c-polysaccharide of *Pneumonococcus* and is known to rise significantly as a marker of generalized inflammation in response to acute or chronic infection or injury. Recently, a high-sensitivity (hs)-CRP assay was developed that allows accurate discrimination in the high normal range associated with chronic inflammatory states *(27)*. The presence and degree of inflammation defined by CRP, fibrinogen, IL-1, IL-6, and TNF-α has been associated with an increased risk of future cardiac events.

The European Concerted Action on Thrombosis and Disabilities Angina Study Group examined 3043 patients with angina who underwent coronary angiography and were followed for 2 yr. After adjustment for the extent of coronary artery disease (CAD) and other risk factors, an increased incidence of MI or sudden death was associated with higher baseline concentrations of fibrinogen, von Willebrand factor antigen, and tissue plasminogen activator antigen. The concentration of CRP was directly correlated with the incidence of coronary events, except when adjusted for fibrinogen concentration. In contrast, low fibrinogen and CRP levels were associated with a low risk of new coronary events, even in patients with elevated cholesterol *(28)*. A nested case–control study of 148 case patients and 296 control patients, drawn from the 12,000 patients enrolled the Multiple Risk Factor Intervention Trial followed for up to 17 yr found that the risk of coronary heart disease (CHD) death in the quartile of patients with the highest baseline levels of CRP (>3.3 mg/L) was 2.8 times that of patients in the lowest quartile of CRP levels (<1.2 mg/L). For smokers, the relative risk of CHD death in the highest quartile of CRP as compared with the lowest quartile was 4.3 (95% confidence interval [CI], 1.74–10.8) *(29)*.

A study from the Physician's Health Study found that in 543 apparently healthy men at baseline, the men in the quartile with the highest baseline CRP values (>2.11 mg/L) had three times the risk of MI. The relationship between CRP and cardiovascular events was independent of other cardiovascular risk factor or homeostatic variables. Additionally, the use of aspirin was associated with significant reductions in the risk of MI among men in the highest quartile but with only small, nonsignificant reductions among those in the lowest quartile of CRP level (Fig. 2) *(30)*. These and other studies comprise fairly convincing evidence that chronic inflammation, as measured by CRP, is related clinically to the development of CAD. The differential treatment effect of aspirin in the Physician's Health Study opens the door to the clinical use of hs-CRP to help guide therapy.

A second, large observational study showing a differential treatment effect based on hs-CRP levels was a nested case–control study of 391 patients with a previous MI in the Cholesterol and Recurrent Events trial of pravastatin therapy, who subsequently developed recurrent nonfatal MI or a fatal coronary event and from an equal number of age- and gender-matched participants who remained free of these events during follow-up. CRP and serum amyloid A (SAA) levels at baseline were higher among cases than among control subjects (for CRP, $p = 0.05$; for SAA, $p = 0.006$), such that individuals with levels in the highest quintile had a relative risk of recurrent events 75% higher than patients with levels in the lowest quintile. The risk reduction with pravastatin was much greater (54%) in patients with an elevated level of CRP than in patients without such an elevation (25%) (Fig. 3), suggesting that a subset of patients who stand to derive particular benefit from hydroxymethylglutaryl (HMG)-coenzyme A (CoA) reductase inhibitor therapy might be predicted based on an elevated hs-CRP level *(31)*. The mechanism behind this interaction is unclear, although it has been proposed that it may be caused by an interaction between inflammatory mediators and the incorporation of ox-LDL, or a result of the anti-inflammatory properties of the HMG-CoA reductase inhibitors *(32,33)*.

Elevated CRP as a Prognostic Factor in Acute Coronary Syndromes

The emergence of inflammation as central in the process of plaque rupture has prompted exploration into the pattern of increases in inflammatory markers in acute coronary syndromes. Of particular relevance to the future use of these markers in a

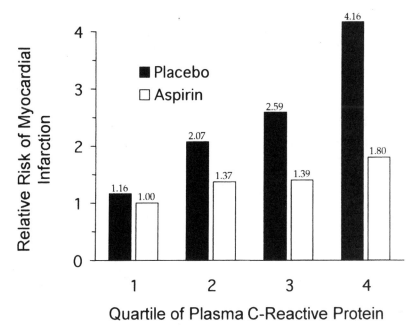

Fig. 2. Relative risk of first myocardial infarction associated with baseline plasma concentrations of C-reactive protein, stratified according to randomized assignment to aspirin or placebo therapy. (From ref. *30*.)

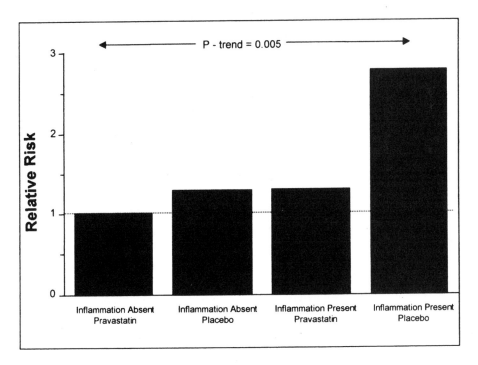

Fig. 3. Relative risk of recurrent events among post-MI patients according to presence (both CRP and SAA levels >90th percentile) or absence (both CRP and SAA levels, <90th percentile) of evidence of inflammation and by randomized pravastatin assignment. (From ref. *31*.)

clinical setting are whether markers such as hs-CRP can aid in the diagnosis of acute coronary syndromes as well as in the determination of the prognosis of developing complications and recurrent events.

It has long been recognized that the CRP *(34–36)* and IL-6 *(37,38)* levels rise with MI, although it was unclear whether this response was anything more than a marker of inflammation associated with myocardial necrosis. Studies that are more recent showed that increases in CRP and IL-6 can occur before elevations in myocardial-specific troponins or isoenzyme of creatine kinase-myocardial band and may indicate a poor prognosis *(39–41)*.

In terms of diagnosis and as a predictor of in-hospital events, Liuzzo and colleagues *(39)* found that the levels of CRP and SAA protein were at least 0.3 mg/dL in 13% of 32 patients with stable angina, in 65% of 31 patients with unstable angina, and in 76% of 29 patients with acute MI. At the time of hospital admission, creatine kinase and cardiac troponin T levels were normal in all the patients. The 20 patients with unstable angina who had levels of CRP and SAA protein of at least 0.3 mg/dL had more in-hospital ischemic episodes and a trend toward higher rates of revascularization, MI, and death than those with levels less than 0.3 mg/dL *(39)*. A study of 195 patents with unstable angina found that the rate of in-hospital death, MI, or emergency revascularization was not higher in patients with a CRP level greater than 0.3 mg/dL *(42)*. In a study of 437 patients with non-ST elevation coronary syndromes enrolled in the Thrombolysis in MI 11A trial, a CRP level of at least 1.55 mg/dL at presentation was correlated with an increase in 14-d mortality, even in patients with a negative rapid qualitative assay for cardiac-specific troponin T *(40)*.

There have also been several studies showing the usefulness of an elevated hs-CRP level as a predictor of recurrent events and late complications after admission for acute coronary syndromes. In a study of 965 patients with unstable angina or non-Q-wave MI enrolled in the Fragmin During Instability in CAD (FRISC) study, stratification by baseline CRP levels showed that there was a gradation of mortality risk at 5 mo with respect to CRP level *(43)*. In a separate study of 102 patients with unstable angina followed for 3 mo, hs-CRP was a predictor of MI in a multivariate model and added incremental prognostic value to the level of troponin T *(44)*.

Several studies have addressed whether CRP levels at discharge may be a more reliable predictor of future instability than those at admission. A study of 54 patients with unstable angina found that a CRP of greater than 3 mg/L at discharge was most predictive of recurrent instability at 1 yr *(45)*. In a similar study of 194 patients with unstable angina including both derivation and validation sets, the CRP level at discharge was more predictive than at admission for the combined endpoint of refractory angina, MI, or death at 90 d. CRP at hospital discharge was the strongest independent marker of an adverse outcome, with a relative risk of 3.16 (95% CI, 2.0–5.2; $p = 0.0001$) (Fig. 4). A cutoff point of 1.5 mg/dL for CRP provided optimum sensitivity and specificity for adverse outcome, based on the receiver operator curves *(46)*.

Although an elevated CRP level in patients with acute non-ST elevation coronary syndromes is fairly well-established as a negative prognostic predictor at this point, the next step is to determine whether this is an indicator of chronic inflammation that could potentially be treated to improve outcome. There have been several reports that the CRP levels are lower in patients who have undergone successful thrombolytic therapy as compared with those with failed thrombolysis or who did not receive reperfusion therapy

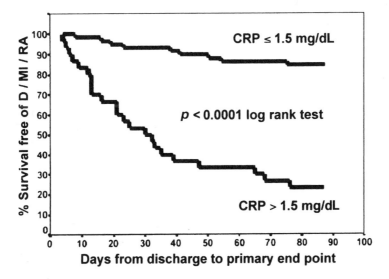

Fig. 4. Kaplan–Meier plot: cumulative freedom from risk of death (D), myocardial infarcion (MI), or refractory angina (RA) within 90 d with CRP levels above or below 1.5 mg/dL. (Adapted from ref. *46.*)

(47–50), although further work is necessary to clarify this relationship. There have not been any published reports of any treatment strategies or pharmacological agents having a differential effect based on CRP levels at the time of admission for acute coronary syndromes, such as those reported with aspirin and HMG-CoA reductase inhibitors in chronic atherosclerotic disease. There are several trials of anti-inflammatory or anticytokine agents in various stages of planning, and several of these may incorporate an elevated CRP level as an enrolling criterion.

DETECTION OF THE VULNERABLE PLAQUE

There has been recent interest in developing technology to localize a vulnerable plaque that may be prone to rupture and cause an acute coronary syndrome. If those patients at increased risk for plaque rupture could be determined by an increased hs-CRP or other inflammatory marker, a search for a vulnerable plaque may lead to a catheter-based treatment to stabilize such a lesion. Human atherosclerotic plaques from carotid end-arterectomy specimens have been shown to display thermal heterogeneity, with areas of increased temperature correlating with clusters of macrophages *(51)*. Macrophages have been shown to produce heat associated with increased glucose metabolism and phago-cytosis *(52)*. Clustering of macrophages occurs at the shoulder region of an atherosclerotic plaque that is most prone to rupture *(23,24,53)*. Macrophages also play a role in restenosis after percutaneous coronary intervention *(54)*, although in a more diffuse manner than in primary plaque rupture. Restenotic lesions are also associated with changes in temperature profile, but these changes are more diffuse and of a smaller magnitude than seen in native atherosclerosis, which is consistent with a more diffuse infiltration of macrophages *(55)*.

It has been suggested that a catheter-based means for measuring coronary artery temperature profile may offer a method of determining which plaques are most active and

either responsible for an acute coronary syndrome or predict those that might cause acute events in the near future. An intravascular catheter for the in vivo thermography of coronary arteries has been developed and is used to show that the temperature heterogeneity between plaque and healthy vessel wall increases progressively from stable angina to unstable angina to acute MI (56). Further preliminary data from this same group suggest that, within each diagnostic class, those percutaneous coronary intervention target sites with increased temperature heterogeneity are associated with worse outcomes (57). Other catheter-based systems using infrared (58) or near-infrared imaging (59) to detect arterial wall temperature profile are in earlier stages of development. The development of this technology is not ready for clinical use at this time, but its development in parallel with studies of plaque stabilization pharmacological agents, which could be used either systemically or locally, is promising.

CASE FOR AN INFECTIOUS COMPONENT TO ATHEROSCLEROSIS

The traditional risk factors of smoking, hypertension, hyperlipidemia, diabetes, and, more recently, hyperhomocysteinemia, only account for approx 30 to 50% of cases of advanced atherosclerosis (60). This implies that there may be an undetermined amount of chronic inflammation contributing to the atherosclerotic process. Several infectious agents that tend to cause chronic inflammatory states—most notably *Chlamydia pnuemoniae* and members of the herpesvirus family have recently been proposed and fervently studied as possible inciting agents in at least a portion of the these unexplained cases of atherosclerosis.

Viral Disease

The theory that infectious agents may play a role in the development of atherosclerosis dates back more than 20 yr. Fabricant and coworkers found that when chickens were infected with Marek's disease virus, an avian herpesvirus, typical atherosclerotic lesions developed in large coronary arteries, aortas, and major aortic branches of infected normocholesterolemic or hypercholesterolemic chickens (61,62). The authors suggested that these results might have an important bearing on our understanding of human arteriosclerosis because there is widespread and persistent infection in humans with up to five different herpesviruses.

Cytomegalovirus

Cytomegalovirus (CMV) antigen has been detected in atherosclerotic plaques (63–65), although this may be caused by an innocent bystander phenomenon. CMV has also been shown to induce arterial changes similar to early atherosclerotic lesions in a rat allograft model (66,67). Although studies have linked CMV seropositivity to arterial disease, most of these studies have shown an association with transplant vasculopathy (68–70), early carotid thickening (71–74), or restenosis after percutaneous intervention (71,75). Although a few studies have associated CMV seropositivity with native coronary disease, these associations have been rather marginal (76,77). There is preliminary evidence that as multiple pathogens (including CMV, hepatitis A, herpesvirus types 1 and 2, and *C. pneumoniae*) that are capable of producing a chronic inflammatory response co-infect a particular patient, the CRP levels increase and the CAD prevalence increases (78–80).

Bacterial Agents

HELICOBACTER PYLORI

The discovery that *Helicobacter pylori* was the causative agents for a large portion of peptic ulcer disease, a disease that for many years was not thought to be infectious or a primary inflammatory disorder, certainly laid the foundation for the theory that bacterial infections could be an etiological agent of atherosclerosis. Several studies have reported an association between seropositivity and atherosclerosis *(81–83)*, although these associations have been weak, and often diminish a role for *H. pylori* even further when controlling for other risk factors. There is some evidence to suggest that if there is an association between CHD and *H. pylori*, it is caused by folate deficiency associated with chronic gastric disease.

C. PNEUMONIAE

C. pneumoniae is a newly discovered third species of *Chlamydia* shown to cause pneumonia, bronchitis, pharyngitis, and sinusitis in humans *(84)*. It was first described by Grayston and coworkers *(85)*. *C. pneumoniae* is an obligate intracellular organism that spends most of its life cycle within macrophages. Most infections are subclinical or cause only benign flu-like symptoms *(86)*. The prevalence of antibodies to *C. pneumoniae* begins in late adolescence and increases with age to at least 50% in middle-aged US adults, and as high as 80% in the elderly *(86,87)*.

Seroepidemiological Studies. A link between *C. pneumoniae* and atherosclerosis was first suggested when Saikku and colleagues reported a small seroepidemiological study showing a much higher rate of seropositivity in patients with acute MI or chronic coronary disease than in patients without such history *(88)*. Saikku discovered this association after testing the antigen detection techniques that he had learned in Dr. Grayston's laboratory on a population that he thought to be normal, those admitted to the coronary intensive care unit, and found the seropositive rate to be much higher than expected. To date, there have been at least 20 studies showing a relationship between seropositivity to *C. pneumoniae* and atherosclerotic disease and events, whereas there have been several which have failed to show a relationship (Fig. 5).

In a case–control study from the Helsinki Heart Study, the 103 patients of the 4081 enrolled who suffered fatal or nonfatal MI or sudden cardiac death during the 5-yr follow-up were compared with matched controls in terms of antibodies against *C. pneumoniae* at study entry. Using a conditional logistic regression model, odds ratios (ORs) for the development of CHD were 2.7 (95% CI, 1.1–6.5) for elevated immunoglobulin A titers; 2.1 (CI, 1.1–3.9) for the presence of immune complexes, and 2.9 (95% CI, 1.5–5.4) for the presence of both factors *(89)*. Recently, a longer-term follow-up was reported on this same cohort with follow-up out to 8.5 yr and including baseline serology to adenovirus, enterovirus, cytomegalovirus, and herpes simplex virus (HSV) as well as to *C. pneumoniae* and *H. pylori*. Antibody levels to HSV-1 and to *C. pneumoniae* were higher in cases than in controls, whereas the distributions of antibodies to other infectious agents were similar. Mean CRP was higher in cases (4.4 vs 2.0 mg/L; $p = 0.001$), and high CRP levels increased the risks associated with smoking and with high antimicrobial antibody levels. The ORs in subjects with high antibody and high CRP levels were 25.4 (95% CI 2.9–220.3) for HSV-1 and 5.4 (95% CI 2.4–12.4) for *Chlamydia* compared with subjects with low antibody levels and low CRP. High antibody levels to either HSV-1 or to *C.*

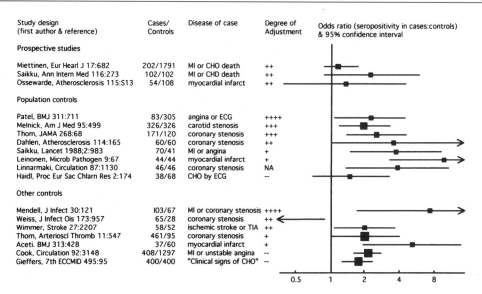

Study design (first author & reference)	Cases/ Controls	Disease of case	Degree of Adjustment	Odds ratio (seropositivity in cases:controls) & 95% confidence interval
Prospective studies				
Miettinen, Eur Hearl J 17:682	202/1791	MI or CHO death	++	
Saikku, Ann Intern Med 116:273	102/102	MI or CHD death	++	
Ossewarde, Atherosclerosis 115:S13	54/108	myocardial infarct	++	
Population controls				
Patel, BMJ 311:711	83/305	angina or ECG	++++	
Melnick, Am J Med 95:499	326/326	carotid stenosis	+++	
Thom, JAMA 268:68	171/120	coronary stenosis	+++	
Dahlen, Atherosclerosis 114:165	60/60	coronary stenosis	++	
Saikku, Lancet 1988;2:983	70/41	MI or angina	+	
Leinonen, Microb Pathogen 9:67	44/44	myocardial infarct	+	
Linnarmaki, Circulation 87:1130	46/46	coronary stenosis	NA	
Haidl, Proc Eur Sac Chlarn Res 2:174	38/68	CHO by ECG	--	
Other controls				
Mendell, J Infect 30:121	I03/67	MI or coronary stenosis	++++	
Weiss, J Infect Ois 173:957	65/28	coronary stenosis	++	
Wimmer, Stroke 27:2207	58/52	ischemic stroke or TIA	++	
Thom, Arterioscl Thromb 11:547	461/95	coronary stenosis	+	
Aceti. BMJ 313:428	37/60	myocardial infarct	+	
Cook, Circulation 92:3148	408/1297	MI or unstable angina	--	
Gieffers, 7th ECCMID 495:95	400/400	"Clinical signs of CHO"	--	

0.5   1   2   4   8

Fig. 5. Odds ratios of epidemiological studies of *C. pneumoniae* seropositivity and vascular disease. (From ref. *88*.)

pneumoniae increased the risk independently of the other, and their joint effect was close to additive *(90)*. These data support the concept that patients with evidence of chronic infection from an infectious agent, or more likely several agents, is at particular risk for events, and may be a population that would benefit from therapeutic intervention, although the details of such a strategy is yet to be worked out.

Another study that showed an association between elevated levels of antibodies to chlamydia and angiographically significant atherosclerosis was a 342-patient case–control study from the Group Health Cooperative in Seattle, WA. After adjusting for age, gender, and calendar quarter of blood drawing, the OR for CAD associated with the presence of antibody was 2.6 (95% CI, 1.4–4.8) *(91)*. Similar to the Helsinki Heart study, there was an association with smoking. In fact, in this study, the association was limited to cigarette smokers, in whom the OR was 3.5 (95% CI, 1.7–7.0). Among never-smokers, the OR was 0.8 (95% CI, 0.3–1.9). Some have suggested that smokers increased susceptibility to respiratory tract infections, such as *C. pneumoniae*, may explain part of the atherosclerotic risk associated with atherosclerosis *(92)*.

A study of particular note that failed to show an association between seropositivity to *C. pneumoniae* comes from the Physician's Health Study, in which, contrary to the association between CRP and events in this population, there was no increase risk for cardiovascular events with *C. pneumoniae (93)*. Note that this study is based on antibody presence at entry into the study, and includes a 12-yr follow-up. It is not known whether seroconversion during the follow-up period occurred more frequently in those suffering events. This study was also controlled for smoking status, hyperlipidemia, and other more traditional cardiovascular risk factors.

Antigen Detection Studies. *C. pneumoniae* or its antigens have been found in atheroma from human aorta *(94)*, carotid arteries *(95)*, and coronary arteries *(96–98)*. Although these studies are intriguing in that they show that *Chlamydia* is able to survive within atherosclerotic plaques, it does not, however, prove a causative role because it could be present as an innocent bystander, because the organism inhabits macrophages that inhabit

atherosclerotic plaque. Conversely, *C. pneumoniae* could have an effect on atherosclerosis without direct infection, because it could induce a chronic inflammatory response caused by chronic infection at a distant site.

   Animal Studies. Although Koch's postulates cannot be fully met in a multifactorial disease such as atherosclerosis, proof for a role of *C. pneumoniae* in the initiation or progression of atherosclerosis, as well as insight into the mechanism of such a role, comes from animal models of chlamydial-facilitated atherosclerosis *(79)*. In apolipoprotein E-deficient mice, *C. pneumoniae* infection accelerates the progression of atherosclerosis in the aortic arch *(99)*. *C. pneumoniae* was detected by direct plating, isolation, and polymerase chain reaction in alveolar macrophages and peripheral blood mononuclear cells, but not plasma, of intranasally inoculated mice *(100)*. Normocholesterolemic rabbits develop intimal alterations when infected with *C. pneumoniae (101,102)*. Additionally, rabbits fed a modestly cholesterol-enhanced diet have been shown by Muhlestein and colleagues *(103)* to develop accelerated aortic atherosclerosis, which is prevented by treatment with the macrolide antibiotic, azithromycin *(104)*. *C. pneumoniae* antigen could be detected in the aortic atheroma in this model, and although treatment ameliorated the accelerated atherosclerosis, *C. pneumoniae* antigen was still detected in the atheroma after treatment. It is unclear whether this represented viable quiescent organism or merely antigenic remnants of killed organism. The coronary arteries of cholesterol-fed minipigs show inflammatory changes including an increased presence of matrix metalloproteinases when infected intranasally with *C. pneumoniae (105)*. These various animal models add convincing evidence that *C. pneumoniae* can contribute to the atherosclerotic process. Continued work with these models will be important to elucidate the mechanisms behind the role of *C. pneumoniae* in atherosclerosis and to elucidate the details regarding potential treatments and their timing.

   The Early Clinical Trials. Two relatively small trials of macrolide antibiotics that are effective against *C. pneumoniae* showed dramatic reductions of coronary events with short courses of therapy. The Roxithromycin Study (ROXIS) Pilot Study was an Argentinean study in which 202 patients with unstable angina or non-Q-wave MI regardless of serology status were randomized to 150 mg roxithromycin or placebo for up to 30 d. At 30 d, there was a statistically significant reduction in the combined endpoint of cardiac death, MI, and severe recurrent ischemia (2 vs 9%; $p = 0.03$) *(106)*. The treatment effect seemed to dwindle over time, however, such that at 3 and 6 mo, although there was still a difference in the combined endpoint, the difference had lost statistical significance (12.5 vs 4.37%, $p = 0.06$ at 3 mo; 14.6 vs 8.69%, $p = 0.26$ at 6 mo) *(107)*. It is unclear whether this loss of treatment effect is because of inadequate length of treatment, or merely a play of chance at 30 d.

   The second preliminary study that drew a considerable amount of attention, despite its small size and several flaws in study design, was performed at a single center in the United Kingdom. In this study, 60 fairly stable post-MI patients who were at least 6 mo from their MI and had persistently positive (>1:64) *C. pneumoniae* antibody titers, were randomized to either 3- or 6-d regimens of oral azithromycin ($n = 40$) or placebo ($n = 20$). In a rather questionable analysis, in which 20 patients who met the study criteria but were not randomized were included in the placebo group, a fivefold reduction in a combined endpoint that included death, MI, or unstable angina requiring intravenous medical therapy or mechanical reperfusion therapy was observed *(108)*.

   When first published in 1997, these two trials generated a considerable amount of enthusiasm and reports of some practitioners beginning to prescribe macrolide antibiot-

ics to their patients with unstable coronary syndromes or a history of MI. The longer-term follow-up from the ROXIS trial and warnings about possible adverse effects helped to temper some of this enthusiasm *(109)*. Even more enthusiasm was lost when the results of the ACADEMIC trial were reported. This single-center randomized trial of 302 patients with CAD was designed to examine the effect of 3 mo of azithromycin therapy on serum markers of inflammation (CRP, IL-1, IL-6, and TNF-α) and *C. pneumoniae* immunoglobulin G titers. Azithromycin reduced a global rank sum score of the four inflammatory markers at 6 mo ($p = 0.011$) but not at 3 mo. Change-score ranks were significantly lower for CRP ($p = 0.011$) and IL-6 ($p = 0.043$). In contrast to the two earlier trials, no reduction in clinical events was observed, although it was not powered to find such results *(110)*.

Ongoing Antibiotic Trials. The encouraging results of the early small-scale treatment trials of the macrolide antibiotics led to the organization of several large-scale multicenter randomized trials. Although *C. pneumoniae* infection has been associated with the initiation and progression of atherosclerosis, results of clinical trials investigating antichlamydial antibiotics as adjuncts to standard therapy in patients with CAD have been inconsistent. In a recent meta-analysis of clinical trials of antichlamydial antibiotic therapy in patients with CAD, investigators reviewed prospective, randomized, placebo-controlled trials of antichlamydial antibiotic therapy in patients with CAD that reported all-cause mortality, MI, or unstable angina. Of the 110 potentially relevant articles identified, 11 studies enrolling 19,217 patients were included. Endpoints of interest included all-cause mortality, MI, and a combined endpoint of MI plus unstable angina. Antibiotic therapy had no impact on all-cause mortality among treated vs untreated patients (4.7 vs 4.6%; OR, 1.02; 95% CI, 0.89–1.16; $p = 0.83$), on the rates of MI (5.0 vs 5.4%; OR, 0.92; 95% CI, 0.81–1.04; $p = 0.19$), or on the combined endpoint of MI plus unstable angina (9.2 vs 9.6%; OR, 0.91; 95% CI, 0.76–1.07; $p = 0.25$). Evidence available to date does not demonstrate an overall benefit of antibiotic therapy in reducing mortality or cardiovascular events in patients with CAD.

CONCLUSIONS

Atherosclerosis is now clearly recognized as a chronic inflammatory disease at a basic level. Recent studies of clinical markers of this specialized inflammatory response have developed rapidly. These clinical markers can now be used to predict those patients who are at increased risk for the development of atherosclerosis or its complications. Chronic infections by several bacterial and viral agents have been shown to be associated with a chronic inflammatory response and with increased atherosclerotic events. In the coming years, studies will be emerging that will incorporate the use of the markers of inflammation to guide therapies aimed at interrupting the development and progression of the chronic infection and inflammation. This is indeed an exciting time in which a true paradigm shift is occurring in the understanding and treatment of atherosclerosis as an inflammatory disease.

REFERENCES

1. Ross R. Atherosclerosis—an inflammatory disease. N Engl J Med 1999;340:115–126.
2. Ross R. Atherosclerosis is an inflammatory disease. Am Heart J 1999;138:S419–S420.
3. McGill HC Jr. George Lyman Duff memorial lecture. Persistent problems in the pathogenesis of atherosclerosis. Arteriosclerosis 1984;4:443–451.

4. Stary HC, Chandler AB, Glagov S, et al. A definition of initial, fatty streak, and intermediate lesions of atherosclerosis. A report from the Committee on Vascular Lesions of the Council on Arteriosclerosis, American Heart Association. Circulation 1994;89:2462–2478.

5. Morrow DA, Ridker PM. Inflammation in cardiovascular disease. In: Topol EJ, ed. Textbook of Cardiovascular Medicine Updates. Lippincott Williams & Wilkins, Cedar Knolls, NJ, 1999, pp. 1–12.

6. Rohde LE, Lee RT, Rivero J, et al. Circulating cell adhesion molecules are correlated with ultrasound-based assessment of carotid atherosclerosis. Arterioscler Thromb Vasc Biol 1998;18:1765–1770.

7. Nakashima Y, Raines EW, Plump AS, Breslow JL, Ross R. Upregulation of VCAM-1 and ICAM-1 at atherosclerosis-prone sites on the endothelium in the apoE-deficient mouse. Arterioscler Thromb Vasc Biol 1998;18:842–851.

8. Talbott GA, Sharar SR, Harlan JM, Winn RK. Leukocyte-endothelial interactions and organ injury: the role of adhesion molecules. New Horiz 1994;2:545–554.

9. Wood KM, Cadogan MD, Ramshaw AL, Parums DV. The distribution of adhesion molecules in human atherosclerosis. Histopathology 1993;22:437–444.

10. Libby P, Sukhova G, Lee RT, Galis ZS. Cytokines regulate vascular functions related to stability of the atherosclerotic plaque. J Cardiovasc Pharmacol 1995;25:S9–S12.

11. Aqel NM, Ball RY, Waldmann H, Mitchinson MJ. Monocytic origin of foam cells in human atherosclerotic plaques. Atherosclerosis 1984;53:265–271.

12. Mantovani A, Sozzani S, Introna M. Endothelial activation by cytokines. Ann NY Acad Sci 1997; 832:93–116.

13. Ip JH, Fuster V, Badimon L, et al. Syndromes of accelerated atherosclerosis: role of vascular injury and smooth muscle cell proliferation. J Am Coll Cardiol 1990;15:1667–1687.

14. Galis ZS, Muszynski M, Sukhova GK, et al. Enhanced expression of vascular matrix metalloproteinases induced in vitro by cytokines and in regions of human atherosclerotic lesions. Ann NY Acad Sci 1995;748:501–507.

15. Amorino GP, Hoover RL. Interactions of monocytic cells with human endothelial cells stimulate monocytic metalloproteinase production. Am J Pathol 1998;152:199–207.

16. Galis ZS, Sukhova GK, Kranzhofer R, Clark S, Libby P. Macrophage foam cells from experimental atheroma constitutively produce matrix-degrading proteinases. Proc Natl Acad Sci USA 1995;92:402–406.

17. Kwon HM, Kang S, Hong BK, et al. Ultrastructural changes of the external elastic lamina in experimental hypercholesterolemic porcine coronary arteries. Yonsei Med J 1999;40:273–282.

18. Newby AC, Southgate KM, Davies M. Extracellular matrix degrading metalloproteinases in the pathogenesis of arteriosclerosis. Basic Res Cardiol 1994;89:59–70.

19. Prescott MF, Sawyer WK, Linden-Reed JV, et al. Effect of matrix metalloproteinase inhibition on progression of atherosclerosis and aneurysm in LDL receptor-deficient mice overexpressing MMP-3, MMP-12, and MMP-13 and on restenosis in rats after balloon injury. Ann NY Acad Sci 1999;878:179–190.

20. Schonbeck U, Mach F, Sukhova GK, et al. Regulation of matrix metalloproteinase expression in human vascular smooth muscle cells by T-lymphocytes: a role for CD40 signaling in plaque rupture? Circ Res 1997;81:448–454.

21. Schoenhagen P, Ziada KM, Kapadia SR, et al. Extent and direction of arterial remodeling in stable versus unstable coronary syndromes: an intravascular ultrasound study. Circulation 1999;101:598–603.

22. Davies MJ. A macro and micro view of coronary vascular insult in ischemic heart disease. Circulation 1990;82:II38–II46.

23. Lendon CL, Davies MJ, Born GV, Richardson PD. Atherosclerotic plaque caps are locally weakened when macrophages density is increased. Atherosclerosis 1991;87:87–90.

24. Moreno PR, Falk E, Palacios IF, et al. Macrophage infiltration in acute coronary syndromes. Implications for plaque rupture. Circulation 1994;90:775–778.

25. Fabunmi RP, Sukhova GK, Sugiyama S, Libby P. Expression of tissue inhibitor of metalloproteinases-3 in human atheroma and regulation in lesion-associated cells: a potential protective mechanism in plaque stability. Circ Res 1998;83:270–278.

26. Galis ZS, Sukhova GK, Lark MW, Libby P. Increased expression of matrix metalloproteinases and matrix degrading activity in vulnerable regions of human atherosclerotic plaques. J Clin Invest 1994;94:2493–2503.

27. Wilkins J, Gallimore JR, Moore EG, Pepys MB. Rapid automated high sensitivity enzyme immunoassay of C-reactive protein. Clin Chem 1998;44:1358–1361.

28. Thompson SG, Kienast J, Pyke SD, et al. Hemostatic factors and the risk of myocardial infarction or sudden death in patients with angina pectoris. European Concerted Action on Thrombosis and Disabilities Angina Pectoris Study Group [see comments]. N Engl J Med 1995;332:635–641.

29. Kuller LH, Tracy RP, Shaten J, Meilahn EN. Relation of C-reactive protein and coronary heart disease in the MRFIT nested case–control study. Multiple Risk Factor Intervention Trial. Am J Epidemiol 1996;144:537–547.

30. Ridker PM, Cushman M, Stampfer MJ, et al. Inflammation, aspirin, and the risk of cardiovascular disease in apparently healthy men. N Engl J Med 1997;336:973–979.

31. Ridker PM, Rifai N, Pfeffer MA, et al. Inflammation, pravastatin, and the risk of coronary events after myocardial infarction in patients with average cholesterol levels. Cholesterol and Recurrent Events (CARE) Investigators. Circulation 1998;98:839–844.

32. Kurakata S, Kada M, Shimada Y, et al. Effects of different inhibitors of 3-hydroxy-3-methylglutaryl coenzyme A (HMG-CoA) reductase, pravastatin sodium and simvastatin, on sterol synthesis and immunological functions in human lymphocytes in vitro. Immunopharmacology 1996;34:51–61.

33. Vaughan CJ, Murphy MB, Buckley BM. Statins do more than just lower cholesterol [see comments; published erratum appears in Lancet 1997;349:214]. Lancet 1996;348:1079–1082.

34. de Beer FC, Hind CR, Fox KM, et al. Measurement of serum C-reactive protein concentration in myocardial ischaemia and infarction. Br Heart J 1982;47:239–243.

35. Kushner I, Broder ML, Karp D. Control of the acute phase response. Serum C-reactive protein kinetics after acute myocardial infarction. J Clin Invest 1978;61:235–242.

36. Voulgari F, Cummins P, Gardecki TI, et al. Serum levels of acute phase and cardiac proteins after myocardial infarction, surgery, and infection. Br Heart J 1982;48:352–356.

37. Ikeda U, Ohkawa F, Seino Y, et al. Serum interleukin 6 levels become elevated in acute myocardial infarction. J Mol Cell Cardiol 1992;24:579–584.

38. Miyao Y, Yasue H, Ogawa H, et al. Elevated plasma interleukin-6 levels in patients with acute myocardial infarction. Am Heart J 1993;126:1299–1304.

39. Liuzzo G, Biasucci LM, Gallimore JR, et al. The prognostic value of C-reactive protein and serum amyloid A protein in severe unstable angina. N Engl J Med 1994;331:417–424.

40. Morrow DA, Rifai N, Antman EM, et al. C-reactive protein is a potent predictor of mortality independently of and in combination with troponin T in acute coronary syndromes: a TIMI 11A substudy. Thrombolysis in myocardial infarction. J Am Coll Cardiol 1998;31:1460–1465.

41. Biasucci LM, Vitelli A, Liuzzo G, et al. Elevated levels of interleukin-6 in unstable angina [see comments]. Circulation 1996;94:874–877.

42. Benamer H, Steg PG, Benessiano J, et al. Comparison of the prognostic value of C-reactive protein and troponin I in patients with unstable angina pectoris. Am J Cardiol 1998;82:845–850.

43. Toss H, Lindahl B, Siegbahn A, Wallentin L. Prognostic influence of increased fibrinogen and C-reactive protein levels in unstable coronary artery disease. FRISC Study Group. Fragmin during instability in coronary artery disease. Circulation 1997;96:4204–4210.

44. Rebuzzi AG, Quaranta G, Liuzzo G, et al. Incremental prognostic value of serum levels of troponin T and C-reactive protein on admission in patients with unstable angina pectoris. Am J Cardiol 1998;82:715–719.

45. Biasucci LM, Liuzzo G, Grillo RL, et al. Elevated levels of C-reactive protein at discharge in patients with unstable angina predict recurrent instability. Circulation 1999;99:855–860.

46. Ferreiros ER, Boissonnet CP, Pizarro R, et al. Independent prognostic value of elevated C-reactive protein in unstable angina. Circulation 1999;100:1958–1963.

47. Pietila K, Harmoinen A, Poyhonen L, et al. Intravenous streptokinase treatment and serum C-reactive protein in patients with acute myocardial infarction. Br Heart J 1987;58:225–229.

48. Pietila K, Harmoinen A, Teppo AM. Acute phase reaction, infarct size and in-hospital morbidity in myocardial infarction patients treated with streptokinase or recombinant tissue type plasminogen activator. Ann Med 1991;23:529–535.

49. Pudil R, Pidrman V, Krejsek J, et al. The effect of reperfusion on plasma tumor necrosis factor alpha and C reactive protein levels in the course of acute myocardial infarction. Acta Med 1996;39:149–153.

50. Pietila K, Harmoinen A, Hermens W, et al. Serum C-reactive protein and infarct size in myocardial infarct patients with a closed versus an open infarct-related coronary artery after thrombolytic therapy. Eur Heart J 1993;14:915–919.

51. Casscells W, Hathorn B, David M, et al. Thermal detection of cellular infiltrates in living atherosclerotic plaques: possible implications for plaque rupture and thrombosis [see comments]. Lancet 1996;347:1447–1451.

52. Loike JD, Silverstein SC, Sturtevant JM. Application of differential scanning microcalorimetry to the study of cellular processes: heat production and glucose oxidation of murine macrophages. Proc Natl Acad Sci USA 1981;78:5958–5962.

53. van der Wal AC, Becker AE, van der Loos CM, Das PK. Site of intimal rupture or erosion of thrombosed coronary atherosclerotic plaques is characterized by an inflammatory process irrespective of the dominant plaque morphology [see comments]. Circulation 1994;89:36–44.

54. Moreno PR, Bernardi VH, Lopez-Cuellar J, et al. Macrophage infiltration predicts restenosis after coronary intervention in patients with unstable angina. Circulation 1996;94:3098–3102.

55. Lauer MA, Zhou ZM, Forudi F, et al. The temperatures of atherosclerotic lesions in the hypercholesterolemic rabbit double injury model are elevated following angioplasty. J Am Coll Cardiol 1999;33:67A.

56. Stefanadis C, Diamantopoulos L, Vlachopoulos C, et al. Thermal heterogeneity within human atherosclerotic coronary arteries detected in vivo: a new method of detection by application of a special thermography catheter. Circulation 1999;99:1965–1971.

57. Stefanadis C, Diamantopoulos L, Vlachopoulos C, et al. Thermal heterogeneity within human atherosclerotic coronary arteries detected in vivo: a new method of detection by application of special thermography catheter. Circulation 1999;99:1965–1971.

58. Guo B, Willerson JT, Bearman G, et al. Application of infrared fiber optic imaging of atherosclerotic plaques. Proc of SPIE 1999;3698:75–82.

59. Moreno PR, Lodder RA, O'Connor WN, et al. Characterization of vulnerable plaques by near infrared spectroscopy in an atherosclerotic rabbit model. J Am Coll Cardiol 1999;33:66A.

60. Ridker PM, Haughie P. Prospective studies of C-reactive protein as a risk factor for cardiovascular disease. J Invest Med 1998;46:391–395.

61. Fabricant CG, Fabricant J, Litrenta MM, Minick CR. Virus-induced atherosclerosis. J Exp Med 1978;148:335–340.

62. Fabricant CG, Fabricant J, Minick CR, Litrenta MM. Herpesvirus-induced atherosclerosis in chickens. Fed Proc 1983;42:2476–2479.

63. Melnick JL, Hu C, Burek J, et al. Cytomegalovirus DNA in arterial walls of patients with atherosclerosis. J Med Virol 1994;42:170–174.

64. Hendrix MG, Salimans MM, van Boven CP, Bruggeman CA. High prevalence of latently present cytomegalovirus in arterial walls of patients suffering from grade III atherosclerosis. Am J Pathol 1990;136:23–28.

65. Hendrix MG, Dormans PH, Kitslaar P, et al. The presence of cytomegalovirus nucleic acids in arterial walls of atherosclerotic and nonatherosclerotic patients. Am J Pathol 1989;134:1151–1157.

66. Lemstrom K, Koskinen P, Krogerus L, et al. Cytomegalovirus antigen expression, endothelial cell proliferation, and intimal thickening in rat cardiac allografts after cytomegalovirus infection. Circulation 1995;92:2594–2604.

67. Lemstrom KB, Bruning JH, Bruggeman CA, et al. Cytomegalovirus infection enhances smooth muscle cell proliferation and intimal thickening of rat aortic allografts. J Clin Invest 1993;92:549–558.

68. McGiffin DC, Savunen T, Kirklin JK, et al. Cardiac transplant coronary artery disease. A multivariable analysis of pretransplantation risk factors for disease development and morbid events. J Thorac Cardiovasc Surg 1995;109:1081–1089.

69. Mangiavacchi M, Frigerio M, Gronda E, et al. Acute rejection and cytomegalovirus infection: correlation with cardiac allograft vasculopathy. Transplant Proc 1995;27:1960–1962.

70. Gao SZ, Hunt SA, Schroeder JS, et al. Early development of accelerated graft coronary artery disease: risk factors and course. J Am Coll Cardiol 1996;28:673–679.

71. Zhou YF, Shou M, Guetta E, et al. Cytomegalovirus infection of rats increases the neointimal response to vascular injury without consistent evidence of direct infection of the vascular wall. Circulation 1999;100:1569–1575.

72. Nieto FJ, Adam E, Sorlie P, et al. Cohort study of cytomegalovirus infection as a risk factor for carotid intimal-medial thickening, a measure of subclinical atherosclerosis. Circulation 1996;94:922–927.

73. Sorlie PD, Adam E, Melnick SL, et al. Cytomegalovirus/herpesvirus and carotid atherosclerosis: the ARIC Study. J Med Virol 1994;42:33–37.

74. Adam E, Melnick JL, Probtsfield JL, et al. High levels of cytomegalovirus antibody in patients requiring vascular surgery for atherosclerosis. Lancet 1987;2:291–293.

75. Zhou YF, Leon MB, Waclawiw MA, et al. Association between prior cytomegalovirus infection and the risk of restenosis after coronary atherectomy. N Engl J Med 1996;335:624–630.

76. Melnick JL, Adam E, DeBakey ME. Possible role of cytomegalovirus in atherogenesis. JAMA 1990;263:2204–2207.

77. Dummer S, Lee A, Breinig MK, et al. Investigation of cytomegalovirus infection as a risk factor for coronary atherosclerosis in the explanted hearts of patients undergoing heart transplantation. J Med Virol 1994;44:305–309.

78. Zhu J, Quyyumi AA, Norman JE, et al. Total pathogen burden contributes incrementally to coronary artery disease risk and to C-reactive protein levels. Circulation 1998;98:I-142.

79. Epstein SE, Zhou YF, Zhu J. Infection and atherosclerosis: emerging mechanistic paradigms. Circulation 1999;100:e20–e28.

80. Wanishsawad C, Zhou YF, Epstein SE. Chlamydia pneumoniae-induced transactivation of the major immediate early promoter of cytomegalovirus: potential synergy of infectious agents in the pathogenesis of atherosclerosis. J Infect Dis 2000;181:787–790.

81. Markus HS, Mendall MA. Helicobacter pylori infection: a risk factor for ischaemic cerebrovascular disease and carotid atheroma. J Neurol Neurosurg Psychiatry 1998;64:104–107.

82. Whincup PH, Mendall MA, Perry IJ, et al. Prospective relations between Helicobacter pylori infection, coronary heart disease, and stroke in middle aged men. Heart 1996;75:568–572.

83. Patel P, Mendall MA, Carrington D, et al. Association of Helicobacter pylori and Chlamydia pneumoniae infections with coronary heart disease and cardiovascular risk factors [see comments; published erratum appears in Br Med J 1995;311:985]. Br Med J 1995;311:711–714.

84. Grayston JT, Aldous MB, Easton A, et al. Evidence that Chlamydia pneumoniae causes pneumonia and bronchitis. J Infect Dis 1993;168:1231–1235.

85. Grayston JT, Campbell LA, Kuo CC, et al. A new respiratory tract pathogen: Chlamydia pneumoniae strain TWAR. J Infect Dis 1990;161:618–625.

86. Saikku P. The epidemiology and significance of Chlamydia pneumoniae. J Infect 1992;25(Suppl 1):27–34.

87. Grayston JT, Wang SP, Kuo CC, Campbell LA. Current knowledge on Chlamydia pneumoniae, strain TWAR, an important cause of pneumonia and other acute respiratory diseases. Eur J Clin Microbiol Infect Dis 1989;8:191–202.

88. Saikku P, Leinonen M, Mattila K, et al. Serological evidence of an association of a novel Chlamydia, TWAR, with chronic coronary heart disease and acute myocardial infarction. Lancet 1988;2:983–986.

89. Saikku P, Leinonen M, Tenkanen L, et al. Chronic Chlamydia pneumoniae infection as a risk factor for coronary heart disease in the Helsinki Heart Study. Ann Intern Med 1992;116:273–278.

90. Roivainen M, Viik-Kajander M, Palosuo T, et al. Infections, inflammation, and the risk of coronary heart disease. Circulation 2000;101:252–257.

91. Thom DH, Grayston JT, Siscovick DS, et al. Association of prior infection with Chlamydia pneumoniae and angiographically demonstrated coronary artery disease. JAMA 1992;268:68–72.

92. Hahn DL, Golubjatnikov R. Smoking is a potential confounder of the Chlamydia pneumoniae-coronary artery disease association. Arterioscler Thromb 1992;12:945–947.

93. Ridker PM, Kundsin RB, Stampfer MJ, et al. Prospective study of Chlamydia pneumoniae IgG seropositivity and risks of future myocardial infarction. Circulation 1999;99:1161–1164.

94. Kuo CC, Gown AM, Benditt EP, Grayston JT. Detection of Chlamydia pneumoniae in aortic lesions of atherosclerosis by immunocytochemical stain. Arterioscler Thrombs 1993;13:1501–1504.

95. Grayston JT, Kuo CC, Coulson AS, et al. Chlamydia pneumoniae (TWAR) in atherosclerosis of the carotid artery. Circulation 1995;92:3397–3400.

96. Kuo CC, Shor A, Campbell LA, et al. Demonstration of Chlamydia pneumoniae in atherosclerotic lesions of coronary arteries. J Infect Dis 1993;167:841–849.

97. Muhlestein JB, Hammond EH, Carlquist JF, et al. Increased incidence of Chlamydia species within the coronary arteries of patients with symptomatic atherosclerotic versus other forms of cardiovascular disease. J Am Coll Cardiol 1996;27:1555–1561.

98. Ramirez JA. Isolation of Chlamydia pneumoniae from the coronary artery of a patient with coronary atherosclerosis. The Chlamydia pneumoniae/Atherosclerosis Study Group. Ann Intern Med 1996;125:979–982.

99. Moazed TC, Campbell LA, Rosenfeld ME, et al. Chlamydia pneumoniae infection accelerates the progression of atherosclerosis in apolipoprotein E-deficient mice. J Infect Dis 1999;180:238–241.

100. Moazed TC, Kuo CC, Grayston JT, Campbell LA. Evidence of systemic dissemination of Chlamydia pneumoniae via macrophages in the mouse. J Infect Dis 1998;177:1322–1325.

101. Fong IW, Chiu B, Viira E, et al. Rabbit model for Chlamydia pneumoniae infection. J Clin Microbiol 1997;35:48–52.

102. Laitinen K, Laurila A, Pyhala L, et al. Chlamydia pneumoniae infection induces inflammatory changes in the aortas of rabbits. Infect Immun 1997;65:4832–4835.

103. Muhlestein JB, Anderson JL, Hammond EH, et al. Infection with *Chlamydia pneumoniae* accelerates the development of atherosclerosis and treatment with azithromycin prevents it in a rabbit model. Circulation 1998;97:633–636.
104. Muhlestein JB, Anderson JL, Hammond EH, et al. Infection with Chlamydia pneumoniae accelerates the development of atherosclerosis and treatment with azithromycin prevents it in a rabbit model. Circulation 1998;97:633–636.
105. Lauer MA, Mawhorter SD, Vince DG, et al. Increase in coronary artery matrix metalloproteinases in minipigs induced by intranasal Chlamydia pneumoniae infection. J Am Coll Cardiol 2000;35:302A.
106. Gurfinkel E, Bozovich G, Daroca A, et al. Randomised trial of roxithromycin in non-Q-wave coronary syndromes: ROXIS Pilot Study. ROXIS Study Group. Lancet 1997;350:404–407.
107. Gurfinkel E, Bozovich G, Beck E, et al. Treatment with the antibiotic roxithromycin in patients with acute non-Q-wave coronary syndromes. The final report of the ROXIS Study [see comments]. Eur Heart J 1999;20:121–127.
108. Gupta S, Leatham EW, Carrington D, et al. Elevated Chlamydia pneumoniae antibodies, cardiovascular events, and azithromycin in male survivors of myocardial infarction. Circulation 1997;96:404–407.
109. Grayston JT. Antibiotic treatment of Chlamydia pneumoniae for secondary prevention of cardiovascular events [editorial; see comments]. Circulation 1998;97:1669–1670.
110. Andraws R, Berger JS, Brown DL. Effects of antibiotic therapy on outcomes of patients with coronary artery disease: a meta-analysis of randomized controlled trials. JAMA. 2005;293:2641–2647.

II

RISK FACTORS AND THEIR MANAGEMENT IN CORONARY ARTERY DISEASE

4 Low-Density Lipoprotein Cholesterol and Coronary Artery Disease

Clinical Evidence and Clinical Implications

JoAnne Micale Foody, MD

CONTENTS

INTRODUCTION

Except for age, dyslipidemia is the most important predictive factor for coronary artery disease (CAD) *(1)*. The strong, independent, continuous, and graded relationship between total cholesterol (TC) levels, or low-density lipoprotein (LDL)-cholesterol (C) level and the risk of CAD events has been clearly demonstrated world wide in men and women and in all age groups *(2–6)*. High cholesterol levels are a major contributor to CAD: 38 million Americans have a TC of more than 240 mg/dL and 96 million are estimated to have levels above 200 mg/dL *(7)*. In general, a 1% increase in the LDL-C level may lead to a 2–3% increase in CAD risk *(3,4)*. Aggressive lipid-lowering drug treatment in high-risk individuals will reduce coronary heart disease (CHD) morbidity and mortality rates and increase overall survival *(8–12)*.

Conclusive evidence from rigorous, large-scale, randomized clinical trials, such as the Scandinavian Simvastatin Survival Study (4S) *(9)*, the Cholesterol and Recurrent Events (CARE) *(8)* trial, the West of Scotland Coronary Prevention Study (WOSCOPS) *(11)*, the Long-Term Intervention with Pravastatin in Ischaemic Disease (LIPID) *(12)* trial and the Air Force/Texas Coronary Atherosclerosis Prevention Study (AFCAPS/TEXCAPS) *(13)* has given new impetus to the practice of preventive cardiology. Recent findings from the Heart Protection Study (HPS) *(14)*, Anglo-Scandinavian Cardiac Outcomes Trial Lipid-

From: *Contemporary Cardiology: Preventive Cardiology:*
Insights Into the Prevention and Treatment of Cardiovascular Disease, Second Edition
Edited by: J. M. Foody © Humana Press Inc., Totowa, NJ

Lowering Arm (ASCOT-LLA) *(15)*, Pravastatin in elderly individuals at risk of vascular disease (PROSPER) *(16)*, Collaborative Atorvastatin Diabetes Study (CARDS) *(17)*, PROVE-IT *(18)*, and Treating to New Targets (TNT) *(19)* have further strengthened the position of lipid lowering strategies in clinical medicine.

Despite national guidelines *(20–22)* emphasizing the importance of lipid lowering, more than two-thirds of patients treated for hyperlipidemia by primary care physicians fail to reach recommended National Cholesterol Education Program (NCEP) targets. More striking is the fact that 80% of patients with established CAD, those at greatest risk, fail to reach the NCEP target *(23)*. This failure is partially because of inconsistent strategies applied toward the management of patients at risk for the development and progression of CAD.

EPIDEMIOLOGICAL AND POPULATION STUDIES

Total Cholesterol

Cholesterol is now viewed as a crucial factor in the development of atherosclerosis *(1)*. Initial work from the Framingham Study *(2)* as well as from the Multiple Risk Factor Intervention Trial (MRFIT) *(5,24)* have demonstrated a continuous and graded positive relationship between the level of TC and CAD mortality.

In the Framingham Study *(2,5,6)*, a stepwise increase in serum cholesterol and the associated increase in 24-yr incidence of CHD were particularly powerful factors in young men but were much less apparent in women. In the Framingham Study, 20% of myocardial infarctions (MIs) occurred within a range of cholesterol that is considered "normal" by the NCEP guidelines (<200 mg/dL). The contribution of LDL to CAD risk in young men was apparent in the Framingham study. In an older population of men and women (aged 50 to 80 yr), LDL-C was associated significantly ($p < 0.05$) with CHD after 7 yr of follow-up.

MRFIT *(5,24)* investigated the effect of risk factor interventions on the development of CHD. A total of 361,662 men were screened for the MRFIT, and a 6-yr mortality rate was calculated in relation to serum cholesterol. Of note, the risk of CAD death increased progressively in men with a serum cholesterol higher than 181 mg/dL. Men with a serum cholesterol level in excess of 253 mg/dL had a relative risk 3.8 times greater than those men with levels lower than 181 mg/dL. Furthermore, serum cholesterol higher than the 90th percentile is often used to define "hypercholesterolemia," yet 54% of the CHD occurred in men whose levels fell below the 85th percentile. In this group of 356,222 men aged 35 to 57 yr, without previous MI, there was no lower threshold below which CAD risk did not occur.

LDL Cholesterol

The dyslipidemia most clearly associated with the development of CAD is hypercholesterolemia, particularly caused by an elevation in LDL-C. Based on the known relationship between LDL-C and CAD, the treatment guidelines of the NCEP *(20–22)* focus on LDL-C reduction for the primary and secondary prevention of CAD events. Numerous clinical trials support the importance of LDL-C lowering in decreasing CAD risk, both in angiographic trials, which measure CAD progression, and in trials that assess morbidity and mortality.

LDL Subclasses and Clinical Implications

It is important to remember that LDL is not a homogeneous particle but consists of a set of discrete subspecies with distinct molecular properties, including size and density. In normal subjects, at least four major LDL subspecies can be identified: LDL-I is the largest and least dense, and, the smallest, LDL-IV, is the most dense. LDL size is a powerful predictor of CAD risk, independent of triglycerides (TG), high-density lipoprotein (HDL)-C, LDL-C, and body mass index (BMI) *(25)*.

Three prospective trials that investigated the predictive nature of LDL size have been reported. The Physicians Health Study investigated the importance of LDL subclass pattern on CAD risk in 14,916 men. In 266 cases and 308 control subjects followed for 7 yr, LDL diameter was related to CAD. The Stanford Five City Project prospectively evaluated the role of LDL size in CAD in 124 matched pairs of cases and control subjects. LDL size was significantly smaller and more dense ($p < 0.001$) among CAD cases compared with control subjects. The association was graded across quintiles of LDL size. This difference was independent of HDL-C, TG, smoking, blood pressure, and BMI. In this study, LDL size was the best discriminator of CAD status. The Quebec Cardiovascular Study was a prospective investigation of CAD risk factors in 2103 asymptomatic men. After 5 yr of follow-up, LDL diameter proved to be an independent predictor of CAD risk. The power of LDL size as a risk predictor was independent of age, BMI, alcohol consumption, smoking, and fasting TG, apolipoprotein (apo)-B, LDL-C, and HDL-C levels.

Although elevated LDL-C increases CAD risk, it seems that an LDL subclass distribution may be a more common and more powerful predictor of risk. It is present in 50% of men with CAD and identifies a group of people that can respond particularly well to appropriate treatment and are good arteriographic responders to treatment. TC and LDL-C are frequently within normal limits in these individuals and, thus, their high-risk state is not identified on routine blood tests *(25)*.

CLINICAL TRIALS IN DYSLIPIDEMIA

LDL-C Modification

Conclusive evidence from rigorous, large scale, randomized clinical trials, such as the 4S study *(9)*, CARE *(8)*, WOSCOPS *(11)*, and the LIPID trial *(12)* has given new impetus to the practice of preventive cardiology. More recent results from the HPS *(14)*, PROVE-IT *(18)*, PROSPER *(16)*, and TNT *(19)*, in combination with landmark secondary prevention trials, have further strengthened the position of lipid-lowering strategies in clinical medicine and created a new paradigm for the management of lipids.

Primary Prevention Trials

Until recently, the literature did not support protecting patients through cholesterol reduction. Early primary prevention trials tested the hypothesis that a decrease in TC leads to a decrease in cardiovascular events (Fig. 1). In the early 1980s, two additional large-scale primary trials were conducted: the Lipid Research Clinics Coronary Primary Prevention Trial *(26–28)* and the Helsinki Heart Study (HHS) *(29,30)*. The Lipid Research Clinics Coronary Primary Prevention Trial was a randomized, double-blind, placebo-controlled trial of diet plus cholestyramine vs diet plus placebo. This landmark study conclu-

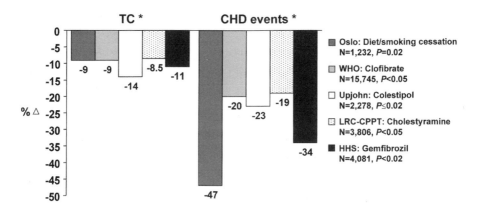

N=number enrolled.

Fig. 1. Early primary-prevention trials: overview. * = net difference between treatment and control groups (*p* values are for events).

sively showed that reducing cholesterol by diet and a pharmacological regimen reduced the risk of CHD in men with hypercholesterolemia. Specifically, a 10 to 15% reduction in serum cholesterol may result in a 20 to 30% reduction in risk for CHD. The HHS was a double-blind, placebo-controlled primary prevention trial that randomized men without CHD to receive either placebo or gemfibrozil. Overall, a 34% reduction in the incidence of CHD was observed. Importantly, the HHS identified a subgroup of patients with high risk for cardiac events. This group was characterized by an LDL-C to HDL-C ratio greater than five and TG greater than 200 mg/dL, and this group experienced a 71% reduction in CHD event rate with treatment. These studies demonstrated significant reductions in lipids and an associated decrease in CHD events. They provide clear evidence of the clinical benefits associated with the primary prevention of CHD.

With the development of hydroxymethylglutaryl (HMG)-coenzyme A (CoA) reductase inhibitors, a new era of lipid-lowering management was begun. These powerful new drugs provided a significant mortality benefit in patients without overt CAD. The landmark WOSCOPS *(11)* was conducted on 6595 men between the ages of 45 and 64 yr, with TC levels greater than 252 mg/dL and LDL-C levels between 174 and 232 mg/dL, but no clinical evidence of heart disease. Study participants were treated with dietary intervention and randomized to receive placebo or 40 mg/d pravastatin. Pravastatin reduced the risk of a first heart attack by 31% and the need for coronary revascularization procedures by 37% (Fig. 2).

More recently, AFCAPS/TEXCAPS *(13)* capitalized on the increased risk of healthy subjects with low HDL and increased TC to HDL-C ratios. Therapy with the cholesterol-lowering drug, lovastatin (Mevacor), reduced the risk of first acute major coronary events in healthy adults with average-to-mildly elevated cholesterol levels and low HDL by 36% (Fig. 3). The trial included 6605 healthy adults aged 45 to 73 yr including a broad spectrum of men and women, including African Americans and Hispanic Americans (997 women, 487 Hispanic Americans, and 206 African Americans). More than 20% were aged 65 yr and older. Inclusion criteria for the study included lack of evidence for CAD, an LDL-C between 130 and 190 mg/dL, HDL less than 45 mg/dL (<47 mg/dL for

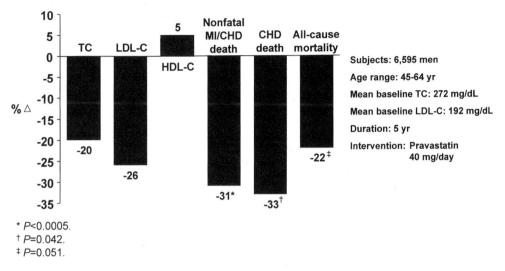

* *P*<0.0005.
† *P*=0.042.
‡ *P*=0.051.

Fig. 2. WOSCOPS: lipid lowering and coronary events. (Adapted from ref. *11*.)

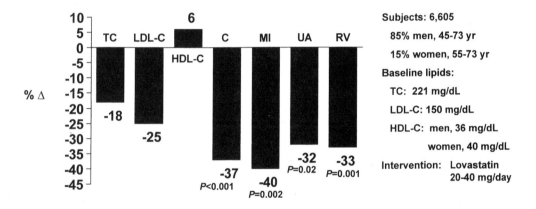

C=coronary events defined as fatal/nonfatal myocardial infarction, sudden death, and unstable angina;
MI=fatal/nonfatal myocardial infarction; UA=unstable angina;
RV=revascularizations.

Fig. 3. AFCAPS/TEXCAPS: LDL-C lowering and coronary events. (Adapted from ref. *13*.)

women), and TG levels less than 400 mg/dL. Therefore, none of the participants had evidence of heart disease; 22% had hypertension, 2% had diabetes, and 12% were smokers. Participants were randomly assigned to receive either lovastatin or a placebo. Dosage of the drug began at 20 mg/d, and in 50% of patients was raised to 40 mg/d to target the LDL-C to less than 100 mg/dL. Before the trial was begun, the average TC level among participants was 221 mg/dL, the LDL level was 150 mg/dL, and the average HDL level was 37 mg/dL. TC levels in the lovastatin group were reduced by 18.4%, LDL levels fell by 25%, and TGs were reduced by 15%.

Preliminary results indicate that patients taking lovastatin had a reduced risk for coronary events. Their risk of first acute coronary event (sudden death, MI, or unstable

angina) was reduced by 36%, risk of first coronary events was reduced by 54% in women, 34% in men, 43% in hypertensive patients and diabetic patients, and 29% in the elderly. Patients in the lovastatin group also had a 33% reduction in procedures such as angioplasty and bypass, and a 34% reduction in hospitalization because of unstable angina.

These results are particularly significant because most of the study participants would not ordinarily have been considered candidates for cholesterol-lowering therapy based on previous NCEP guidelines. This group, however, represent the majority of persons who eventually develop heart disease. This study represents a significant advance in our understanding of the role of reducing cholesterol in preventing new onset of heart disease in apparently healthy persons.

Although the WOSCOPS study demonstrated that treatment of relatively high-risk men with profoundly elevated cholesterol levels significantly reduced risk of heart attack and death from heart disease, the AFCAPS/TEXCAPS study has demonstrated benefit in those with more typical risk profiles, including lower cholesterol values. It has been suggested that AFCAPS/TEXCAPS expands the number of possible candidates for cholesterol-lowering drug therapy in the United States by more than 8 million people. The participants in AFCAPS/TEXCAPS would not ordinarily have been considered candidates for cholesterol-lowering therapy based on previous NCEP guidelines.

HIGH-RISK PRIMARY PREVENTION TRIALS

Heart Protection Study (14). The HPS explored the role of lipid lowering in individuals with diabetes or at high risk for vascular events. Although it is known that people with diabetes are at increased risk of cardiovascular morbidity and mortality, their plasma concentrations of LDL-C are similar to those in the general population. Existing evidence regarding the effects of lowering cholesterol in people with diabetes was limited, and most diabetic patients do not receive cholesterol-lowering therapy despite their increased risk. Given these issues, the HPS sought to determine the role of lipid lowering in 5963 adults (aged 40–80 yr) known to have diabetes, and an additional 14,573 adults with occlusive arterial disease (but no diagnosed diabetes). Patients were randomly allocated to receive 40 mg simvastatin daily or matching placebo. The primary outcome of interest was first major coronary event (i.e., nonfatal MI or coronary death) and first major vascular event (i.e., major coronary event, stroke, or revascularization) at 5 yr. There were highly significant reductions in the first event rate for major coronary events, for strokes, and for revascularizations. For the first occurrence of any of these major vascular events among participants with diabetes, there was a 22% (95% confidence interval [CI], 13–30) reduction in the event rate (601 [20.2%] simvastatin allocated vs 748 [25.1%] placebo allocated; $p < 0.0001$), which was similar to that among the other high-risk individuals studied. There were also highly significant reductions, of 33% (95% CI, 17–46; $p = 0.0003$) among the 2912 diabetic participants who did not have any diagnosed occlusive arterial disease at entry, and of 27% (95% CI, 13–40; $p = 0.0007$) among the 2426 diabetic participants whose pretreatment LDL-C concentration was below 3.0 mmol/L (116 mg/dL). The HPS study provides direct evidence that cholesterol-lowering therapy is beneficial for people with diabetes even if they do not already have manifest coronary disease or high cholesterol concentrations. Allocation to 40 mg simvastatin daily reduced the rate of first major vascular events by 22% in a wide range of diabetic patients studied. Based on the results of the HPS, statin therapy should now be considered routinely for all diabetic patients at sufficiently high risk of major vascular events, irrespective of their initial cholesterol concentrations.

Collaborative Atorvastatin Diabetes Study *(17)*. This study was the first large primary prevention study to focus entirely on the role of lipid lowering in patients with type 2 diabetes without evidence of cardiovascular disease (CVD). This trial randomized 2383 diabetic patients aged 40 to 75 yr to either 10 mg of atorvastatin or placebo. The trial was stopped early at 4 yr, demonstrating a 37% relative risk reduction ($p < 0.001$) for 10 mg atorvastatin in the primary endpoint of heart disease death, fatal or nonfatal MI, unstable angina requiring hospitalization, cardiac arrest, coronary revascularization, or stroke. Benefits were consistent irrespective of initial LDL-C levels. Consistent with the HPS, CARDS demonstrates improvements in outcomes in diabetics treated with statin therapy irrespective of initial LDL levels.

Anglo-Scandinavian Cardiac Outcomes Trial Lipid-Lowering Arm *(15)*. This study sought to establish the benefits of lowering lipids in well-controlled hypertensive patients who were not conventionally considered dyslipidemic. In this study of 19,342 hypertensive patients (aged 40 to 79 yr) with at least three cardiovascular risk factors, participants were randomized to one of two antihypertensive regimens in the ASCOT trial. In 10,305 of these participants with nonfasting TC less than 160 mg/dL, additional randomization to either 10 mg atorvastatin or placebo occurred. These patients comprised the lipid-lowering arm of the study. The primary outcome of interest was nonfatal MI and fatal CHD at 5 yr. This trial was stopped early at 3.3 yr. At that time, atorvastatin therapy was associated with a 36% reduction in primary events compared with placebo. Based on the results of ASCOT-LLA, statin therapy should be considered in hypertensive patients with multiple risk factors irrespective of their initial cholesterol values.

Pravastatin in Elderly Individuals at Risk of Vascular Disease *(16)*. PROSPER was another randomized, placebo-controlled trial designed to test the benefits of statin treatment in 2804 men and 3000 women between 70 and 82 yr of age with, or at high risk for, CVD. The mean age of the patients was 75.3 yr. This was one of the few statin trials that enrolled similar numbers of men and women, and treated elderly individuals at risk for CVD. The primary endpoint was the composite of coronary death, nonfatal MI, and fatal or nonfatal stroke after 3.2 yr of follow-up. For the entire study population, statin therapy decreased LDL-C by 34%, and this was associated with 408 events in the pravastatin group and 473 in the placebo group, for a hazard ratio of 0.85, which was statistically significant ($p = 0.014$). There was also a reduced risk for the secondary endpoints of coronary death and nonfatal MI ($p = 0.006$) or coronary death alone ($p = 0.043$).

The PROSPER investigators also analyzed the primary endpoint according to sex because reduction of risk for coronary death, nonfatal MI, and fatal or nonfatal stroke seemed to be more pronounced in men than in women, based on the 186 events in women and 229 events in men compared with the events in the respective placebo groups (194 and 272 events). The hazard ratio for this endpoint was 0.96 in women and 0.77 in men, but a test for interaction revealed no significant differences between the genders. PROSPER was unable to detect an effect of statin treatment specifically on the incidence of stroke in this population. The investigators offered that the study may have lacked the statistical power to detect an effect on stroke, or that the duration of follow-up, 3.2 yr, was too short to see an effect. In addition, there were more new cancer diagnoses in the pravastatin group ($p = 0.02$).

SECONDARY PREVENTION TRIALS

Regression Trials. A number of smaller trials have evaluated the effect of aggressive lipid lowering on actual vessel blockage. These so-called regression trials (Tables 1 and 2)

Table 1
Lipid Lowering and Plaque Regression: Monotherapy Studies

Study	Treatment group		Δ% Stenosis (p)	Event reduction (%)
	Regimen	LDL-C		
NHLBI II	D + R	↓31	—	33
STARS	D + R	↓36	↓7.7(<0.01)	89
Heidelberg	D + E	↓8	↓4.0 (0.05)	–29[a]
CCAIT	D + L	↓29	↓1.2 (0.039)	—
MARS	D + L	↓38	↓0.6	—
BECAIT	D + F	↓3	↓2.55	77
LCAS	D + FI	↓24	↓2.0 (0.043)	33
Post-CABG	D + L	↓14	↓5.4 (0.001)	—

Data from refs. *31–34* and *52–54*.
[a]A 27% reduction means a 27% increase (not significant).
D, diet; R, resin; E, exercise program; F, fibrate-type drug; FI, fluvastatin; L, lovastatin.

Table 2
Lipid Lowering and Plaque Regression: Combination Therapy Studies

Study	Treatment group		Δ% Stenosis (p)	Event reduction (%)
	Regimen	LDL-C		
CLAS I	D + R + N	↓43	—	25
POSCH (5 y)	D + PIB ± R	↓42	—	35 (62)
Lifestyle	V + M + E	↓37	↓2.2 (0.001)	—
FATS (N + C)	D + R + N	↓32	↓0.9 (0.005)	80
FATS (L + C)	D + R + L	↓46	↓0.7 (0.02)	70
CLAS II	D + R + N	↓40	—	43
USCF-SCOR	D + R + ± L	↓39	↓1.5 (0.04)	—
SCRIP	D + (R + N + L +F) + E, BP	↓21	—	50
HARP	D + P + N + C + F	↓41	↑2.1	33
Post-CABG	D + L + C	↓37–40	↓0.054	29

Data from refs. *33* and *34*.
C, cholestyramine; D, diet; E, exercise program; F, fibrate-type drug; L, lovastatin; M, relaxation techniques; N, nicotinic acid; P, pravastatin; PIB, partial ileal bypass; R, resin; V, vegetarian diet.

assessed the degree of atherosclerotic progression and regression by either ultrasonography of the carotid arteries or, more often, by coronary angiography *(31,34)*. The Multicenter Anti-Atheroma Study (MAAS) *(31)* was a double-blind clinical trial that randomized 381 patients with documented CHD to receive dietary treatment plus 20 mg/d simvastatin or placebo during a 48-mo trial duration. Angiographic analysis showed a decreased rate of progression of luminal stenosis in the simvastatin group, with a divergence between the plotted curves of the simvastatin and placebo groups.

The St. Thomas' Arteriographic Regression Study *(32)* followed coronary arteriography in 90 men whose TCs were between 232 and 386 mg/dL and were randomized to a control group, to a group treated with a low-fat, high-fiber (3.6 g/1000 kcal pectin) diet,

or to a group treated with the low-fat, high-fiber diet plus 16 g/d cholestyramine. No substantial differences were reported among the groups for HDL-C. Arteriographically defined progression was reported to have occurred in 54% of the control group, compared with 19% of the diet group and 17% of the diet plus cholestyramine group, respectively. Regression occurred in 4% of the control group, compared with 42% of the diet group and 38% of the diet plus cholestyramine group. Dense LDL reduction was reported to be the best predictor of arteriographic change.

The Cholesterol-Lowering Atherosclerosis Study *(33)* involved 162 postcoronary bypass patients randomly assigned to placebo or treatment with colestipol and niacin. After 2 yr of treatment, the average number of lesions that progressed was significantly lower ($p = 0.03$) in the drug-treatment group. The number of subjects who showed new atheroma formation in native coronary arteries ($p = 0.03$) and changes in bypass grafts ($p = 0.04$) was also significantly lower. Atherosclerosis regression was reported to have occurred in 16.2% of the drug-treated patients ($p = 0.002$). Drug treatment resulted in a 43% reduction in LDL-C, a 22% reduction in TGs, and a 37% increase in HDL-C. The mean LDL-C levels in the treatment and control groups were 97 and 160 mg/dL, respectively. Subjects with lower TGs received no arteriographic benefit compared with the control group, despite substantial blood lipid changes.

The Post Coronary Artery Bypass Study *(34)* investigated the effect of aggressive LDL-C reduction (a goal of LDL-C of 60–85 mg/dL) vs moderate LDL-C reduction (a goal of LDL-C of 130–140 mg/dL) for 4 yr, in 1351 subjects who had a previous coronary artery bypass graft (CABG). Of the moderate treatment group, 35% had substantial progression of their grafts compared with 24% in the aggressive treatment group ($p < 0.001$) (Table 3). Although this indicates benefit from aggressive treatment, it also indicates that 24% of Coronary Artery Bypass Study patients who achieved LDL-C levels of less than 100 mg/dL continued to show arteriographic progression.

The Regression Growth Evaluation Statin Study *(35)* treated 885 hypercholesterolemic men with either pravastatin or a placebo for 2 yr. The mean segment diameter worsened by 0.10 mm in the placebo group and worsened by 0.06 mm in the pravastatin group, which represents a significant ($p = 0.02$) reduction in the rate of progression. The Pravastatin Limitation of Atherosclerosis in the Coronary Arteries study *(36)* treated 408 CAD patients with either pravastatin or placebo for 3 yr. There was a trend for decreased progression ($p = 0.07$) and a significant reduction in progression for lesions of less than 50% at baseline ($p < 0.04$). The Canadian Coronary Artery Intervention Trial *(37)* used lovastatin in 331 CAD patients to reduce LDL-C and impact CAD progression. Progression with no regression occurred in 48 of 146 (32.9%) of the lovastatin-treated patients and in 76 of 153 (49.7%) placebo-treated patients. Lovastatin slowed the progression of CAD in patients with a mean baseline LDL-C of 173 mg/dL, but there was no significant effect on regression. The Monitored Atheroma Regression Study *(38)* was similar to Canadian Coronary Artery Intervention Trial in the treatment of CAD patients with lovastatin or placebo. After 2 yr of treatment, the lovastatin group had a 38% reduction in LDL-C and a trend for reduced arteriographic progression (increased 2.2% in placebo-treated group and increased 1.6% in the lovastatin-treated group; $p < 0.20$) but was significantly reduced for lesions that were more than 50% obstructed.

The Stanford Coronary Risk Intervention Project *(39)* used quantitative coronary arteriography to assess the effect of 4 yr of multifactorial risk intervention in a group of 300 subjects who had documented CAD, randomized to a usual-care group and a special-intervention group. The special-intervention group received diet, exercise, weight reduc-

Table 3
Post-CABG Angiographic Outcomes

| | MRE | | Difference | |
	Moderate	Aggressive	(%)	p Value
Progression	39	28	28	<0.001
new occlusions	16	10	40	<0.001
New lesions	21	10	52	<0.001
Mean lumen change in mm				
Minimum diameter	−0.38	−0.20	48	<0.001
Mean diameter	−0.34	−0.16	52	<0.001

From ref. *34*.
MRE, mean per-patient percentage of grafts.

tion, and smoking cessation advice. Bile acid-binding resins, nicotinic acid, gemfibrozil, and lovastatin were used to achieve an LDL-C goal of 110 mg/dL. Baseline plasma lipids were representative of a typical CAD population. The LDL-C was reduced approx 18% more, and HDL-C increased approx 7% more in the special-intervention group than the usual-care group. A significantly greater ($p < 0.01$) annualized rate of minimum diameter change for diseased vessels appeared in the usual-care group (0.046 mm/yr), compared with the special-intervention group (0.022 mm/yr). CAD regression was reported to be significantly greater ($p < 0.025$) in the special-intervention group (21%) than in the usual-care group (10%). For the final 3 yr of the study, significantly fewer deaths ($p < 0.006$) and nonfatal MIs occurred in the special intervention group ($n = 2$) than in the usual-care group ($n = 13$).

Two important observations have been made from these trials. First, although lesion regression was uncommon, the rate of lesion progression was often slowed appreciably. Second, the small changes in luminal narrowing observed with lowering TC are unlikely to be the principal mechanism by which lipid lowering achieves a reduction in clinical events and revascularization rates. Endothelium-dependent vasomotor function, and the cellular characteristics of plaques that seem to be intimately related to rupture and thrombosis, are factors that might explain the clinical success from correcting the dyslipidemias.

CLINICAL OUTCOMES TRIALS

The 4S *(9)* included 4444 men and women with CAD and TC levels of 212–309 mg/dL to treatment with 20–40 mg simvastatin or placebo for up to 6.2 yr. The mean LDL level at baseline was 188 mg/dL, with a range of 130–266 mg/dL. The number of patients with major coronary events (coronary deaths or nonfatal MI) was 622 (28%) in the placebo group and 431 (19%) in the simvastatin group ($p < 0.00001$). To demonstrate the sustained efficacy and safety of simvastatin, the 4S investigators designed and implemented a 2-yr extension of 4S. During the combined study period (7.4 yr), total mortality in the placebo group was 15.8 vs 11.4% among patients treated with simvastatin ($p = 0.0001$) (Fig. 4). After completion of the original study, all patients in the placebo group were offered therapy with simvastatin. Nonetheless, the curves continued to separate, and patients treated with simvastatin were found to benefit during the full study period. Simvastatin maintained the reduction in risk of total mortality by 30% ($p = 0.00001$) *(24)*.

A recent analysis presented vascular event curves during the duration of the 4S trial, including intermittent claudication, carotid bruits, angina, and cerebrovascular events *(25)*. Note that the curves separate at 2 yr and beyond (Fig. 5), except perhaps for carotid bruits, which seems to separate earlier.

Meanwhile, the CARE study was a randomized controlled trial *(8)* designed to evaluate the effects of treatment with pravastatin in 4159 subjects who had experienced an acute MI 3 to 20 mo before randomization and had moderately elevated TC levels (mean = 209 mg/dL). Patients were randomized to either 40 mg/dL pravastatin or placebo; in addition, they followed the NCEP-recommended guidelines for diet therapy, and, if their LDL levels were persistently elevated (>175 mg/dL), they received cholestyramine. Results were encouraging: during a 5-yr period, TC levels were reduced by 20%, LDL levels dropped by 28%, TG declined by 14%, and HDL increased by 5% (Fig. 6). The incidence of primary combined endpoint of CHD death or nonfatal MI was reduced by 24% ($p < 0.002$) (Fig. 7). CARE was not statistically powered to observed differences in mortality. Importantly, the benefits of pravastatin therapy in preventing recurrent coronary events were similar in the subset analysis of age, sex, ejection factor, hypertension, diabetes mellitus, and smoking.

This secondary prevention trial suggests that risk reduction in this large portion of the population with only moderately elevated TC could have positive public health implications. It remains to be determined whether treatment for lower levels of LDL will be beneficial.

The LIPID trial is a secondary prevention study *(12)* performed in New Zealand and Australia. It was a double-blind, randomized placebo-controlled study with 9014 subjects (1511 of whom were women, one-third were older than 65 yr, and 777 had diabetes) using 40 mg/d pravastatin. Subjects aged 31–75 yr, who experienced an acute MI or unstable angina within the previous 3 mo to 3 yr, and had TC values from 155 to 270 mg/dL, and TG less than 445 mg/dL, were eligible for participation. A significant medical or surgical event, significant heart failure, renal or hepatic disease, uncontrolled endocrine disorders, or use of cyclosporine and/or lipid-lowering agents excluded the patients from being recruited.

Baseline levels of lipids included TC of 219 mg/dL; LDL, 150 mg/dL; TG, 139 mg/dL; and HDL, 37 mg/dL. Of the participants, 82% were taking aspirin, whereas 47% were taking β-blockers. Despite the local discretion permitted within the protocol, intent-to-treat analyses found a 25% reduction in LDL values according to original recruitment assignments. The primary endpoint, coronary mortality, was reduced by 24% ($p < 0.0005$). Secondary objectives, total mortality (reduced by 23%; $p < 0.0001$), and overall cardiac events (23% reduction; $p < 0.0001$) were also met, with demonstrated positive results. The risk reduction in MI incidence was 29%, $p < 0.00001$. Procedure rates of CABG and percutaneous transluminal coronary angioplasty (PTCA) were also reduced by 24% and 18%, respectively. Stroke incidence was reduced by 20% ($p = 0.022$).

There were no major safety biochemical differences between the placebo and drug groups. Liver enzymes (aspartate aminotransferase [AST] and alanine aminotransferase [ALT]) were mildly higher in the pravastatin group ($p = 0.01$), but not clinically significant. It was concluded that one cardiovascular event could be prevented through the treatment for 6 yr of 20 LIPID-equivalent patients. Furthermore, the safety of providing this medication was clear. The LIPID study was designed to determine the benefits of pravastatin in the majority of people with heart disease.

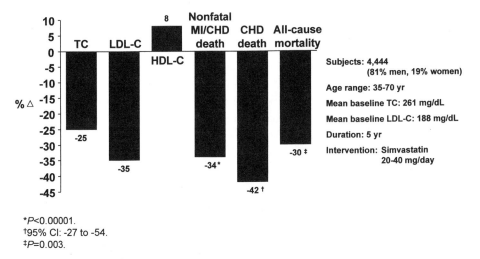

*P<0.00001.
†95% CI: -27 to -54.
‡P=0.003.

Fig. 4. 4S: effect of LDL-C lowering and coronary events. (Adapted from ref. *9.*)

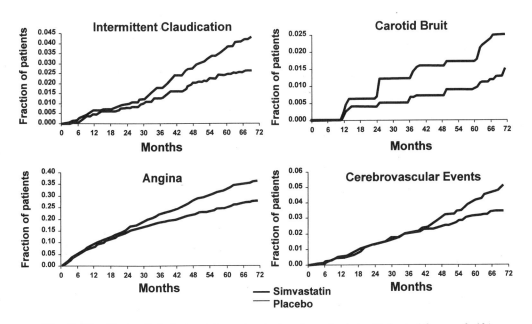

Fig. 5. 4S: effects of cholesterol-lowering ischemic endpoints. (Adapted from ref. *40.*)

Although the 4S trial was the first secondary prevention trial to clearly demonstrate a reduction in total mortality, the LIPID trial had significant differences in design and hypotheses. Of the LIPID enrollees, 80% were not candidates for 4S based on their cholesterol level, age, or history of CAD. LIPID included patients:

1. Older than the age of 70 yr.
2. A greater proportion of patients with diabetes.
3. A lower baseline cholesterol range.
4. Physician discretion in lipid management.

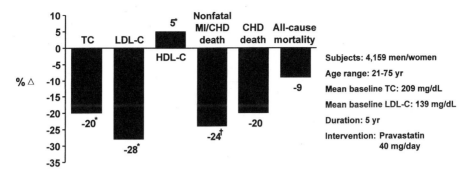

*As compared to placebo.
†P=0.003.

Fig. 6. CARE: effect of lipid lowering on lipids and coronary events. (Adapted from ref. *8*.)

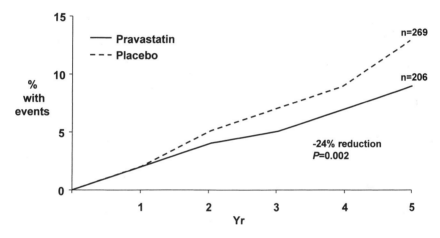

Fig. 7. CARE: fatal CHD or nonfatal MI. (Adapted from ref. *8*.)

LIPID is the first study to examine the use of an HMG-CoA reductase inhibitor in patients with a history of unstable angina. The LIPID study provides new data on noncoronary mortality (stroke) and on other groups, such as women and diabetic patients, who, to date, were underrepresented in clinical trials.

The Atorvastatin vs Revascularization Treatment (AVERT) study *(42)* provides intriguing data on the role of lipid lowering in the management of patients with mild coronary atherosclerosis. It is known that lipid lowering has been effective in the reduction of percutaneous revascularization rates. In the 4S trial, PTCA was reduced by 37% with aggressive lipid lowering ($p = 0.00001$). Studies of PTCA vs standard therapy have failed to demonstrate a significant reduction in coronary events. It was, therefore, hypothesized that, in a population with mild-to-moderate CAD under consideration for coronary revascularization via PTCA, aggressive lipid lowering would provide a significant reduction in clinical events and improved outcomes.

The AVERT Trial randomized 341 patients with CAD (one lesion of at least 50% stenosis), LDL-C greater than 115 mg/dL, left ventricular ejection fraction greater than

40% to either PTCA plus standard care, or to medical management and aggressive lipid lowering with 80 mg/dL atorvastatin. Patients with left main CAD or its equivalent of three-vessel CAD were excluded.

The AVERT trial showed a trend toward improved outcomes with medical therapy and aggressive lipid lowering compared with PTCA and standard medical care. There was a 13% ischemic event rate in individuals receiving atorvastatin vs a 21% ischemic event rate in individuals randomized to PTCA. This represented a 36% reduction in events in the group treated with high-dose atorvastatin, although this did not represent a statistically significant difference ($p = 0.048$). In general, high-dose atorvastatin was well-tolerated, with only a 2.4% incidence of AST or ALT abnormalities (greater than three times normal). The AVERT trial is a small, underpowered trial with a short follow-up time. It represents a highly selected population that may not have clinical relevance. It does, however, serve as an interesting hypothesis-generating trial that adds insights into the role of lipid lowering in patients undergoing revascularization and points to the potential therapeutic benefits in this subset.

The Myocardial Ischemia Reduction with Aggressive Cholesterol Lowering trial *(43)* tested the hypothesis that lipid lowering in unstable angina or non-Q-wave MI would reduce myocardial ischemia and recurrent events. This study randomized 3086 patients with unstable angina or non-Q-wave MI to 80 mg/d atorvastatin or placebo, beginning within 1 to 4 d of hospitalization and continuing for 16 wk of follow-up. The primary outcome measure was the time to occurrence of an ischemic event, defined as death, nonfatal MI, resuscitated cardiac arrest, or recurrent symptomatic myocardial ischemia with emergency rehospitalization. Atorvastatin therapy was associated with a 2.6% absolute reduction in the risk of the primary endpoint (14.8 vs 17.4%; relative risk, 0.84; 95% CI, 0.70–1.00; $p = 0.48$). This reduction was driven predominantly by a 2.2% absolute reduction in the incidence of emergent rehospitalization for symptomatic myocardial ischemia.

The REVERSAL study *(44)* was designed to provide insight into the response of the atheroma to lipid lowering. The REVERSAL study was a multicenter, double-blind, comparative, parallel trial involving 654 patients, 502 of whom had evaluable intravascular ultrasound examinations at baseline and after 18 mo of treatment. Patients were randomly assigned to receive a moderate lipid-lowering regimen consisting of 40 mg of pravastatin or an intensive lipid-lowering regimen consisting of 80 mg of atorvastatin. The primary outcome was the percentage change in atheroma volume (follow-up minus baseline). In this study, baseline LDL-C level (mean, 150.2 mg/dL [3.89 mmol/L] in both treatment groups) was reduced to 110 mg/dL (2.85 mmol/L) in the pravastatin group and to 79 mg/dL (2.05 mmol/L) in the atorvastatin group ($p < 0.001$). C-reactive protein decreased 5.2% with pravastatin and 36.4% with atorvastatin ($p < 0.001$). The primary endpoint (percentage change in atheroma volume) showed a significantly lower progression rate in the atorvastatin (intensive) group ($p = 0.02$). Similar differences between groups were observed for secondary efficacy parameters, including change in total atheroma volume ($p = 0.02$), change in percentage atheroma volume ($p < 0.001$), and change in atheroma volume in the most severely diseased 10-mm vessel subsegment ($p < 0.01$). For the primary endpoint, progression of coronary atherosclerosis occurred in the pravastatin group (2.7%; 95% CI, 0.2–4.7%; $p = 0.001$) compared with baseline. Progression did not occur in the atorvastatin group (–0.4%; 95% CI, –2.4 to 1.5%; $p = 0.98$) compared with baseline. Thus, the REVERSAL study demonstrates that, for patients

with CHD, intensive lipid-lowering treatment with atorvastatin reduced progression of coronary atherosclerosis compared with pravastatin. Compared with baseline values, patients treated with atorvastatin had no change in atheroma burden, whereas patients treated with pravastatin showed progression of coronary atherosclerosis.

The recently published PROVE-IT *(18)* study assessed the role of intensive lipid lowering vs more moderate lipid lowering in the setting of acute coronary syndromes. This study enrolled 4162 patients who were recently hospitalized with acute coronary syndrome within the past 10 d. Patients were randomized to 40 mg of pravastatin (moderate arm) or 80 mg of atorvastatin (intensive arm). The primary endpoint of interest was a composite of death, MI, documented unstable angina requiring hospitalization, revascularization, and stroke. The study follow-up averaged 24 mo. Participants in the study achieved a median LDL-C level of 95 mg/dL in the moderate arm and a median level of 62 mg/dL in the intensive arm. The rate of the primary endpoint was 26.3% in the moderate arm compared with 22.4% in the intensive arm, a 16% relative risk reduction in favor of intensive therapy ($p = 0.005$). Thus, in this study of patients with recent acute coronary syndrome, early and intensive lipid lowering provided great protection against death, cardiovascular events, and rehospitalization. Of note, these findings support the aggressive lowering of lipids in patients with acute coronary syndromes to levels well below current recommended targets.

Recent trials have demonstrated that lowering LDL-C below currently recommended guidelines is beneficial in patients with acute coronary syndromes. TNT sought to determine the role of lipid lowering in patients with stable CHD. In this study, a total of 10,001 patients with clinically diagnosed CHD and LDL-C levels of less than 130 mg/dL were randomized to receive either 10 mg or 80 mg atorvastatin. Patients were followed for 4.9 yr for the occurrence of first major cardiovascular event defined as CHD death, nonfatal MI, cardiac arrest, or fatal and nonfatal stroke. The mean LDL-C levels achieved in this study was 77 mg/dL. The primary event rate was 8.7 and 10.9% in the 80 mg and 10 mg atorvastatin arms, respectively, representing a 2.2% absolute risk reduction and a 22% relative risk reduction. In this study of patients with stable CHD, intensive lipid lowering with 80 mg atorvastatin was associated with greater clinical benefit, although transaminase levels were higher in the intensive arm.

GUIDELINES FOR THE MODIFICATION OF LIPIDS

A national consensus panel concluded that the risk of coronary disease could be defined by dividing the population into three relative risk groups according to age- and sex-specific percentiles. The second report of the NCEP *(20)* chose to define a similar set of relative risk groups, using single-cutoff values for the entire adult population, as did the third report of the NCEP published in 2001 *(21)*. Since the publication of the most recent NCEP Adult Treatment Panel (ATP) III, however, six major clinical trials of statin therapy with clinical outcomes have been published. These data were not integrated into ATP II. In view of this, the coordinating committee of the NCEP issues a statement reviewing the results of these recent trials and assessing their implications for clinical management of lipids *(22)* (Table 1).

A new paradigm has emerged, whereby a patient's risk is assessed rather than strict lipid levels. Our challenge is to determine "vascular risk" to identify individuals at high risk of coronary events who would be appropriate candidates for intensive medical intervention, which would include lifestyle changes, statin therapy, aspirin, antihypertensive

medications, and other proven interventions. In this model, all CAD risk factors are first integrated into an assessment form, such as the Framingham risk factor algorithm. The algorithm incorporates several risk factors, some of which are binary, such as presence or absence of smoking and presence or absence of hypertension, with others that are continuous, such as TC, HDL-C, and age. By integrating these risk factors, you can achieve additional incremental power to predict who is at risk for CAD events. That is the approach taken by the NCEP ATP III. They have indicated risk factors for intermediate or high risk and recommended using the Framingham risk factor algorithm to quantitate them and determine which individuals need therapy. If an individual has more than one risk factor by the NCEP guidelines, the Framingham risk factor algorithm should be applied (http://www.nhlbi.nih.gov/guidelines/cholesterol/index.htm). There are some limitations to the Framingham risk assessment, however. The model is based on classic risk factors, such as age, TC, HDL-C, and smoking. We have become much more sophisticated in the past decade or so and know that other risk factors are involved.

The Framingham risk factor algorithm does not account for predisposing risk factors, such as obesity, physical inactivity, and socioeconomic status. These risk factors are complex and interact with each other and with classic risk factors. The algorithm also does not account for conditional risk factors; that is, risk factors that assume more or less importance given genetic and standard risk factors. Examples of these are hypertriglyceridemia, which may be more important in a patient with low HDL-C or in a patient with central adiposity, but less important in patients with high HDL-C. Lipoprotein little A antigen [Lp(a)], we know, is only a weak independent predictor of CHD, but when LDL-C is even mildly elevated, the importance of Lp(a) becomes clinically important. Other conditional risk factors, such as particle size, homocysteine, and high sensitivity C-reactive protein levels, also are not included in the Framingham risk factor algorithm.

The Framingham assessment also underestimates the risks associated with highly abnormal individual risk factors, such as very high TC or blood pressure, or very low HDL-C. Framingham addresses only short-term risk—10 yr—and does not take family history into account. Finally, the algorithm is very dependent on age, which trumps all of the other risk actors. Imaging may provide us with information to fill some of the gaps in risk assessment that the Framingham tool overlooks.

Despite its limitations, however, the Framingham risk score serves as an efficient means by which to risk stratify patients and determine intensity of clinical interventions. Based on the Framingham risk score, individuals can be stratified into appropriate risk groups, and lipid-lowering targets can be determined. Based on emerging clinical data, a growing number of individuals are of sufficient risk and garner significant enough clinical benefit to warrant lipid-lowering therapy—often irrespective of lipid values.

Treatment of Hyperlipidemia

DIET

NCEP and American Heart Association (AHA) guidelines promote a diet in which fat composes only 30% or less of the day's total calories. The committee on nutrition from the AHA, based on recommendations from the World Health Organization, suggests that fat calories constitute no less than 15% of total calories. The Step I and Step II AHA diets (Table 4) use dietary therapy to reduce the intake of saturated fat and cholesterol to lower the LDL-C. The first step in dietary therapy, usually the Step I diet, parallels the NCEP recommendations. A change from the average American diet to the Step I diet of less than

Table 4
Step I and Step II Diet Recommendations

	Step I diet (% of total calories)	Step II diet (% of total calories)
Total	<30%	<30%
Saturated fat	8–10%	<7%
Polyunsaturated fat	Up to 10%	Up to 10%
Monounsaturated	Up to 15%	Up to 15%
Carbohydrates	50–60%	50–60%
Protein	15%	15%
Cholesterol	<300 mg/d	<200 mg/d

10% saturated fatty acids and less than 300 mg/d of cholesterol reduces serum cholesterol levels by approx 7%, whereas further restriction to less than 7% saturated fatty acids and less than 200 mg/d cholesterol (Step II diet) should reduce cholesterol levels by an additional 3 to 7%.

EXERCISE

Many large epidemiological investigations have failed to demonstrate consistently a correlation between reported physical activity and lipid values in populations not specifically selected for hyperlipidemia. A paucity of cross-sectional studies have investigated physical activity and hypercholesterolemia. Yet, it is generally accepted that exercise improves the spectrum of lipid abnormalities, in conjunction with a healthy diet and weight loss.

PHARMACOTHERAPY

The NCEP ATP III and the AHA–American College of Cardiology guidelines for modifying cholesterol levels in persons without CHD indicate that the goal of therapy is an LDL-C less than 130 mg/dL; and, in persons with documented CHD, the goal of therapy is to reduce LDL-C levels to below 100 mg/dL.

The guidelines also recommend that an HMG-CoA reductase inhibitor or statin be the initial therapy in patients with TG levels lower than 400 mg/dL. Optional goals of 100 mg/dL and 70 mg/dL, respectively, may be deemed appropriate in high-risk individuals, as outlined in the proposed modifications to the ATP III (5).

Statins (HMG-CoA Reductase Inhibitors)

HMG-CoA reductase inhibitors competitively inhibit the rate-limiting enzyme in hepatic cholesterol synthesis, 3-hydroxy-3-methylglutaryl–coenzyme A. This results in a compensatory increase in hepatic LDL receptor activity and seems to have some effect on LDL production rates. The Food and Drug Administration (FDA) has approved Lovastatin (Merck), pravastatin (Bristol–Myers Squibb), simvastatin (Merck), fluvastatin (Hoest Marion Roussel), atorvastatin (Pfizer), and rosuvastatin (AstraZeneca) for use in the United States.

INDICATIONS

HMG-CoA reductase inhibitors are included by the NCEP ATP III among first-line alternatives for the treatment of hypercholesterolemia. The category includes six drugs:

lovastatin, simvastatin, pravastatin, fluvastatin, atorvastatin, and the newest agent, rosuvastatin. The HMG-CoA reductase inhibitors are indicated as an adjunct to diet for reduction of elevated TC in patients with hypercholesterolemia (types IIa and IIb) when nonpharmacological measures, such as diet, are inadequate. Although HMG-CoA reductase inhibitors may be effective in lowering total and LDL-C in patients with mixed hyperlipidemias (elevated cholesterol and TGs), the agents have not been extensively studied in subjects with lipoprotein lipase functional impairment with severe elevation in TGs (types I), remnant clearance abnormalities caused partially by an abnormal apoE isoform, and accompanied by both high TG and cholesterol values (type III), isolated elevations in TGs and reductions in HDL (type IV), and profound increases in TGs predominantly from an intestinal origin (type V).

In patients who have hypercholesterolemia, these compounds can achieve reductions of 30 to 60%, and, when combined with a resin, reductions of 60 to 70% are possible. They have a small effect on reducing fasting plasma triglyceride concentrations, but this masks a significant reduction in postprandial triglyceridemia. Like the resins, these agents are useful in treating patients who have elevations in LDL-C, but are not the agents of choice for treating hypertriglyceridemia. They seem to have little effect on Lp(a). Recommendations vary on what time of day to take the medication and whether the medication should be taken in conjunction with meals.

Efficacy and Safety Profile. HMG-CoA reductase inhibitors are extremely effective in reducing LDL-C in most patients with primary hypercholesterolemia. The HMG-CoA reductase inhibitors decrease TC in the range of 15 to 60%, LDL-C by 20 to 60%, and increase HDL-C by 5 to 15%. Declines in apoB commensurate with LDL reductions have been also demonstrated. TGs have been reduced by 10 to 25%. TG lowering parallels LDL lowering, in that higher doses of more potent agents produce TG reductions of more than 40%. The HMG-CoA reductase inhibitors seem to have minimal effects on apoAI, apoAII, and Lp(a).

The currently available HMG-CoA reductase inhibitors (atorvastatin, fluvastatin, lovastatin, pravastatin, and simvastatin) are well-tolerated, efficacious, and approximately equivalent with respect to safety profiles during monotherapy within trials. Cerivastatin was withdrawn from the market because of a dramatic increase in rhabdomyolysis, particularly when combined with fibrates. The safety and efficacy of rosuvastatin has not been determined in large clinical trials. Given their similar drug class, there is no reason to believe this agent will not perform as effectively and safely as the earlier statins, however, rosuvastatin has no clinical outcome data at this time. Fewer than 5% of patients in controlled clinical trials report side effects with HMG-CoA reductase inhibitors, the most common of which are mild gastrointestinal (GI) disturbances (nausea, abdominal pain, diarrhea, constipation, flatulence), which rarely warrant therapy discontinuation. Headache, fatigue, pruritus, and myalgia are other minor side effects that seldom prompt treatment termination.

ADVERSE EFFECTS

Liver Function Test Abnormalities. Mild transient elevations in liver enzymes have been reported with all HMG-CoA reductase inhibitors. Elevations in serum amino transferases three times the upper limit of normal have occurred in less than 2% of patients in controlled clinical trials. At the usual midrange dosing, the frequency is less than 1%. In general, for each doubling of statin dose, there is a 0.6% increase in risk for transami-

nase elevation. Therapy should be discontinued when a greater than threefold elevation occurs. Enzyme levels typically return to normal within 2 wk, and either lower doses of the same medication can be reinstituted or a different HMG-CoA can be used. Monitoring of hepatic aminotransferase levels is recommended for those taking HMG-CoA reductase inhibitors at 6 to 8 wk after drug initiation. Because of the excellent safety profiles of pravastatin and simvastatin, the FDA recommends discontinuing hepatic enzyme monitoring after 3 mo for pravastatin, and after 6 mo of continuous same-dose therapy for simvastatin.

Myopathy. Myopathy, a rare but potentially serious side effect of HMG-CoA reductase inhibitors, occurs with muscle symptoms and serum creatine kinase (CK) elevations to more than 10 times the upper limit of normal. CK measurements are not required unless symptoms are present. When statins are used in combination with certain pharmaceutical agents, for example, erythromycin, gemfibrozil, azole antifungals, cimetidine, methotrexate, and/or cyclosporine, the risk of CK elevation and myositis increases. Pravastatin and fluvastatin combinations are considered relatively safe, because they do not use the cytochrome P450 3A4 microsomal pathways. These drug combinations should either be avoided, or used judiciously with interval measurements of CK levels and liver function tests.

COST EFFECTIVENESS OF STATINS

Cost effectiveness studies in patients with established CHD are consistent in demonstrating that intervention with lipid-lowering drugs is highly cost effective. The incremental cost of intervention may be negative or cost saving in some instances. The cost of cholesterol lowering is less than the cost of doing nothing and allowing the patient to proceed to another event.

Initial data from the 4S study indicate that, in patients with established CHD, the addition of simvastatin to the treatment of 100 patients with CHD during 6 yr could be expected to prevent 4 of 9 deaths, 7 of 21 nonfatal MIs, and 6 of 19 bypass procedures. Formal analysis of the cost effectiveness of simvastatin indicated a total cost of hospitalization in the placebo group of 52.8 million Swedish kronor compared with 36.0 million Swedish kronor in the simvastatin group. This amounted to a 32% reduction per patient.

HMG-CoA Reductase Inhibitors and Combination With Other Agents

One-third of patients with hypercholesterolemia do not respond adequately to monotherapy alone. The statins' high efficacy in LDL-C lowering and few side effects make them an attractive choice for patients with or without established CHD. Nonetheless, the target level of 100 mg/dL or below may be difficult to attain. Consequently, combination therapy is often required. The best combination is one of a statin with a bile acid sequestrant or the newer agent, ezetimibe, because these provide little added toxicity. Moreover, the LDL-C-lowering required may not necessitate the full dosage. Combining a statin with niacin may also enhance LDL-C lowering, but also increases the risk of drug-induced myopathy. Because patients may have a risk of myopathy as high as 3% when taking this drug combination, all patients should be instructed to report any muscle pain, and to discontinue drug use should this occur until a medical evaluation and CK levels are determined. Patients with low HDL-C, high TG, and high LDL-C levels may benefit from the combination of a statin with either niacin or gemfibrozil. When a statin is used with gemfibrozil, the report of myopathy may be as high as 5%. Occasionally,

triple-drug therapy is necessary to lower LDL-C levels to less than 100 mg/dL. These patients require careful monitoring for liver and muscular toxicity.

In a few cases, poor response represents poor absorption of the medications. More often, failures involve subjects with LDL values greater than 160 mg/dL, and primarily those greater than 190 mg/dL. The latter cases are often associated with inherited disorders of metabolism, e.g., familial hypercholesterolemia, familial defective apoB, or familial combined hyperlipidemia. If the patient has an LDL more than 160 mg/dL, a polygenic form of hyperlipidemia should be considered. Before the release of atorvastatin and cerivastatin, a majority of CHD subjects required two or three agents to maintain their LDL values less than 100 mg/dL. This may be somewhat easier with the availability of progressively more potent agents. Combination therapy may be required in only the most extreme cases.

STATINS PLUS RESINS

In the isolated forms of LDL elevation, HMG-CoA reductase inhibitors and bile acid resins exhibit highly complementary mechanisms of action in combination therapy, and are, therefore, useful for the treatment of severe hypercholesterolemia. By disrupting the enterohepatic recirculation of bile acids, the sequestrants induce a compensatory rise in conversion of hepatic cholesterol to bile acids, as well as a secondary rise in hepatic cholesterol synthesis. This phenomenon consequently upregulates hepatic LDL receptor expression and, thereby, decreases LDL serum concentration. Adding an HMG-CoA reductase inhibitor blocks the secondary rise in cholesterol synthesis and, therefore, produces a further increase in hepatic LDL receptors. This combination has been found to be additive in altering LDL levels. Because the HMG-CoA reductase inhibitor acts systemically, whereas the resin is nonsystemic, systemic drug interactions are minimized.

Combination therapy reduces LDL by 30 to 55%. This combination was initially administered to familial hypercholesterolemic subjects, using high doses of both statins and resins. More recently, the issues of lower-dose preparations using resins and statins have been reviewed, favoring the addition of low-dose resins rather than the doubling of ongoing statin agents. Usually, the addition of 4 to 8 g of a resin to an ongoing statin regimen will result in greater LDL lowering than doubling the statin dose. The marginal value of adding resin to a statin will likely diminish as the potency of available statin agents increases. The angiographic trial Lipoprotein and Coronary Atherosclerosis Study used fluvastatin alone, or a combination of fluvastatin and resin when LDL was greater than 160 mg/dL. Similar angiographic benefits were observed in monotherapy and combined cohorts, suggesting that LDL lowering is the relevant parameter, not the means by which it is achieved.

In some patients with combined or mixed hyperlipidemias, resin may not be advocated because of its triglyceride-elevating effect, and statin therapy alone may not be adequate to lower LDL-C.

Bile Acid-Binding Resins

Bile acid-binding resins have been used for longer than 25 yr. Intestinal binding of bile salts by the resin decreases bile salt resorption through the enterohepatic recirculation route. Hepatic cholesterol, HMG-CoA reductase activity, and hepatic cholesterol synthesis are increased. Inhibition of normal bile salt resorption also has been hypothesized as

the cause of increased plasma triglyceride concentrations by enhanced activity of phosphatidic acid phosphatase. In type II hyperlipidemia patients, resin therapy can result in LDL-C reductions of approx 72 mg/dL, or 27%, and an HDL-C increase of 2 to 3 mg/dL, or 4%. There seems to be little effect on Lp(a).

INDICATIONS

Because of their long history for safety and efficacy, and because of their nonsystemic nature, bile acid-binding resins are the first-line drugs of choice for reduction of plasma LDL-C.

Resins are useful for patients who have a mild elevation in plasma LDL-C and who do not fall within the classic hyperlipidemia definition (90th percentile), and, in whom, reduction is warranted because of high-CAD risk from other factors. In this group, it is important to note that low-dose resin therapy can have a significant effect on LDL-C reduction. One-half the recommended full dose of six packets per day can achieve approx 75% of the full-dose LDL-C reduction. A colestipol dose of 5 g/d (16% full dose) can achieve 50% of the LDL-C reduction as that of a 50% dose. Approximately 50% of moderately hypercholesterolemic subjects can achieve the US NCEP goal of an LDL-C of less than 130 mg/dL with less than 50% of the full resin dose. It is no longer necessary to dose patients two of three times per day. Once-a-day dosing achieves nearly the same effect as twice-a-day dosing.

COMPLIANCE

Common patient complaints include difficulty in ingesting the resins, GI distress, and constipation. Several tricks are available to enhance compliance. First, for all diet, exercise, weight reduction, and drug therapies, compliance can be enhanced greatly by effective use of a dedicated nurse. Second, the resins can be mixed in various liquid media, including juices and semisolid foods, such as applesauce. Third, combining either mineral oil or supplemental fiber can reduce constipation complaints, and some fibers can further reduce LDL-C by approx 10%. Bowel gas can be reduced by using simethicone.

Nicotinic Acid

Nicotinic acid is a B vitamin that affects the lipoprotein system mediated through nicotinamide adenine dinucleotide, or nicotinamide adenine dinucleotide phosphate, by the inhibition of adenylate cyclase. Only nicotinic acid or its glycine conjugate (nicotinuric acid) has an antilipolytic effect. Nicotinamide is inactive regarding lipoprotein change. Nicotinic acid inhibits endogenous cholesterol synthesis, increases catabolism, and reduces the plasma concentrations of nonesterified fatty acids by its action at the level of the adipocyte. Rapid release of prostaglandins from platelets is thought to be responsible, in part, for the vasodilation and flush response. Similar to other medications, nicotinic acid has pharmacological effects that may benefit atherosclerosis that are not reflected in plasma lipoprotein measurements. These effects include prostaglandin/thromboxane perturbations, platelet aggregation inhibition, and fibrinolysis. A long-acting, once-a-day niacin that is dosed at bedtime was recently approved by the FDA. This niacin has a significant effect in reducing small dense LDL, and, in LDL pattern B subjects, achieves a mean 40% reduction in LDL-C.

INDICATIONS

Nicotinic acid is useful in patients who have elevated TGs, TG-rich lipoproteins, LDL-C, reductions in HDL-C, and LDL subclass pattern B. Effects on lipids are commonly

seen after the renal threshold is exceeded, which generally is around 1500 mg/d. The response of plasma lipoproteins is dose dependent within the range of approx 1500 to 6000 mg/d. Unmodified or time-release nicotinic acid can result in 10 to 25% reductions in daily doses of 1500 to 3000 mg. Nicotinic acid is one of the few lipid medications that seems to have some effect on Lp(a). Nicotinic acid can suppress expression of LDL subclass pattern B when TG levels are reduced below approx 140 mg/dL.

COMPLIANCE

Nicotinic acid is the lipid-altering drug with the most potential for side effects and, consequently, adherence problems. Because of nicotinic acid's great potential benefit, it is worth expending extra effort on achieving compliance. Individual variability exists in the side effects to such an extent that it often can be attributed to differences in formulation. For this reason, obtaining several brands and testing each for individual tolerance can be helpful. Slowly titrating the dose from 100 to 500 mg three times a day during a 1-mo period can ease the patient into a therapeutic dose range. The prostaglandin-mediated flush can be ameliorated in part by ingesting 81 mg of aspirin 15 min before the niacin dose. Avoiding alcohol, monosodium glutamate, hot beverages, and spicy foods also can help ameliorate the flush. GI distress can be reduced by ingesting niacin with food. The most important tool to enhance adherence is a dedicated lipid nurse.

Niaspan® (KOS Pharmaceutical) is a new once-a-night niacin preparation dosed from 500 to 3000 mg/d. Niaspan has been compared with immediate-release niacin and found to have comparable benefits with fewer side effects. The new formulation of this product, as well as the evening dosing, reduces the apparent flushing episodes. LDL reductions of 10, 18, and 20% are found with 1, 2, and 3 g of Niaspan, respectively. Parallel to these changes, HDL increases by 15, 25, and 30%, whereas TGs decrease by 10, 35, and 45%. The reduction in Lp(a) was found to be 10, 25, and 30% for the 1-, 2-, and 3-g doses. Glucose increases by an average of 6%, uric acid increases by 34%, and some decrease in phosphorus (−16%) was also noted. Overall, an approx 10% of study participants had increased AST levels over baseline, but only 2% had increases to two times the upper limit of normal, the latter consistent with that found in the placebo group. Long-term, 2-yr studies resulted in 2 patients out of 500 discontinuing Niaspan because of liver function elevations (<0.5%), with less than 1% of patients having AST and ALT elevations beyond two times the upper limit of normal. Concomitant statin therapy reduced LDL another 14% on the average, but seemed to modestly reduce the Lp(a) benefit (not significant). Niaspan is a good alternative to regular niacin preparations, with 70% of patients not reporting flushing. Given some of the foregoing trials, niacin or one of its analogs should perhaps be administered more often in "mixed" phenotype patients. It is noted to decrease dense LDL particle concentration in such subjects. Statin–niacin outcome trials are clearly needed.

Fibric Acid Derivatives

Fibric acid derivatives enhance lipoprotein lipase activity and hepatic bile secretion and reduce hepatic TG production. TG and LDL-C response to these agents depends on the lipoprotein abnormality and specific fibric acid derivative used. TG reductions between 8 and 72%, LDL-C reductions between 0 and 35%, and HDL-C increases between 0 and 25% have been reported. Generally, the greatest benefit is seen in patients who have elevations in plasma TG, although fenofibrate has been reported to produce significant

LDL-C reduction (~1.2 mmol/L) in type IIa patients. In hypertriglyceridemic patients who initially have low or normal LDL-C, gemfibrozil treatment may result in an increase in LDL-C, perhaps because of an increase in LDL production or a decrease in fractional LDL clearance rates. This response suggests the presence of a second lipoprotein abnormality that often requires two-drug therapy.

INDICATIONS

Fibric acid derivatives are useful in the treatment of hypertriglyceridemia and in selected patients who have elevated LDL-C levels in combination with elevated TGs. The HDL-C level often is reported to increase significantly when initial HDL-C is low or when it is associated with reduction of TGs. These agents are the drugs of choice in type III hyperlipidemia. In the HHS, 600 mg gemfibrozil twice daily resulted in an overall 42% reduction in TGs, a 10% reduction in LDL-C, and a 10% increase in HDL-C.

COMPLIANCE

Fibric acid derivatives generally are well-tolerated. Occasionally, mild GI distress (nausea) is experienced in the first week. To reduce this potential side effect, it can be useful to start therapy with one-half the normal dose for several days before increasing to a full dose.

FENOFIBRATE

Fenofibrate is a fibric acid derivative, dosed at 200 or 400 mg/d. It is absorbed and rapidly converted into fenofibric acid, the active metabolite. The vast majority of the drug is protein bound, with a 4-h time-to-peak plasma levels. Elimination half-life is approx 20 h. The micronized form of fenofibrate—smaller particles and an absorption rate that is almost twice as fast as regular fenofibrate (200 mg/d)—was administered in 1334 subjects with serum TG above 200 mg/dL and TC greater than 250 mg/dL. LDL was decreased by 27%, TG by approx 50%, and HDL increased overall by 15% (increased by 30% in those subjects whose baseline values were <35 mg/dL). LDL lowering is dependent on the baseline LDL value, with 10% reductions at a baseline of 150 mg/dL, and 25% reduction at a baseline of 190 mg/dL. Combination statin–fenofibrate therapy reduces LDL in an additive fashion. Fenofibrate seems to decrease the density of LDL, and to upregulate both lipoprotein lipase and apoCIII, thereby enhancing the catabolism of TG-rich particles. These alterations, including the increase in HDL-associated apoAI and apoAII production, is related to fenofibrate-induced activation of the peroxisome proliferator-activated receptors. This superfamily of nuclear hormone receptor genes operate as transcription factors, and can secondarily result in upregulation of several lipoprotein-related enzymes and proteins. Furthermore, fenofibrate can produce reductions in both fibrinogen (7–23%) and in Lp(a) (>7%).

Fenofibric acid is excreted primarily through the kidney, and, therefore, needs a dosing modification in renal failure. It is recommended that coumadin be dosed at one-third its standard dose when administered with fenofibrate, with careful follow-up of protimes. Glucose tolerance is not affected by this agent, and no lithogenic potential has been observed. Creatine phosphokinase elevations are noted in 0.6 to 1.1% of cases, but seem to be usually associated with renal failure. Liver enzymes increase in less than 2% of cases, whereas GI disturbances (constipation, dyspepsia, and diarrhea) account for well over 50% of side effects and lead to greater than 3.5% discontinuation rates.

Comparatively, fenofibrate generally reduces LDL by at least 5 to 10% more than gemfibrozil, with a modest enhanced effect on HDL and TGs. Clinical outcomes data with fenofibrate are scant.

Ezetimibe

Statins inhibit cholesterol synthesis by inhibiting HMG-CoA reductase, a key step in the biosynthesis of cholesterol. By inhibiting cholesterol production in the liver, statins reduce hepatic cholesterol stores. The liver upregulates LDL receptors and clears more cholesterol from the blood. Cholesterol secreted by the liver into the bile, as well as cholesterol ingested from food, is absorbed in the small intestine. On average, approx 50% of total intestinal cholesterol is reabsorbed. In view of this, it seems appropriate to develop complementary lipid-lowering strategies that would inhibit the multiple pathways of cholesterol synthesis and absorption.

Ezetimibe (Zetia) is in a class of lipid-lowering compounds that selectively inhibits the intestinal absorption of cholesterol and related phytosterols. The chemical name of ezetimibe is 1-(4-fluorophenyl)-3(R)-[3-(4-fluorophenyl)-3(S)-hydroxypropyl]-4(S)-(4-hydroxyphenyl)-2-azetidinone. Ezetimibe, administered alone or in combination with an HMG-CoA reductase inhibitor (statin), either separately or in a combined formulation with simvastatin (Vytorin), is indicated as adjunctive therapy to diet for the reduction of elevated TC, LDL-C, and apoB levels in patients with primary (heterozygous familial and nonfamilial) hypercholesterolemia when diet alone is not enough. By virtue of targeting a lipid-lowering pathway other than the HMG-CoA reductase pathway, ezetimibe is an attractive add-on to statin therapy in patients who may be intolerant to higher doses of statins or in those not at target on maximum statin doses. The effect of this strategy on cardiovascular outcomes, however, has not been determined.

The recently published Vytorin vs Atorvastatin study *(45)* assessed the efficacy and safety of ezetimibe plus simvastatin vs atorvastatin monotherapy across their respective dose ranges in patients with hypercholesterolemia in a prospective multicenter 10-wk trial. Patients with hypercholesterolemia greater than the LDL-C goal defined by NCEP ATP III guidelines were randomized by an equal allocation to eight treatment arms: 10/10 mg, 10/20 mg, 10/40 mg, and 10/80 mg doses of ezetimibe/simvastatin, and 10, 20, 40, and 80 mg doses of atorvastatin. Men and women, 18 to 79 yr, with an LDL-C level at or above drug-treatment thresholds established by NCEP ATP III were eligible for enrollment if they met the following criteria: established CHD or CHD risk equivalent, with an LDL-C level at least 130 mg/dL; no established CHD or CHD risk equivalent, with at least two risk factors conferring a 10-yr risk for CHD between 10% and 20%, and an LDL-C level of at least 130 mg/dL; no established CHD or CHD risk equivalent, with at least two risk factors conferring a 10-yr risk for CHD less than 10%, and an LDL-C level of at least 160 mg/dL; and no established CHD or CHD risk equivalent, with fewer than two risk factors, and with LDL-C level of at least 190 mg/dL. In this study, 10/20 mg Vytorin decreased LDL-C by 51 vs 36% for 10 mg atorvastatin and vs 44% for 20 mg atorvastatin. The 10/40 mg dose of Vytorin decreased LDL-C by 57 vs 48% for 40 mg atorvastatin. The 10/80 mg dose of Vytorin reduced LDL-C by 59 vs 53% for 80 mg atorvastatin. All between-treatment differences in LDL-C levels were statistically significant at $p < 0.001$.

Ezetimibe is generally well-tolerated. Adverse experiences were reported in at least 2% of patients treated with Ezetimibe, and at an incidence greater than placebo in pla-

cebo-controlled studies of Ezetimibe, regardless of causality. When Ezetimibe was coadministered with a statin, consecutive elevations in serum transaminases (>3 times the upper limit of normal) were slightly higher (1.3%) than those of statins alone (0.4%). Liver function tests should be performed according to statin recommendations when Ezetimibe is added to statin therapy. In postmarketing experience with Ezetimibe, cases of myopathy and rhabdomyolysis have been reported regardless of causality. Most patients who developed rhabdomyolysis were taking a statin before initiating Ezetimibe. However, rhabdomyolysis has been reported very rarely with Ezetimibe monotherapy or with the addition of Ezetimibe to agents associated with increased risk of rhabdomyolysis, such as fibrates. The safety and effectiveness of Ezetimibe with fibrates have not been established; therefore, coadministration with fibrates is not recommended until use in patients is studied. The effects of Ezetimibe, either alone or in addition to a statin, on the risk of cardiovascular morbidity and mortality have not been established, nor has the independent effect of raising HDL-C or lowering TG on the risk of coronary and cardiovascular morbidity and mortality been determined.

CLINICAL EFFICACY IN SPECIAL POPULATIONS

Statins and Stroke

Although the link between elevated cholesterol and CAD is well-established, the link between elevated cholesterol and stroke was less convincing. Recent clinical trials *(46)* and meta-analyses *(47,48)* of HMG-CoA reductase inhibitors have demonstrated a significant reduction in ischemic stroke in patients with a history of CAD, both with and without elevated cholesterol (Table 5). Both the 4S and CARE studies strongly suggest that statin therapy results in a decrease in the risk for stroke.

In a recent meta-analysis *(47)* of 16 published trials testing statins from 1985–1995, statins had a clear benefit on stroke and total mortality. In 29,000 subjects considered in the meta-analysis, the average reductions in total and LDL-C achieved were large—22 to 30%, respectively. A total of 454 strokes and 1175 deaths occurred. Individuals assigned statin drugs had a 29% decrement in stroke (95% CI, 14–41%) as well as a reduction in total mortality of 22% (95% CI, 12–31%). Additional data regarding non-CVD mortality and cancer indicate no enhanced risk with the use of statins in these trials.

In a meta-analysis *(46)* looking at 12 trials of both primary and secondary prevention (n = 7,808 primary; n = 11,710 secondary), a 27% risk reduction was seen in the group receiving statins for secondary prevention (p = 0.001) but not in the primary prevention group. In the statin group, 182 strokes were observed, whereas 248 were observed in the placebo group followed for a mean of 4 yr (Fig. 8). In a meta-analysis of 28 trials, Bucher and coworkers *(28)* noted a 20% risk reduction in stroke with the use of statins. Twenty other trials using alternative cholesterol-lowering approaches were also examined. Resins that reduced death from CHD by 31%, equivalent to that of statins, as well as diet and fibrates, demonstrated no stroke benefits.

The LIPID *(12)* trial recently reported a significant decrease in stroke mortality with the use of statins. A 23% reduction in stroke was found with a 25% lowering of LDL-C through the use of pravastatin. The basis for this benefit could be the reduction in CVD, and, therefore, a reduction in cardiac sources of embolic phenomenon, or perhaps more probable, a direct effect on vasoregulation in the cerebral vasculature. Carotid internal medial thickness measurements were reduced in the pravastatin group for the full 4- to 5-yr period of the LIPID trial. Other studies using other statins have reported similar benefits.

Table 5
Effect of Cholesterol Lowering on Stroke Events: A Meta-Analysis of Statin Trials

Investigators	Statin	LDL-C (% ↓)	Sample size	Event rates[a] placebo/drug
First-degree prevention				
Shepherd et al.	P	26	3302	3.2/2.8
Salonen et al.	P	29	224	6.0/3.0
Mercuri et al.	P	22	151	0.0/0.0
Furberg et al.	L	28	231	1.4/0.0
Second-degree prevention				
PMSGCRP[b]	P	26	530	11.3/0.0
Pitt et al.	P	28	206	3.3/0.0
Crouse et al.	P	28	75	13.2/4.4
Jukema et al.	P	28	450	4.6/2.2
Sacks et al.	P	32	2081	7.5/5.2
Blankenhorn et al.	L	32	134	0.0/0.0
Waters et al.	L	29	165	0.0/6.1
4S	S	38	2221	7.6/5.6

From ref. 46.
[a]Annual rate per 10,000 patients.
[b]Pravastatin Multinational Study Group for Cardiac Risk Patients.
L, lovastatin; P, pravastatain; S, simvastatin.

Importantly, fewer cerebrovascular events occurred among those patients treated in the 4S, CARE, LIPID, and AFCAPS/TEXCAP studies. These results, and the uniformity in results from the three aforementioned meta-analyses recently reported, provide a clear basis for statin therapy to decrease the incidence of stroke. Even though we await subanalyses of these investigations, this finding may require a rethinking of lipid-lowering therapy in the elderly toward a more aggressive posture.

Cardiac Transplant Recipients

Transplant-associated atherosclerosis is a major cause of cardiac allograft failure after the first year after transplantation (49). Several distinct features are unique for atherosclerosis that develops after transplantation as compared with the commonly occurring disease. The pathological process involves the coronaries in a concentric fashion and often involves the epicardial and intramyocardial branches (49). Although the role of conventional risk factors in the development of transplant-associated atherosclerosis has not yet been defined, it seems logical to control those that are amenable to treatment.

Greater than 60% of transplant patients are observed to have hypercholesterolemia (50). Because vascular disease is a major cause of ultimate transplantation failure, and cholesterol reduction in CHD patients has been profoundly successful, serious efforts at cholesterol lowering have been made within the transplantation population. At the present time, lovastatin, pravastatin, and simvastatin are the only pharmaceutical agents that have demonstrated a benefit toward reducing rejection after human cardiac transplantation and decreasing the level of vasculopathy (51–56).

The Kobashigawa study (56) included 47 transplant subjects who initiated 20 mg pravastatin 1 to 2 wk after surgery (increased to 40 mg within 8 wk), and 50 transplant

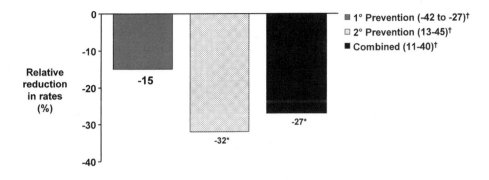

*P=0.001.
†95% confidence interval of percentage of relative reduction.

Fig. 8. Effects of statins on stroke events: a meta-analysis of primary- and secondary-prevention trials. (Adapted from ref. *26*.)

subjects who did not have statin agents administered. Baseline characteristics were generally similar. Cholesterol values at 12 mo were 193 mg/dL vs 248 mg/dL for pravastatin vs placebo, respectively. One-year survival was 94 vs 78% ($p = 0.025$), cardiac rejection with hemodynamic compromise 3 vs 14% ($p = 0.005$), and intravascular ultrasound-defined maximal intimal thickness was 0.11 vs 0.23 mm ($p = 0.002$).

In a 4-yr prospective randomized study *(57)* with heart transplant recipients (35 cases, 37 control subjects), the efficacy of simvastatin was assessed. The simvastatin group had significantly lower LDL-C concentrations (115 vs 156 mg/dL; $p = 0.002$), an improved long-term survival (88.6 vs 70.3%; $p = 0.05$) and a lower incidence of accelerated graft vessel disease (16.6 vs 42.3%; $p = 0.045$). The results of this trial show that simvastatin decreased the incidence of transplant atherosclerosis and reduced mortality from graft failure caused by acute rejection, confirming earlier reports by Kobashigawa.

However, although the hypothesis tested was a reasonable one based on clinical trial data related to cholesterol lowering, the mechanism of benefit in transplant patients remains unclear. In the Kobashigawa study, LDL lowering did not specifically correlate with vascular benefits, and, in the Wenke study *(57)*, no suggestion of this correlation was reported. Thus, some of the immune-related activity of HMG-CoA reductase inhibitors, rather than LDL lowering *per se*, may be relevant to the observed benefits. Wenke notes that a large percentage of cyclosporin is bound to LDL, so that LDL reduction could lead to an increase in free cyclosporin availability to ward off rejection.

Cyclosporine-induced alterations in the metabolism of HMG-CoA reductase inhibitor as well as steroid-derived lipoprotein metabolic abnormalities critically impact the treatment and expected benefit of lipid-lowering agents toward vascular disease *(51,58,59)*. Because of the metabolic compromise of statins by cyclosporine, toxicity may be observed at higher statin doses. An increase in serum levels has been documented for all of the available HMG-CoA reductase inhibitors when coadministered with cyclosporine. Therefore, the use of these agents in cardiac transplantation has been of concern because of the possibility of myositis and potential rhabdomyolysis. Most of the recent studies in transplanted patients have, therefore, been carried out using relatively low doses of statins. This paradigm may change as more sites begin to use fewer lipid-targeted agents,

e.g., tacrolimus. Statins are successful in reducing LDL values, and seem more potent potentially because of the consequences of medication use and/or discontinuation as described. Specifically, these agents include lovastatin, simvastatin, and pravastatin for lowering cholesterol in heart transplant recipients treated with cyclosporine and prednisone. Although the mechanisms of action remain to be elucidated, the survival benefit demonstrated suggests the importance of prophylactic statin use in all transplant candidates.

Lipid-Lowering Therapy After Coronary Artery Bypass Surgery

Atherosclerotic lesions develop at an accelerated rate in saphenous vein grafts (SVGs) compared with native coronary arteries, and thrombosis also contributes to occlusion. In a follow-up study of 82 patients, 10 yr after coronary artery bypass surgery, subjects who demonstrated progression or inception of coronary artery narrowing had higher values of very low-density lipoprotein and LDL, and lower values for HDL, even though standard traditional risk factors, such as cigarette use, blood pressure, and diabetes, were equivalent *(60)*. On multivariate analyses, the HDL value and the LDL-related apoB concentration were the best variables to predict who would progress. Subsequently, in a seminal work by Blankenhorn and colleagues *(61)*, beneficial effects of cholesterol lowering on atherosclerosis in saphenous vein grafts in a randomized intervention trial in 162 men younger than 60 yr of age who took niacin and colestipol or placebo for 2 yr was reported. Both LDL-C and the TG/HDL-C component of the lipid profile were profoundly improved. The post-CABG *(34)* study has furthered the findings of this original work, having been carried out during a longer period, with more carefully defined measures of quantitative angiography and a broader range of patients.

A total of 1351 patients were randomized, 92% men, with a mean age at entry of 61.5 yr. In addition to a Step I diet, patients were randomly assigned to receive one of two different lipid lowering regimens: the aggressive treatment arm (targeting an LDL goal of 60–85 mg/dL) included treatment starting with 40 mg/d lovastatin, whereas the moderate treatment arm (targeting an LDL goal of 130–140 mg/dL) started with 2.5 mg/d lovastatin. Cholestyramine was added if it was required to meet the goal.

The post-CABG study, in which patients were recruited who had undergone CABG 1 to 11 yr before randomization, was designed to evaluate whether aggressive lowering of LDL would be more effective than moderate lowering in reducing the progression of atherosclerotic lesions in SVGs. The trial was blinded to intensity of treatment. Participants who were men had at least two patent SVGs (at least one in women) and LDL levels of 130–175 mg/dL after diet therapy. The primary endpoint was significant worsening of the atherosclerosis (progression of at least 0.6 mm) during a 4.5-yr time period, and secondary endpoints including new occlusions, new lesions, and luminal narrowing.

A mean LDL level of 95 mg/dL was achieved in the aggressive arm and a 135 mg/dL LDL value in the moderate treatment arm. Analyses of the 1192 follow-up angiograms showed less progression of atherosclerosis in the SVGs of patients who underwent aggressive vs moderate LDL-lowering therapy. A modified ratio estimate statistic was used to calculate the mean percentage of grafts per patient showing progression (defined as a decrease in lumen diameter of at least 0.6 mm), which was the primary endpoint. The modified ratio estimate statistic for the combined endpoint of progression or death was 27% in the aggressive group vs 39% in the moderate treatment group ($p < 0.001$). New lesions occurred in 10% of the patients in the aggressive group and in 21% of the moderate

group. Occlusion occurred in 6% of patients in the aggressive group and in 11% of patients in the moderate group. Low-dose warfarin treatment, one arm of the study, showed no statistically significant benefit over placebo in any of the angiographic or clinical measures.

Although the trial was not powered to detect differences in clinical events, the rate of revascularization procedures (repeat bypass surgery or angioplasty) was 6.5% in the aggressive cholesterol treatment group and 9.2% in the moderate treatment group ($p = 0.03$), a 29% reduction.

These results suggest at least one of two positions: a 35% LDL reduction is more advantageous than simply a 15% reduction, or that it is important to target LDL levels to less than 100 mg/dL. Whether the conclusion is one or both, aggressive cholesterol lowering in patients with SVGs can reduce the progression of atherosclerotic narrowing of grafts, occlusion of grafts, and the need for repeat coronary bypass surgery or balloon angioplasty. The post-CABG and Blankenhorn data strongly suggest use of LDL-lowering agents after these procedures.

CONCLUSIONS

Treatment of hypercholesterolemia with HMG-CoA reductase inhibitors has revolutionized therapy for the prevention of CAD. New provocative trials have greatly expanded the role of statins in the primary and secondary prevention of CAD. Dramatic reductions in cardiovascular morbidity and mortality could be achieved with the implementation of preventive strategies, including the aggressive use of statins in the management of patients at risk for CAD. Statins provide the clinician with powerful new agents to prevent and potentially reverse CAD.

A greater understanding of the pathophysiological mechanisms leading to acute coronary syndromes as well as an elucidation of lipid metabolism has lead to the development of powerful lipid-lowering therapies. These agents have afforded clinicians the opportunity to arrest and potentially reverse CAD. New agents directed at defined metabolic pathways may offer attractive therapies for lipid lowering in select patient populations. Elucidating of the molecular mechanisms involved in lipoprotein metabolism and its relation to acute coronary syndromes will lead to improved therapies and potentially new classes of drugs for the targeted treatment of CAD.

REFERENCES

1. Simon LA. Interrelations of lipids and lipoproteins with coronary artery disease mortality in 19 countries. Am J Cardiol 1986;57:5–10.
2. Kannel WB, Castelli WD, Gordon T, McNamara PM. Serum cholesterol, lipoproteins and risk of coronary artery disease: The Framingham Study. Ann Intern Med 1971;74:1–12.
3. Kannel WB, Castelli WP, Gordon T. Serum cholesterol lipoproteins and risk of coronary heart disease. Ann Intern Med 1971;74:1–12.
4. Kannel WB. Lipids, diabetes, and coronary heart disease: insights from the Framingham Study. Am Heart J 1985;110:110–116.
5. Kannel WB, Neaton JD, Wentworth D, et al. Overall and coronary heart disease mortality rates in relation to major risk factors in 325,348 men screened for MRFIT. Am Heart J 1986;112:825–836.
6. Kannel WB. Cholesterol and risk of coronary heart disease and mortality in men. Clin Chem 1988;341B:B53–B59.
7. 1997 Heart and Stroke Statistical Update. Dallas: American Heart Association, 1996.
8. Pfeffer M, Sacks F, Lemuel A, et al. Cholesterol and recurrent events: a secondary prevention trial for normolipidemic patients. Am J Cardiol 1995;76:98C–106C.

9. Scandinavian Simvastatin Survival Study Group. Randomised trial of cholesterol lowering in 4444 patients with coronary heart disease: the Scandinavian Simvastatin Survival Study (4S). Lancet 1994;344:1383–1389.

10. Group SSSS. Baseline serum cholesterol and treatment effect in the Scandinavian Simvastatin Survival Study (4S). Lancet 1995;345:1274–1275.

11. Shepherd J, Cobbe SM, Ford I, et al. Prevention of coronary heart disease with pravastatin in men with hypercholesterolemia. N Engl J Med 1995;333:1301–1307.

12. Tonkin A. Management of the Long-Term Intervention with Pravastatin in Ischaemic Disease (LIPID) study after the Scandinavian Simvastatin Survival Study (4S). Am J Cardiol 1995;107C–112C.

13. Downs J, Beere P, Whitney E, et al. Design and rationale of the Air Force/Texas Coronary Atherosclerosis Prevention Study (AFCAPS/TexCAPS). Am J Cardiol 1997;80:287–293.

14. Collins R, Armitage J, Parish S, et al. MRC/BHF Heart Protection Study of cholesterol-lowering with simvastatin in 5963 people with diabetes: a randomised placebo-controlled trial. [see comment]. Lancet 2003;361:2005–2016.

15. Sever PS, Dahlof B. Poulter NR, et al. Prevention of coronary and stroke events with atorvastatin in hypertensive patients who have average or lower-than-average cholesterol concentrations, in the Anglo-Scandinavian Cardiac Outcomes Trial—Lipid Lowering Arm (ASCOT-LLA): a multicentre randomised controlled trial. Lancet 2003;361:1149–1158.

16. Shepherd J, Blauw G, Murphy M, et al. Pravastatin in elderly individuals at risk of vascular disease (PROSPER): a randomised controlled trial. Lancet 2002;360:1623–1630.

17. Colhoun HM, Betteridge DJ, Durrington PN, et al. Primary prevention of cardiovascular disease with atorvastatin in type 2 diabetes in the Collaborative Atorvastatin Diabetes Study (CARDS): multicentre randomised placebo-controlled trial. Lancet 2004;364:685–696.

18. Cannon C, Braunwald E, McCabe C, et al. Comparison of intensive and moderate lipid lowering with statins after acute coronary syndromes. N Engl J Med 2004;350.

19. LaRosa JC, Grundy SM, Waters DD, et al. Intensive lipid lowering with atorvastatin in patients with stable coronary disease. N Engl J Med 2005;352:1425–1435.

20. Expert Panel on Detection, Evaluation, and Treatment of High Blood Cholesterol in Adults. Summary of the second report of the National Cholesterol Education Program (NCEP) expert panel on detection, evaluation, and treatment of high blood cholesterol in adults (Adult Treatment Panel-II). JAMA 1993;269:3015–3023.

21. Executive Summary of the Third Report of the National Cholesterol Education Program (NCEP) Expert Panel on Detection, Evaluation, and Treatment of High Blood Cholesterol in Adults (Adult Treatment Panel III). JAMA 2001;285:2486–2497.

22. Grundy SM, Cleeman JI, Merz CNB, et al. Implications of recent clinical trials for the National Cholesterol Education Program Adult Treatment Panel III guidelines. Circulation 2004;110:227–239.

23. Stafford R, Blumenthal D, Pasternak R. Variations in cholesterol management practices of U.S. physicians. J Am Coll Cardiol 1997;29:139–146.

24. MRFIT Research Group. Multiple risk factor changes and mortality results. JAMA 1982;248:1465–1477.

25. Superko H. What can we learn about dense low density lipoprotein and lipoprotein particles from clinical trials? Curr Opin Lipidol 1996;7:363–368.

26. Family Study Committee for the Lipid Research Clinics Program. The collaborative Lipid Research Clinics Program Family Study. I. Study design and description of data. Am J Epidemiol 1984;119:931–943.

27. Family Study Committee for the Lipid Research Clinics Program Family Study. The collaborative Lipid Research Clinics Program Family Study. Bivariate path analysis of lipoprotein concentration. Genet Res 1983;42:117–135.

28. Lipid Research Clinics Program. The Lipid Research Clinics Coronary Primary Prevention Trial results. II. The relationship of reduction in incidence of coronary heart disease to cholesterol lowering. JAMA 1984;251:365–374.

29. Frick MH, Elo O, Haapa K, et al. Helsinki Heart Study. Primary-prevention trial with gemfibrozil in middle-age men with dyslipidemia. N Engl J Med 1987;317:1235–1245.

30. Manninen V, Elo MO, Frick MH, et al. Lipid alterations and decline in the incidence of coronary heart disease in the Helsinki Heart Study. JAMA 1988;260:641–651.

31. Effect of simvastatin on coronary atheroma: the Multicentre Anti-Atheroma Study (MAAS). Lancet 1994;344:633–638. Erratum in: Lancet 1994;344:762.

32. Watts GF, Lewis B, Brunt JN, et al. Effects on coronary artery disease of lipid-lowering diet, or diet plus cholestyramine, in the St Thomas' Atherosclerosis Regression Study (STARS). Lancet 1992;339:563–569.

33. Cashin-Hemphill L, mack WJ, Pogoda JM, Sanmarco ME, Azen SP, Blankenhorn DH. Beneficial effects of colestipol-niacin on coronary atherosclerosis. A 4-year follow-up. JAMA 1990;264:3013–3017.

34. The Post Coronary Artery Bypass Graft Trial Investigators. The effect of aggressive lowering of low-density lipoprotein cholesterol levels and low-dose anticoagulation on obstructive changes in saphenous-vein coronary-artery bypass grafts. N Engl J Med 1997;336:153–162.

35. Jukema JW, Burschke AV, van Boven AJ, et al. Effects of lipid lowering by pravastatin on progression and regression of coronary artery disease in symptomatic men with normal to moderately elevated serum cholesterol levels. The Regression Growth Evaluation Statin Study (REGRESS). Circulation 1995;91:2528–2540.

36. Pitt B, Mancini GB, Ellis SG, Rosman HS, Park JS, McGovern ME. Pravastatin limitation of atherosclerosis in the coronary arteries (PLAC I): reduction in atherosclerosis progression and clinical events. PLAC I investigation. J Am Coll Cardiol 1995;26:1133-1139.

37. Waters D, Higginson L, Gladstone P, Boccuzzi SJ, Cook T, Lesperance J. Effects of cholesterol lowering on the progression of coronary atherosclerosis in women. A Canadian Coronary Atherosclerosis Intervention Trial (CCAIT) substudy. Circulation 1995;92:2404-2410.

38. Blankenhorn DH, Azen SP, Kramsch DM, et al. Coronary angiographic changes with lovastatin therapy. The Monitored Atherosclerosis Regression Study (MARS). Ann Intern Med 1993;119:969-976.

39. Haskell WL, Alderman EL, Fair JM, et al. Effects of intensive multiple risk factor reduction on coronary atherosclerosis and clinical cardiac events in men and women with coronary artery disease. The Stanford Coronary Risk Intervention Project (SCRIP).Circulation 1994;89:975-990.

40. Pedersen TR, Kjekshus J, Pyorala K, et al. Effect of simvastatin on ischemic signs and symptoms in the Scandinavian simvastatin survival study (4S). Am J Cardiol 1998;81:333–335.

41. Tonkin AM, Colquhoun D, Emberson J, et al. Effects of pravastatin in 3260 patients with unstable angina: results from the LIPID study. Lancet 2000;356:1871-1875.

42. Pitt B, Waters D, Brown WV, et al. Aggressive lipid-lowering therapy compared with angioplasty in stable coronary artery disease. Atorvastatin versus Revascularization Treatment Investigators. N Engl J Med 1999;341:70-76.

43. Schwartz GG, Olsson AG, Ezekowitz MD, et al. Effects of atorvastatin on early recurrent ischemic events in acute coronary syndromes: the MIRACL study: a randomized controlled trial. JAMA 2001;285:1711-1718.

44. Nissen SE, Tuzcu EM, Schoenhagen P, et al. Effect of intensive compared with moderate lipid-lowering therapy on progression of coronary atherosclerosis: a randomized controlled trial. JAMA 2004;291:1071-1080.

45. Ballantyne CM, Abate N, Yuan Z, King TR, Palmisano J. Dose-comparison study of the combination of ezetimibe and simvastatin (Vytorin) versus atorvastatin in patients with hypercholesterolemia: the Vytorin Versus Atorvastatin (VYVA) study. Am Heart J 2005;149:464-473. Erratum in: Am Heart J 2005;149:882.

46. Crouse JR, Byington RP, Hoen HM, Furberg CD. Reductase inhibitor monotherapy and stroke prevention. Arch Intern Med 1997;157:1305–1310.

47. Hebert PR, Gaziano JM, Chan KS, Hennekens CH. Cholesterol lowering with statin drugs, risk of stroke, and total mortality. An overview of randomized trials. JAMA 1997;278:313–321.

48. Bucher HC, Griffith LE, Guyatt GH. Effect of HMGcoA reductase inhibitors on stroke. A meta-analysis of randomized, controlled trials. Ann Intern Med 1998;128:89–95.

49. Billingham ME. Cardiac transplant atherosclerosis. Transplant Proc 1987;19:19–25.

50. Gamba A, Mamprin F, Fiocchi R, et al. The risk of coronary artery disease after heart transplantation is increased in patients receiving low-dose cyclosporine, regardless of blood cyclosporine levels. Clin Cardiol 1997;20:767–772.

51. Vanhaecke J, Van Cleemput J, Van Lierde J, et al. Safety and efficacy of low dose simvastatin in cardiac transplant recipients treated with cyclosporine. Transplantation 1994;58:42–45.

52. PFCheung AK, De Vault GA Jr, Gregory MC. A prospective study on treatment of hypercholesterolemia with lovastatin in renal transplant patients receiving cyclosporine. J Am Soc Nephrol 1993;3:1884–1891.

53. Kuo PC, Kirshenbaum JM, Gordon J, et al. Lovastatin therapy for hypercholesterolemia in cardiac transplant recipients. Am J Cardiol 1989;64:631–635.

54. Ogawa N, Koyama I, Shibata T, et al. Pravastatin prevents the progression of accelerated coronary artery disease after heart transplantation in a rabbit model. Transplant Int 1996;9:S226–S229.
55. Kobashigawa JA, Murphy FL, Stevenson LW, et al. Low-dose lovastatin safely lowers cholesterol after cardiac transplantation. Circulation 1990;82:IV281–IV283.
56. Kobashigawa JA, Katznelson S, Laks H, et al. Effect of pravastatin on outcomes after cardiac transplantation. N Engl J Med 1995;333:621–627.
57. Wenke K, Meiser B, Thiery J, et al. Simvastatin reduces graft vessel disease and mortality after heart transplantation: a four-year randomized trial. Circulation 1997;96:1398–1402.
58. Vathsala A, Weinberg RB, Schoenberg L, et al. Lipid abnormalities in cyclosporine–prednisone-treated renal transplant recipients. Transplantation 1989;48:37–43.
59. Kasiske B, Tortorice K, Heim-Duthoy K, et al. The adverse impact of cyclosporine on serum lipids in renal transplant recipients. Am J Kidney Dis 1991;17:700–707.
60. Campeau L, Enjalbert M, Lesperance J, et al. The relation of risk factors to the development of atherosclerosis in saphenous-vein bypass grafts and the progression of disease in the native circulation. A study 10 years after aortocoronary bypass surgery. N Engl J Med 1984;311:1329–1332.
61. Blankenhorn DH, Nessim SA, Johnson RL, et al. Beneficial effects of combined colestipol-niacin therapy on coronary atherosclerosis and coronary venous bypass grafts. JAMA 1987;257:3233–3240.

5

High-Density Lipoprotein Cholesterol, Triglycerides, and Coronary Artery Disease
Clinical Evidence and Clinical Implications

JoAnne Micale Foody, MD

INTRODUCTION

Epidemiological studies have identified high-density lipoproteins (HDLs) and triglycerides (TGs) as independent risk factors that modulate cardiovascular disease (CVD) risk *(1)*. During the past decade, clinical trials of low-density lipoprotein (LDL)-lowering drugs have clearly established that reductions in LDL are associated with a 30 to 45% reduction in clinical events. However, despite lowered LDL levels, many patients continue to have cardiac events. This implies that a greater improvement could be achieved through further interventional measures, including therapy that modifies lipids other than LDL. Indeed, low HDL and high TG levels are often present in high-risk patients with CVD. In fact, a low level of HDL-cholesterol (C), rather than a high level of LDL-C, is currently the most common lipid abnormality in patients with coronary artery disease (CAD) in the United States. As a result, a great deal of research interest recently has been focused on raising plasma HDL levels as well as lowering TG levels by dietary, pharmacological, or genetic manipulations, as a potential strategy for the treatment of CVD. In addition to epidemiological studies, other lines of evidence suggest that modifying HDL and TG levels would reduce the risk of CVD.

From: *Contemporary Cardiology: Preventive Cardiology:*
Insights Into the Prevention and Treatment of Cardiovascular Disease, Second Edition
Edited by: J. M. Foody © Humana Press Inc., Totowa, NJ

EPIDEMIOLOGICAL AND POPULATION STUDIES
HDL Cholesterol

Although LDL-C is considered the predominant atherogenic lipoprotein in the development of CAD, there is significant variability in the clinical expression of CAD at any given LDL concentration. HDL also exerts significant positive effects on the process of coronary atherosclerosis. The National Cholesterol Education Program (NCEP) identifies a low HDL-C (<35 mg/dL) as a major independent risk factor for CAD. Consistent evidence of an inverse and continuous relationship between HDL-C and CAD exists.

In 1951, Barr et al. *(1)* first reported that patients with CAD had lower HDL levels than healthy men. In a later prospective study, Goffman and colleagues *(2)* demonstrated that patients who developed CAD had lower HDL levels than those who did not. The Framingham Heart Study produced compelling epidemiological evidence that a low level of HDL was an independent predictor of CAD *(3)*. In fact, at all levels of LDL-C, the level of HDL-C influences the risk of developing CAD. The recent Veterans Administration HDL Intervention Trial and the Bezafibrate Intervention Trial (BIP) trials *(4)* have demonstrated that increasing HDL decreases CAD. In addition, the Lipid Research Clinics Coronary Primary Prevention Trial *(5–8)* (using cholestyramine) and the Helsinki Heart Study (using gemfibrozil) both demonstrated that increasing HDL lowered CAD events independent of the effect on LDL lowering. The Adult Treatment Panel III of the NCEP identifies low HDL-C as a major risk factor for CAD and recommends that all healthy adults be screened for both total cholesterol and HDL-C levels.

The observation that low HDL-C was associated with CAD was verified by the Framingham Study *(3)*, which revealed HDL-C to have the strongest standard lipoprotein relation (inverse) to CAD. In men who have HDL-C levels lower than 25 mg/dL, the CAD incidence during 4 yr was 180 in 1000 compared with 25 in 1000 in men who had HDL-C levels in excess of 64 mg/dL. Furthermore, this relationship persisted above the age of 60 yr.

In the Tromso Heart Study *(9)*, 6595 young men (20–49 yr) were followed for 2 yr. Seventeen suffered myocardial infarctions (MIs), and each case was matched with two control subjects for age, residence, ethnic origin, and physical activity. The HDL-C made a threefold greater contribution to the prediction of coronary heart disease (CHD) events than LDL-C in the "young" population. Total cholesterol and TG levels were not different between the groups. Mean LDL-C was 222 mg/dL and 190 mg/dL in the MI patients and control subjects, respectively; and HDL-C was 25.6 mg/dL and 39.4 mg/dL, respectively.

Data from the Framingham Heart Study *(3)*, the Lipid Research Clinics Prevalence Mortality Follow-Up Study *(7)*, the Lipid Research Clinics Coronary Primary Prevention Trial Placebo Group *(8)*, and the Multiple Risk Factor Intervention Trial are consistent. In general, a 1 mg/dL increase in HDL-C was associated with a significant reduction in CAD risk of 2% in men and of 3% in women. In the Lipid Research Clinics Prevalence Mortality Follow-Up Study, in which only fatal endpoints were documented, a 1 mg/dL increase in HDL-C was associated with a significant reduction of fatal endpoints of 3.7% in men and 4.7% in women. The HDL-C level was unrelated to non-CVD mortality *(8)*.

Triglycerides

The independent relationship between plasma TG levels and CAD has now been established *(10)*. It is likely that the defective lipoprotein metabolism involved in hypertriglyceridemia may create a vascular environment predisposed to atherogenesis.

Elevated fasting plasma TG is a hallmark of insulin-resistance syndrome, a metabolic disorder characterized by hyperinsulinemia, glucose intolerance, decreased HDL-C, and possibly central obesity and increased production of atherogenic small, dense LDL particles.

Data from the observational Prospective Cardiovascular Muenster *(11)* study showed that CHD risk is high when TG levels exceed 200 mg/dL and the total cholesterol (TC) to HDL-C ratio is high (>5) because of low HDL-C (<35 mg/dL). In this 8-yr prospective study of 4639 German men, aged 40–65 yr, the incidence of major coronary events steadily increased to 132 in 1000 events per year in patients with TG levels less than 800. There were 258 total events in the entire population of subjects. Patients with TG greater than 200 mg/dL had at least twice the coronary event rate as patients with entirely normal TG levels. Coronary events seem to increase in proportion to TG levels, with the exception of the small number of subjects having TG greater than 800 mg/dL. Within this same population, increased lipoprotein little A antigen [Lp(a)] levels were also an independent risk factor for coronary disease. Patients with increased levels of this lipoprotein had nearly twice the coronary event rate as outpatients with normal levels of Lp(a) *(11)*.

In the observational Paris Prospective Study *(12)*, fasting plasma TG concentration was the only significant predictor of CHD death rate on multivariate analysis in 943 middle-aged men with diabetes or impaired glucose tolerance followed for 11 yr. Variables in the analysis were fasting plasma cholesterol, fasting plasma TG, age, systolic blood pressure, smoking, body mass index, and insulin and glucose concentrations. HDL-C concentrations were not measured. The mean annual CHD mortality rate was approximately three times higher in men who had TG levels above the median (123 mg/dL, 1.39 mmol/L) and TC levels above the median (220 mg/dL, 5.7 mmol/L) than men with values below the medians. The mean annual CHD mortality rate was approximately three times higher in men who had TG levels above the median (123 mg/dL) and TC levels above the median (220 mg/dL) than in patients with values below the median. TG concentrations less than 123 mg/dL seemed to obliterate the harmful effects of hypercholesterolemia; but with TG greater than 123 mg/dL, harmful effects became noticeably worse, not only for those with elevated plasma cholesterol, but also for those with a normal cholesterol concentration.

The Helsinki Heart Study *(13)*, conducted in hyperlipidemic men, demonstrated that increased fasting TG levels in conjunction with a high LDL-C to HDL-C ratio was associated with markedly increased risk for a CHD event. Increased risk was observed for men with elevated TG (>200 mg/dL, 2.3 mmol/L) and men with low HDL-C (<42 mg/dL, 1.08 mmol/L); however, the highest risk occurred in the subgroup of men with elevated TG (>200 mg/dL) and a high LDL-C to HDL-C ratio (>5). These results demonstrate the interdependence among the lipoprotein abnormalities—elevated TG, low HDL-C, and elevated LDL-C—for predicting CHD risk *(13)*.

Hypertriglyceridemia is almost always associated with increased coronary risk on univariate analysis. In some studies, it is also associated with increased risk on multivariate analysis, although not in other studies. This risk for CHD associated with hypertriglyceridemia may be a direct result of the influence of TG-rich lipoprotein accumulation in the circulation on the course of atherosclerotic plaque formation. Alternatively, it may be that hypertriglyceridemia, a central feature of the insulin-resistance syndrome, is a simple marker for coronary risk owing to other associated conditions of insulin resistance, such as evolving type 2 diabetes, isolated low HDL-C levels, and obesity. This may explain the decline in the significance of hypertriglyceridemia on multivariate analysis.

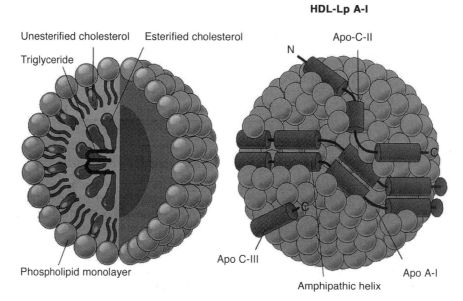

Fig. 1. Structure of HDL.

PATHOPHYSIOLOGY

HDL Cholesterol

HDL is a heterogeneous molecule and has diverse biological roles. More than 50% of HDL weight is from apolipoproteins, more than 90% of which are apolipoprotein (Apo)A-I and ApoA-II. Other constituents include ApoCs and ApoE, lecithin cholesterol acyltransferase, and paroxonases (Fig. 1). HDL particles can be categorized into several subclasses based on their shape, density, size, and other variables, including phospholipids. Small discoidal particles known as nascent or pre-β-HDL are formed when ApoA-I combines with phospholipids. When these lipid-poor particles absorb cholesterol and additional apolipoproteins, they become the more spherical particles called HDL3, which subsequently become the larger HDL2. According to some epidemiological studies, the risk of CHD may be increased when the proportion of HDL2 particles is decreased relative to HDL3 particles.

Although our understanding of how HDL protects against CVD is still incomplete, there is evidence that HDL contributes to:

1. Reversing cholesterol transport.
2. Inhibiting the oxidation of LDL-C.
3. Inhibiting the expression of adhesion molecules.
4. Providing protective effects on endothelial cells.

HDL-C is an important contributor to reverse cholesterol transport, the process by which cholesterol from peripheral tissues is transported to the liver, where it can be disposed of in bile. HDL-mediated efflux of cholesterol from cholesterol-loaded macrophages or foam cells is a well-established anti-atherogenic function of HDL. Cholesterol efflux from macrophages to HDL can occur by passive diffusion, by interaction with the SR-BI receptor, or by binding to the adenosine triphosphate-binding cassette protein A1 (ABCA1) transporter. In reverse cholesterol transport, foam cells give up cholesterol

to nascent HDL particles by way of the ABCA1. The preferred acceptor for the ABCA1 transporter-mediated cholesterol efflux is poorly lipidated ApoA-I, which is converted to mature, cholesterol ester-enriched spherical HDL particles. After accepting excess cellular cholesterol from arterial macrophages and other peripheral tissues, HDL transports the excess cholesterol to the liver for disposal, either directly through uptake by the hepatic SR-BI receptor, or indirectly, by first transferring cholesterol to very low-density lipoprotein (VLDL) or LDL-C particles via cholesterol ester transfer protein. The VLDL and LDL particles, in one of their normal metabolic roles, can then be taken up by the liver via LDL receptors and, in the process, dispose of the HDL-donated cholesterol. HDL is, thus, an integral component of the atheroprotective reverse cholesterol transport process, functioning as a carrier of excess cellular cholesterol from peripheral tissues to the liver, where it is excreted from the body as bile acids and cholesterol.

Antioxidant and anti-inflammatory properties of HDL contribute to the anti-atherogenic potential of these lipoproteins. Atherosclerosis is an inflammatory disorder initiated by an accumulation and subsequent oxidation of LDL in the arterial intima. HDL seems to exert some of its anti-atherogenic effects by inhibiting the oxidation of LDL-C. HDL particles have a high content of lipophilic antioxidants, such as α-tocopherol. In addition, ApoA-I acts as an antioxidant by virtue of its methionine groups, which can be converted to methionine sulfoxides. By scavenging reactive oxygen species, these antioxidants prevent lipid hydroperoxides and oxidized cholesterol esters, which are responsible for several harmful effects associated with oxidized LDL, from forming. Oxidized or modified LDL, unlike normal LDL, is readily taken up by the scavenger receptor, SR-A, or by CD36 on macrophages, resulting in cholesterol ester accumulation with foam cell formation. Macrophages also express a range of cytokines, some of which stimulate endothelial cells to express adhesion proteins. This leads to binding of blood monocytes to the endothelium before their recruitment into the artery wall by monocyte chemoattract protein-1. HDLs have the potential to impact at several points in this process.

In vitro, HDL particles have also been found to block the oxidized LDL-induced adhesion of monocytes to endothelial cells and to inhibit the cytokine-induced expression of adhesion molecules. HDL inhibits the expression of the adhesion molecules E-selectin (which enables tethering and rolling of monocytes along the endothelial surface), vascular adhesion molecule-1, and intercellular adhesion molecule-1. Adhesion of monocytes to the endothelium is an important early step in the development of atherosclerosis. The ability of HDL to inhibit these molecules and adhesion of monocytes is an additional atheroprotective mechanism.

Endothelial dysfunction is an early marker of atherosclerosis. In vitro studies have demonstrated that HDL prevents endothelial dysfunction that is mediated by oxidized LDL. Oxidized LDL inhibits vasodilation mediated by acetylcholine, and HDL reverses this inhibition. The presence of HDL has been shown to prevent impairment of nitric oxide production by oxidized LDL. Both HDL and ApoA-I also have important direct effects on endothelial cells and decrease endothelial cell death induced by oxidized LDL.

Diabetic Dyslipidemia

Patients with type 2 diabetes have a dyslipidemia comprised of elevated TG levels and decreased HDL levels. The mean concentration of LDL in those with type 2 diabetes is not significantly different than that seen in individuals without diabetes, but patients with diabetes tend to have a greater proportion of small, dense LDL particles. Because these particles are more susceptible to oxidation, they may, therefore, increase cardiovascular risk.

The pathobiology of the atherogenic dyslipidemia associated with diabetes is linked to insulin resistance. Insulin resistance is a hallmark of type 2 diabetes and central to the dyslipidemia associated with it. Insulin resistance at the level of the fat cell leads to increased free fatty acids in the circulation. The increased flux of free fatty acids to the liver stimulates the production and release of VLDL, which results in hypertriglyceridemia. In turn, in the presence of cholesterol ester transfer protein, VLDL exchanges its TGs for cholesteryl esters from both HDL and LDL, producing cholesterol-rich VLDL particles and TG-rich HDL and LDL particles. When hepatic lipase hydrolyzes the TGs in these HDL particles, ApoA-I dissociates from HDL and is then quickly cleared from the plasma, in part by excretion by the kidney, leaving less ApoA-I and HDL available in the circulation. As a result, fewer HDL particles are available for reverse cholesterol transport. Meanwhile, lipase-mediated hydrolysis of TG-rich LDL particles results in small, dense LDL particles.

CLINICAL INTERVENTION TRIALS IN LOW HDL

Clinical intervention trials have, until recently, focused on lowering LDL-C. Even with the best LDL-lowering therapies available, only one-third of heart disease risk is eliminated. It is clear that CAD is caused by the combination of multiple cardiovascular risks and that a low HDL may be an important contributor to the overall progression of CAD. No large scale clinical trials have focused on lowering TGs specifically.

Two prospective morbidity and mortality studies have recently tested the hypothesis that HDL is an independent risk factor for CAD. The BIP (4), a randomized, placebo-controlled clinical trial, assessed the effects of bezafibrate vs placebo in 8000 people with known CAD. BIP determined whether bezafibrate reduced the endpoints of CAD death and nonfatal MI in 3122 patients with CAD who had a "normal" serum total cholesterol level (180–250 mg/dL) and HDL-C levels less than 45 mg/dL. Diabetics were essentially excluded from this trial. There was a 15% increase in HDL-C and an 18% decrease in TGs at 1 yr of follow-up. However, there was no significant difference in CAD events between the two groups ($p = 0.27$). Although a divergence of the Kaplan-Meier curves occurred at approx 3 yr, this was not statistically significant (4).

Another clinical trial exploring the role of HDL reduction in the secondary prevention of CAD events was the Veterans Administration HDL Intervention Trial. This study (14) compared the effect of gemfibrozil vs placebo on CAD endpoints of CHD death or nonfatal MI in men who had low HDL-C (<40 mg/dL) and "normal" or low LDL-C (<140 mg/dL). This lipid profile is thought to comprise approximately one-quarter of all CAD patients, including patients with diabetes and patients with the constellation of symptoms associated with the metabolic syndrome X. In total, 2531 patients were randomized to gemfibrozil or placebo and followed for a mean of 5.1 yr; 25% of patients were diabetic, 57% were hypertensive, and 61% had a previous MI. Baseline TC was 175 mg/dL, HDL-C was 32 mg/dL, LDL-C was 111 mg/dL, and TG was 161 mg/dL. At 1-yr follow-up, there was a 7.5% increase in HDL-C and a 22% decrease in the primary endpoint of CHD death or MI, a 22% reduction in CHD death alone, a 22% reduction in nonfatal MI alone, and a 27% reduction in stroke ($p = 0.05$ for all).

These data provide powerful evidence that raising low HDL-C in patients with CAD improves outcomes. Importantly, these two new clinical trials extend the benefits of lipid modulation to new subsets of patients: those with low LDL and low HDL and diabetic patients with isolated low HDL and elevated TGs.

More recently, the benefits of administration of an HDL mimetic were assessed in a randomized clinical trial. ApoA-1 Milano is a variant of ApoA-I identified in individuals in Italy who exhibit virtually no coronary disease despite very low HDL levels. In animal models, infusion of this recombinant ApoA-1 Milano produced rapid regression of atheroma. In this randomized, placebo-controlled clinical trial of 123 subjects, investigators compared the effect of a 5-wk, weekly infusion of ETC-216 (recombinant ApoA-1 Milano) or placebo on coronary atheroma, as measured by intravascular ultrasound. The main outcome of interest was change in percent atheroma volume and average maximal atheroma thickness. In the ETC group, the mean percent atheroma volume decreased by −1.06% compared with an increase of 0.14% in the placebo group. Although promising and suggestive that a recombinant ApoA-1 Milano complex can reverse atheroma, these results require confirmation in a larger clinical trial with clinical outcomes. These combined results provide support for the concept that raising HDL may represent an additional therapeutic target for prevention of CVD *(15)*.

Several additional new classes of drugs are now in development that have purported HDL-raising effects. The most advanced are the cholesteryl ester transfer protein (CETP) inhibitors. CETP plays an important role in cholesterol metabolism, being responsible for the transfer of cholesteryl esters from HDL to VLDLs and LDLs. The observation that Japanese populations with CETP deficiency exhibited high levels of HDL-C has led to the concept that drugs targeting CETP activity may elevate HDL-C levels and potentially decrease cardiovascular risk. Support of this proposition has been obtained in rabbits in which inhibition of CETP activity is markedly antiatherogenic. Two CETP inhibitors are in late-stage clinical development: torcetrapib (Pfizer) and JJT-705 (Japan Tobacco). Phase 2 results with torcetrapib have recently been published, showing significant increases in HDL (of up to 100%; refs. *15–17*).

In a recent small single-blind, placebo-controlled study of 19 subjects with low HDL, investigators assessed the effects of torcetrapib, a potent inhibitor of CETP, on plasma lipoprotein levels. In this study, treatment with 120 mg of torcetrapib daily increased plasma concentrations of HDL cholesterol by 61% ($p < 0.001$) and 46% ($p = 0.001$) in the atorvastatin and non-atorvastatin cohorts, respectively, and treatment with 120 mg twice daily increased HDL cholesterol by 106% ($p < 0.001$). Torcetrapib significantly altered the distribution of cholesterol among HDL and LDL subclasses, resulting in increases in the mean particle size of HDL and LDL in each cohort. In this small preliminary study of subjects with low HDL cholesterol levels, CETP inhibition with torcetrapib markedly increased HDL cholesterol levels and also decreased LDL cholesterol levels, both when administered as monotherapy and when administered in combination with a statin *(16)*. However, many uncertainties remain regarding the CETP inhibitors. Animal models have provided conflicting results with inhibition of CETP and some studies have demonstrated harm and more atherosclerosis. Further outcome studies are required to fully delineate the role of these agents in clinical practice.

MANAGEMENT OF HDL AND TGs

Diet

NCEP and American Heart Association guidelines promote a diet in which fat composes only 30% or less of the day's total calories. The committee on nutrition from the American Heart Association, based on recommendations from the World Health Organization, suggests that fat calories constitute no less than 15% of total calories. The first

step in dietary therapy, usually the Step I diet, parallels NCEP recommendations. A change from the average American diet to the Step I diet of less than 10% saturated fatty acids and less than 300 mg/d of cholesterol reduces serum cholesterol levels by approx 7%, whereas further restriction to less than 7% saturated fatty acids and less than 200 mg/ d cholesterol (Step II diet) should reduce cholesterol levels by an additional 3 to 7%.

Exercise

Many large epidemiological investigations have failed to demonstrate consistently a correlation between reported physical activity and lipid values in populations not specifi- cally selected for hyperlipidemia. A paucity of cross-sectional studies has investigated physical activity and hypercholesterolemia, particularly its role in raising HDL and low- ering TG. Yet, it is generally accepted that exercise improves the spectrum of lipid abnormalities in conjunction with a healthy diet and weight loss.

Pharmacotherapy (see also *Chapter 4*)

Currently, LDL remains the principle target for intervention, and efforts to reduce cardiovascular risk should first focus on reducing LDL-C to guideline-based recommen- dations. After addressing LDL, HDL and TGs should be addressed, often through com- bination therapy with a statin. Unfortunately, based on the paucity of clinical trials addressing either HDL raising or TG lowering, little guidance is provided clinicians regarding optimal approaches. The mainstays of therapy are limited to nicotinic acid, fibric acid derivatives, and fish oil.

Nicotinic Acid

Nicotinic acid is a B vitamin that affects the lipoprotein system mediated through nicotinamide adenine dinucleotide, or nicotinamide adenine dinucleotide phosphate, by the inhibition of adenylate cyclase. Only nicotinic acid or its glycine conjugate (nicoti- nuric acid) has an antilipolytic effect. Nicotinamide is inactive regarding lipoprotein change. Nicotinic acid inhibits endogenous cholesterol synthesis, increases catabolism, and reduces the plasma concentrations of nonesterified fatty acids by its action at the level of the adipocyte. Rapid release of prostaglandins from platelets is thought to be respon- sible, in part, for the vasodilation and flush response. Similar to other medications, nicotinic acid has pharmacological effects that may benefit atherosclerosis that are not reflected in plasma lipoprotein measurements. These effects include prostaglandin/throm- boxane perturbations, platelet aggregation inhibition, and fibrinolysis. A long-acting, once-a-day niacin that is dosed at bedtime was recently approved by the Food and Drug Administration. This niacin has a significant effect in reducing small, dense LDL, and, in LDL pattern B subjects, achieves a mean 40% reduction in LDL-C.

INDICATIONS

Nicotinic acid is useful in patients who have elevated TGs, TG-rich lipoproteins, and LDL-C; reductions in HDL-C; and LDL subclass pattern B. Effects on lipids are com- monly seen after the renal threshold is exceeded, which generally is approx 1500 mg/d. The response of plasma lipoproteins is dose dependent within the range of approx 1500 to 6000 mg/d. Unmodified or time-release nicotinic acid can result in 10 to 25% reduc- tions in daily doses of 1500 to 3000 mg. Nicotinic acid is one of the few lipid medications that seems to have some effect on Lp(a). Nicotinic acid can suppress expression of LDL subclass pattern B if TGs are reduced below approx 140 mg/dL.

COMPLIANCE

Nicotinic acid is the lipid-altering drug with the most potential for side effects and, consequently, for adherence problems. Because of nicotinic acid's great potential benefit, it is worth expending extra effort on achieving compliance. Individual variability exists in the side effects to such an extent that it often can be attributed to differences in formulation. For this reason, obtaining several brands and testing each for individual tolerance can be helpful. Slowly titrating the dose from 100 to 500 mg three times daily during a 1-mo period can ease the patient into a therapeutic dose range. The prostaglandin-mediated flush can be ameliorated in part by ingesting 81 mg of aspirin 15 min before the niacin dose. Avoiding alcohol, monosodium glutamate, hot beverages, and spicy foods also can help ameliorate the flush. Gastrointestinal (GI) distress can be reduced by ingesting niacin with food. The most important tool to enhance adherence is a dedicated lipid nurse.

Niaspan® (KOS Pharmaceutical) is a new once-a-night niacin preparation that is dosed from 500 to 3000 mg/d. Niaspan has been compared with immediate-release niacin and found to have comparable benefits with fewer side effects. The new formulation of this product as well as the evening dosing reduces the apparent flushing episodes. LDL reductions of 10, 18, and 20% are found with 1, 2, and 3 g of Niaspan, respectively. Parallel to these changes, HDL increases by 15, 25, and 30%; whereas TGs decrease by 10, 35, and 45%. The reduction in Lp(a) was found to be 10, 25, and 30% for the 1-, 2-, and 3-g doses. Glucose increases by an average of 6%, uric acid increases by 34%, and some decrease in phosphorus (–16%) was also noted. Overall, an approx 10% of study participants increased their aspartate transaminase level from baseline, but only 2% went above two times the upper limit of normal, the latter consistent with that found in the placebo group. Long-term, 2-yr studies resulted in 2 patients out of 500 discontinuing Niaspan because of liver function elevations (<0.5%), with less than 1% having aspartate transaminase or alanine transaminase elevations beyond two times the upper limit of normal. Concomitant statin therapy reduced LDL another 14%, on average, but seemed to modestly reduce the Lp(a) benefit (not significant). Niaspan is a good alternative to regular niacin preparations, with 70% of patients not reporting flushing. Given some of the foregoing trials, niacin or one of its analogs should perhaps be administered more often in "mixed" phenotype patients. It is noted to decrease dense LDL particle concentration in such subjects. Statin–niacin outcome trials are clearly needed.

Fibric Acid Derivatives

Fibric acid derivatives enhance lipoprotein lipase activity and hepatic bile secretion and reduce hepatic TG production. TG and LDL-C response to these agents depends on the lipoprotein abnormality and specific fibric acid derivative used. TG reductions between 8 and 72%, LDL-C reductions between 0 and 35%, and HDL-C increases between 0 and 25% have been reported. Generally, the greatest benefit is seen in patients who have elevations in plasma TG, although fenofibrate has been reported to produce significant LDL-C reduction (~1.2 mmol/L) in type IIa patients. In hypertriglyceridemic patients who initially have low or normal LDL-C, gemfibrozil treatment may result in an increase in LDL-C, perhaps because of an increase in LDL production or a decrease in fractional LDL clearance rates. This response suggests the presence of a second lipoprotein abnormality that often requires two-drug therapy.

INDICATIONS

Fibric acid derivatives are useful in the treatment of hypertriglyceridemia and in selected patients who have elevated LDL-C in combination with elevated TGs. The HDL-C level often is reported to increase significantly when initial HDL-C is low or when it is associated with reduction of TGs. These agents are the drugs of choice in type III hyperlipidemia. In the Helsinki Heart Study, gemfibrozil (600 mg twice daily) resulted in an overall 42% reduction in TGs, a 10% reduction in LDL-C, and a 10% increase in HDL-C.

COMPLIANCE

These drugs generally are well-tolerated. Occasionally mild GI distress (nausea) is experienced in the first week. To reduce this potential side effect, it can be useful to start therapy with one-half the normal dose for several days before increasing to a full dose.

FENOFIBRATE

Fenofibrate is a fibric acid derivative, dosed at 200 or 400 mg/d. It is absorbed and rapidly converted into fenofibric acid, the active metabolite. The vast majority of the drug is protein bound, with a 4-h time to peak plasma levels. Elimination half-life is approx 20 h. The micronized form of fenofibrate—smaller particles and an absorption rate that is almost twice as fast as regular fenofibrate (200 mg/d)—was used in 1334 subjects with serum TGs greater than 200 mg/dL and total cholesterol greater than 250 mg/dL. LDL levels decrease by 27%, TG levels by approx 50%, and HDL levels increase overall by 15% (increased by 30% in those subjects whose baseline values were <35 mg/dL). LDL lowering is dependent on the baseline LDL value, with 10% reductions at a baseline of 150 mg/dL, and 25% reduction at a baseline of 190 mg/dL. Combination statin–fenofibrate therapy reduces LDL in an additive fashion. Fenofibrate seems to decrease the density of LDL, and to upregulate both lipoprotein lipase and ApoC-III, thereby, enhancing the catabolism of TG-rich particles. These alterations, including the increase in HDL-associated ApoA-I and ApoA-II production, are related to fenofibrate-induced activation of the peroxisome proliferator-activated receptors. This superfamily of nuclear hormone receptor genes operate as transcription factors, and can secondarily result in upregulation of several lipoprotein related enzymes and proteins. Furthermore, fenofibrate can produce reductions in both fibrinogen (7–23%) as well as in Lp(a) (>7%).

Fenofibric acid is excreted primarily through the kidney, and, therefore, needs a dosing modification in renal failure. It is recommended that coumadin be dosed at one-third its standard dose when administered with fenofibrate, with careful follow-up of protimes. Glucose tolerance is not affected by this agent, and no lithogenic potential has been observed. Creatine phosphokinase elevations are noted in 0.6 to 1.1% of cases, but seem to be usually associated with renal failure. Liver enzymes increase in less than 2% of cases, whereas GI disturbances (constipation, dyspepsia, and diarrhea) account for more than 50% of side effects and lead to greater than 3.5% discontinuation rates.

Comparatively, fenofibrate generally reduces LDL by at least 5 to 10% more than gemfibrozil, with a modest enhanced effect on HDL and TGs. Clinical outcomes data with fenofibrate are scant.

ω-3 Fatty Acids (Fish Oil)

A number of investigators have reported on beneficial effects of increased ω-3 fatty acid (contained in fish oil) intake in patients with CAD. The mechanism by which fish oil may provide beneficial effects include reductions in TG levels as well as reductions

in susceptibility to arrhythmia, decreases in platelet aggregation, lowering of blood pressure, promotion of nitric oxide-induced endothelial relaxation, and anti-inflammatory effects. Fish and fish oils contain long-chain polyunsaturated ω-3 fatty acids, more specifically, eicosapentaenoic acid (EPA) and docosahexanoic acid (DHA). Researchers have demonstrated that fish oil supplementation is highly effective in reducing TG levels and lowering the TG to HDL ratio. One study demonstrated that taking eight fish oil capsules daily (providing 2.4 g of EPA and 1.6 g of DHA) reduced TG levels by approx 26% and the TG to HDL ratio by 28% in women. Another study found an average reduction of 38% in TG levels and an increase in HDL levels of 24%, in both men and women consuming fish on a daily basis. The average American diet contains only approx 100 to 200 mg/d of EPA and DHA. The American Heart Association recommends that people in general increase their intake of long-chain polyunsaturated ω-3 oils from fish or directly from fish oil supplements, approx 1 g/d of EPA and DHA combined.

Statins in Patients With Hypertriglyceridemia

Recent clinical trials have proven that statin therapy causes a marked reduction CAD risk in patients with hypercholesterolemia. It remains to be determined whether stain therapy will decrease serum TGs and reduce risk in this population. In patients with normal TG levels, statin therapy decreases TG levels to a lesser percent than LDL levels. In patients with hypertriglyceridemia, percentage reductions in LDL and TG are similar. This implies a common mechanism of action of statins on both LDL and TGs. Whereas the absolute reduction in TG dose is proportional to the statin dose, the percent of TG lowering relative to LDL reduction remains constant across all statins and all doses. Atorvastatin provides the ability to significantly lower both LDL and TGs. It has been shown to decrease TGs by 27 to 46% across its dosing range.

One approach to the risk reduction in patients with hypertriglyceridemia is to decrease the concentrations of atherogenic TG-rich lipoproteins. This can be achieved through the use of statins, thereby simultaneously decreasing TG and LDL-C. Statins seem to be the first line of therapy in patients with combined elevations of LDL-C and moderate elevations of TGs. No trials have been performed using statins as the primary therapy for hypertriglyceridemia. Clinical efficacy can be extrapolated from the large body of evidence accumulated across broad populations with different forms of dyslipidemia.

There are insufficient trial data to justify the use of statins as first-line therapy in the treatment of hypertriglyceridemia. However, in selected high-risk patients, TG-lowering medications in combination with a statin may be used. Risk reduction with combination therapy of a TG-lowering agent and statin has not been achieved in a clinical trial.

CONCLUSIONS

Epidemiological studies have identified HDLs and TGs as independent risk factors that modulate CVD risk. Low HDL and high TG levels are often present in high-risk patients with CVD. As a result, a great deal of research interest recently has been focused on raising plasma HDL levels as well as lowering TG levels by dietary, pharmacological, or genetic manipulations as a potential strategy for the treatment of CVD. In addition to epidemiological studies, other lines of evidence suggest that modifying HDL and TG levels would reduce the risk of CVD. For now, a prudent strategy is to first address LDL-C levels according to guidelines, then aggressively raise HDL and reduce TGs through available interventions, as we await clinical data on newer strategies in patients with combined dyslipidemia.

REFERENCES

1. Barr DB, Russ EM, Eder HA. Protein–lipid relationship in human plasma: II. In atherosclerosis and related conditions. Am J Med 1951;11:480–493.
2. Goffman JW, Young W, Tandy R. Ischemic heart disease, atherosclerosis, and longevity. Circulation 1966;34:679–697.
3. Castelli WP, Garrison RJ, Wilson WF, et al. Incidence of coronary heart disease and lipoprotein cholesterol levels: the Framingham Study. JAMA 1986;256:2835–2838.
4. Secondary prevention by raising HDL cholesterol and reducing triglyceride in patients with coronary artery disease: the Bezafibrate Infarction Prevention Study. Circulation 2000, July 4;102:21–27.
5. Family Study Committee for the Lipid Research Clinics Program. The collaborative Lipid Research Clinics Program Family Study. I. Study design and description of data. Am J Epidemiol 1984;119:931–943.
6. Family Study Committee for the Lipid Research Clinics Program Family Study. The collaborative Lipid Research Clinics Program Family Study. Bivariate path analysis of lipoprotein concentration. Genet Res 1983;42:117–135.
7. Lipid Research Clinics Program. The Lipid Research Clinics Coronary Primary Prevention Trial results. II. The relationship of reduction in incidence of coronary heart disease to cholesterol lowering. JAMA 1984;251:365–374.
8. Namboodiri KK, Green PP, Kaplan EB, et al. Family aggregation of high density lipoprotein cholesterol. Collaborative Lipid Research Clinics Program Family Study. Arteriosclerosis 1983;3:616–626.
9. Miller NE, Thelle DS, Forde OH, Mjos OD. The Tromso heart-study. High-density lipoprotein and coronary heart-disease: a prospective case-control study. Lancet 1977;1:965-968.
10. Assmann G, Schulte H. Role of triglycerides in coronary artery disease: lessons from the Prospective Cardiovascular Muenster Study. Am J Cardiol 1992;70:10H–13H.
11. Assman G, Schulte H. Obesity and hyperlipidemia: results from the Prospective Cardiovascular and Muenster (PROCAM) study. In: Bjorntorp P, Brodoff B, eds. Obesity. JB Lippincott, New York, 1992, pp. 502–511.
12. Fontbonne A, Charles MA, Thilbult N, et al. Hyperinsulinemia as a predictor of coronary heart disease mortality in a healthy population: The Paris Prospective Study, 15 year follow-up. Diabetologia 1991;34:356–361.
13. Manninen V, Tenkanen L, Koskinen P, Huttunen JK, et al. Joint effects of serum triglycerides and LDL cholesterol and HDL cholesterol concentrations on coronary heart disease risk in the Helskinki Heart Study—implications for treatment. Circulation 1992;85:37–45.
14. Rubins HB, Robins SJ, Collins D, et al. Gemfibrozil for the secondary prevention of coronary heart disease in men with low levels of high-density lipoprotein cholesterol. Veterans Affairs High-Density Lipoprotein Cholesterol Intervention Trial Study Group. N Engl J Med 1999;341:410–418.
15. Nissen SE, Tsunoda T, Tuzcu EM, et al. Effect of recombinant ApoA-I Milano on coronary atherosclerosis in patients with acute coronary syndromes: a randomized controlled trial. JAMA 2003;290:2292–2300.
16. Brousseau ME, Schaefer EJ, Wolfe ML, et al. Effects of an inhibitor of cholesteryl ester transfer protein on HDL cholesterol. N Engl J Med 2004;350:1505–1515.
17. Clark RW, Sutfin TA, Ruggeri RB, et al. Raising high-density lipoprotein in humans through inhibition of cholesteryl ester transfer protein: an initial multidose study of torcetrapib. Arterioscler Thromb Vasc Biol 2004;24:490–497.

6 Management of Hypertension
Implications of JNC 7

Gregory M. Singer, MD and John F. Setaro, MD

INTRODUCTION

Recent recommendations by the Joint National Committee on the Detection, Evaluation, and Treatment of High Blood Pressure (JNC) 7 reflect a paradigm shift in the classification and treatment of hypertension. Incorporating findings of current clinical trials and surveys, JNC 7 reoriented the focus of hypertension management toward an intensive delineation of risk and concentration on goal achievement. This chapter analyzes the evolution of risk stratification, improvement of treatment strategies, and identification of modifiable risk patterns that affect blood pressure (BP) goal achievement. We will survey the components of evaluation and identify potential barriers to successful goal-oriented hypertension management.

DEVELOPMENT OF GOALS

As understanding of the cardiovascular (CV) consequences of elevated BP developed alongside evolving antihypertensive pharmacotherapeutics, early recommendations recognized a threshold of risk. Before thiazide diuretics were introduced in 1957, only hypertensive patients with life-threatening levels of BP were candidates for treatment.

From: *Contemporary Cardiology: Preventive Cardiology:*
Insights Into the Prevention and Treatment of Cardiovascular Disease, Second Edition
Edited by: J. M. Foody © Humana Press Inc., Totowa, NJ

Sympathectomy or poorly tolerated and toxic drugs (ganglionic blockers, peripheral adrenergic blockers, and vasodilators) were too risky for use in less ill patients. However, later, using a fixed dose combination of thiazide diuretic, peripheral sympathetic blocker, and vasodilator, the Veterans Affairs trials demonstrated the efficacy and tolerability of newer antihypertensive therapies and enlarged the scope of patients who could be treated safely (1,2). Subsequently, more effective and better-tolerated medications were introduced, offering the hypertensive patient potential for normalized BP with a lower risk of medication complications (3).

Based on results from Task Force I of the National High Blood Pressure Education Program (4), the National Heart, Lung, and Blood Institute commissioned the first JNC to set criteria for hypertension evaluation and management. Despite data from the Framingham Heart Study in 1971 showing that systolic BP (SBP) was a *better* determinant of risk than diastolic BP (DBP), especially in older people (5), DBP targets were the first goals established. As trial data accumulated, risk reduction became evident at both lower SBP and DBP targets. By 1988, the fourth JNC report redefined criteria for hypertension, incorporating SBP in the treatment goal of less than 140/90 mmHg (6). Convincing results from the Systolic Hypertension in the Elderly Program pilot and main trials (1984, 1991) demonstrated a 32% risk reduction for all CV morbidity and mortality with active treatment (thiazide-like diuretic plus β-adrenergic blocker [BB], if needed) vs placebo (7). The Systolic Hypertension in the Elderly Program goals mandated SBP reduction by 20 mmHg, if SBP was between 160 and 179 mmHg at entry, or to a value below 160 mmHg, if SBP was at least 180 mmHg at entry (8). These targets were founded on evidence from Veterans Affairs trials in the 1960s and 1970s, as well as the Hypertension Detection and Follow-Up Program (1972–1979) that showed a 20.3% mortality reduction and a significant cerebrovascular and CV event reduction in treating hypertension (1,2,9).

Although the Working Group on Hypertension in Diabetes further underscored the vulnerability of patients with both diagnoses by citing an ideal BP below 140/90 mmHg, JNC 4 did not formally recommend a lower goal for these patients (10). Evidence for intensive treatment of high-risk diabetic hypertensive patients was established by the United Kingdom Prospective Diabetes Study (UKPDS 38), which proved benefit using a "tight" BP goal (<150/85 mmHg) vs a "less tight" control (≤180/105 mmHg) (11,12). Subsequently, the Hypertension Optimal Treatment (HOT) study randomized 18,790 volunteers to three DBP goals (<80 mmHg vs <85 mmHg vs <90 mmHg), and found benefit of intensive therapy in the diabetic subgroup. Diabetic patients treated to DBP less than 80 mmHg had 51% fewer CV events compared with diabetic patients treated to DBP less than 90 mmHg (13).

In the 2003 report, JNC 7 presented a new structure in defining the management of high BP. Revising the classification of hypertension, the previous "high normal" or normal BP (120–139/80–89 mmHg) was now recategorized as "prehypertension" (Table 1). This reclassification underscored the continuum of escalating risk for men and women as BP rises from clearly normal levels (<120/80 mmHg) to definitely hypertensive values (≥140/90 mmHg) (14). The new JNC 7 system was influenced by a meta-analysis of more than 1 million volunteers in observational studies showing that CV risk begins at 115/75 mmHg and doubles with each increment of 20/10 mmHg (15), JNC 7 continued the approach of JNC 6, focusing on attaining goal BP, but updated the goals in parallel with newer data-derived guidelines. Although no new trials yet supported the lower goal

Table 1
Classifications of Blood Pressure and Treatment Recommendations of JNC 7

	SBP (mmHg)[a]		DBP (mmHg)[a]	Lifestyle modification	Initial drug therapy
Normal	<120	and	<80	Counsel	None, unless compelling indications present[b]
Prehypertension	120–139	or	80–89	Yes	
Stage 1 hypertension	140–159	or	90–99	Yes	Thiazide-type for most unless compelling indication present
Stage 2 hypertension	≥160	or	≥100	Yes	Two-drug combination (usually including thiazide-type diuretic unless compelling indication present)

Adapted from JNC 7 *(14)*.
[a]Treatment determined by highest BP category.
[b]Goals for compelling indications such as diabetes or chronic kidney disease is less than 130/80 mmHg.
SBP, systolic blood pressure; DBP, dystolic blood pressure.

of less than 130/80 mmHg for diabetic patients or patients with chronic kidney disease (CKD; defined by either depressed glomerular filtration rate less than 60 mL/min/1.73 m² [corresponding approximate serum creatinine values >1.5 mg/dL in men and >1.3 mg/dL in women], or the presence of albuminuria [>300 mg/d or >200 mg albumin/g creatinine]), JNC 7 chose to also recommend this target. JNC 7 further emphasized the importance of titrating to BP goal, and cited all classes of antihypertensives acceptable for initial therapy as fundamentally equivalent, although selection could be modified based on compelling indications for patients with complicated hypertension.

RISK STRATIFICATION OF HYPERTENSIVE PATIENTS WITH MULTIPLE CV RISK FACTORS

Despite extensive evidence of the benefits of BP regulation, hypertension remains a prevalent and uncontrolled modifiable CV risk factor for approx 50 million Americans. Although awareness has improved during the last 30 yr, the majority of treated hypertensive patients demonstrate BP values above recommended guidelines. Data from the 1999–2000 series of the third National Health and Nutrition Examination Survey (NHANES) identified increasing awareness of hypertension from 68 to 70% compared with NHANES III (phase 2, 1991–1994), and treatment improving from 54 to 59% among hypertensive subjects. However, only one-third of patients achieve goal SBP of less than 140 mmHg and DBP of less than 90 mmHg (Table 2) *(14)*.

Mortality associated with CV disease has declined during the past 30 yr, and attention to modifiable risk factors, such as cholesterol, BP, and smoking among those of highest risk, diabetic patients, has improved. However, the proportion of patients with multiple CV risk factors continues to escalate. Estimated by NHANES III, 63% of men and 55% of women in America are overweight (body mass index [BMI] > 25) or obese (BMI > 30), with a prevalence of comorbidities of hypertension, insulin resistance, and hyperlipidemia

Table 2
Trends in Awareness, Treatment, and Control of High Blood Pressure in Adults
With Hypertension Aged 18 to 74 Yr

	II (1976–1980)	III (Phase 1, 1988–1991)	III (Phase 2, 1991–1994)	1999–2000
National Health and Nutrition Examination Survey, weighted %				
Awareness	51	73	68	70
Treatment	31	55	54	59
Control	10	29	27	34

Table 3
Definition of the Metabolic Syndrome—Patients With Three or More of the Following
Criteria

Abdominal obesity	Waist circumference > 102 cm in men and > 88 cm in women
Hypertriglyceridemia	≥150 mg/dL (1.69 mmol/L)
Low high-density lipoprotein cholesterol	<40 mg/dL (1.04 mmol/L) in men and <50 mg/dL (1.29 mmol/L) in women
High BP	≥130/85 mmHg
High fasting glucose	≥110 mg/dL (≥6.1 mmol/L)

correlating with increasing weight (16). The metabolic syndrome (Table 3) is becoming more prevalent. Age-adjusted frequency in the NHANES III (1988–1994) sample was 23.7%, representing an estimated 47 million Americans when applied to the 2000 US census (17). Increased recognition of compounding CV risk as patients accumulate comorbidities has resulted in greater attention to these markers (18). As more evidence defines risk reduction at more stringent targets, the number of at-risk individuals, both lean and obese, is increasing.

In the Framingham Heart Study, Kannel et al. described a geometric acceleration of 10-yr probability of a CV event in patients with mild systolic hypertension (SBP 150–160 mmHg) as risk factors accumulated. Clustering of two or more risk factors among hypertensive subjects appeared in approx 55% of patients, a frequency twice the expected rate, and at four times higher than expected by chance when three or more risk factors were prevalent (19). Similarly, the presence of obesity followed not only the development of hypertension, but also the tendency to cluster associated risk factors. Because obesity predisposes to insulin resistance, dyslipidemia, and hypertension, it is not clearly an independent risk factor, yet it remains an identifiable marker for increased CV risk.

Lifetime risk of developing hypertension for normotensive individuals at age 55 is 90%, based on Framingham data (20). Assessment of lifestyle and other CV risk factors is paramount in directed treatment of high BP. The presence of associated compelling conditions may influence therapeutic strategy (Table 4). Additionally, evidence of target-organ damage should intensify goal-directed therapy (Table 5). Lessons learned from recent clinical trials demonstrate that specific drug selection for patients with uncomplicated hypertension is less important than BP control itself. Condition-specific drug selection can be made according to compelling indications.

Table 4
Drug Class Recommendations for High-Risk Conditions With Compelling Indications by JNC 7

	Diuretic	BB	ACE-I	ARB	CCB	Aldosterone Antagonist
Heart failure	√	√	√	√		√
After myocardial infarction		√	√			√
High coronary disease risk	√	√	√			√
Diabetes	√	√	√	√	√	
Chronic kidney disease			√	√		
Recurrent stroke prevention	√		√			

BB, β-adrenergic blocker; ACE-I, angiotensin-converting enzyme-inhibitor; ARB, angiotensin receptor blocker; CCB, calcium channel blockers.

Table 5
Components for Cardiovascular Risk Stratification in Patients With Hypertension

Major risk factors	Target-organ damage
Hypertension	Heart
Cigarette smoking	Left ventricular hypertrophy
Obesity (BMI ≥30)	Angina or prior myocardial infarction
Physical inactivity	Prior coronary revascularization
Dyslipidemia	Heart failure
Diabetes mellitus	Brain
Microalbuminuria or estimated GFR <60 mL/min	Stroke or transient ischemic attack
Age (>55 yr for men, >65 yr for women)	Chronic kidney disease
Family history of premature cardiovascular disease	
(<55 yr for men, <65 yr for women)	Peripheral arterial disease
	Retinopathy

BMI, body mass index; GFR, glomerular filtration rate.

PATIENT EVALUATION AND EXAMINATION

Evaluation of patients with documented hypertension includes assessment for other risk factors, compelling indications, or evidence of target-organ damage that affect treatment strategies (Tables 4 and 5). Proper assessment of causes or contributors, either endogenous or exogenous (Table 6), is indicated as well.

Accurate BP Measurement

Careful measurement of BP should include avoidance of caffeine or nicotine for at least 30 min because of transient hypertensive effects. The patient should be seated with the arm at heart level, feet on the floor, and should rest for 5 min before the measurement is performed. A cuff of adequate size should be used, with the bladder encompassing two-thirds of the circumference of the arm. The recorded SBP value is the point at which the first of greater than two sounds is heard (Korotkoff phase 1) and the DBP value corresponds to the disappearance of sound (Korotkoff phase 5).

If initial values are elevated, BP should be measured at two subsequent office visits, although immediate treatment is appropriate if the first assessment shows a SBP value

Table 6
Contributors to Hypertension

Endogenous	Exogenous
Sleep apnea	Excess sodium intake
Chronic kidney disease	Nonsteroidal anti-inflammatory agents
Primary aldostereonism	Oral contraceptive therapy
Renovascular disease	Chronic steroid therapy
Pheochromocytoma	Licorice (or similarly flavored chewing tobacco)
Coarctation of the aorta	Cyclosporine/tacrolimus
Thyroid or parathyroid disease	Erythropoietin
Cushing's syndrome	Cholestyramine (or other resin-binding agents)
Insulin resistance/hyperinsulinemia	Antidepressants (monoamine oxidase inhibitors and some tricyclics [Venlafaxine])
Obesity	Sympathomimetic compounds (nasal decongestants containing phenylpropanolamine or pseudoephedrine, inhaled adrenergic antibronchospastic agents, amphetamines, appetite suppressants, cocaine, and herbal preparations containing ephedra)
	Selected over-the-counter dietary supplements and herbal remedies (e.g., bitter orange and yohimbine)
	Excess alcohol intake

greater than 160 mmHg or DBP above 105 mmHg. Typically, a number of patients will have lower or even normal readings at later visits, or during a home or 24-h ambulatory BP study. Such patients have been termed office or white-coat hypertensive patients, requiring close follow-up even if treatment is not begun at first. White-coat hypertension patients do not have as serious a prognosis as those who are hypertensive throughout daily life (21,22). However, they do not enjoy the same favorable outlook as those whose home and office readings are normal, and white-coat hypertensive patients may have elevated vascular resistance and other important cardiac risk factors as well (23). This group should receive dietary and lifestyle modification advice, and should be followed very closely, particularly in that long-term assessment of BP risk has been based largely on office or clinic determinations. Twenty-four hour ambulatory BP monitoring is a useful research technique and has clinical application in cases of unexplained symptoms, white-coat hypertension, paroxysmal hypertension, or resistant hypertension, and has been proposed as an adjunct to titration of multidrug therapy (22). However, it is expensive and not recommended for routine initial assessment. A useful alternative is properly performed home or workplace measurement, which can provide multiple recordings under a variety of conditions of daily life (24).

Physical Exam

In addition to patient history, physical exam assessment should focus on multiple systems. In general, height and weight should be listed, and obesity noted. In particular, android or truncal obesity in men or women raises the possibility of high-risk metabolic syndrome consisting of hypertension, increased insulin resistance, hyperinsulinemia, hypertriglyceridemia, and reduced high-density lipoprotein cholesterol. Truncal obesity,

flushing, excess body or facial hair, and pigmented striae could indicate a hyperadrenal state. Obesity may be a contributor to a syndrome of sleep apnea. Anxiety and tremor point to the possibility of hyperthyroidism or pheochromocytoma. Funduscopic exam is imperative because arteriolar narrowing and arteriovenous crossing changes signal chronic hypertension with target-organ injury present in small cerebral vessels. Hemorrhages and exudates point to accelerated hypertension, and papilledema reflects malignant hypertension.

In the neck, the thyroid should be palpated for size, masses, and tenderness. Jugular vein elevation suggests hypertensive target-organ damage in the form of congestive heart failure (CHF). The finding of a delayed upstroke or bruit in the examination of the carotid arteries is significant for target-organ disease in the form of obstructive atherosclerosis.

Cardiopulmonary exam may demonstrate cardiomegaly, tachycardia, abnormal rhythm, murmurs, gallops, rales, or pleural effusions, suggesting sequelae of CHF. Bronchospastic findings should lead to the use of alternatives to BBs.

Abdominal exam may reveal a high-pitched systolic bruit with a diastolic component located over the right or left epigastrium, suggesting renal artery stenosis. A soft flank mass may reflect polycystic kidney disease. An enlarged, central pulsatile mass may represent an abdominal aortic aneurysm, an advanced complication of hypertension and tobacco use.

Diminished peripheral pulses suggest coarctation of the aorta that has escaped undetected into adulthood, or advanced atherosclerotic peripheral vascular disease in older patients. In the former case, measurement of lower extremity BP is diagnostically useful. In the latter, auscultation of the femoral arteries may disclose bruits, reflecting generalized vascular disease. If arterial obstructive disease is present in multiple distributions, the examiner should consider renal artery disease. Peripheral edema may be evident in hypertensive patients who have CHF, renal impairment, primary hyperaldosteronism, or hypothyroidism.

Routine Laboratory Tests

Several routine laboratory tests are recommended for all hypertensive patients (Table 7) to assess risk, establish cause, screen for common asymptomatic diseases, and guide appropriate therapy. More extensive laboratory evaluation is not necessary unless the BP is resistant to treatment.

Lifestyle Modification

Prehypertensive patients are at risk for developing clinically significant hypertension and, therefore, need effective lifestyle modification to prevent stage I hypertension. Trends of increasing total calories, portion sizes, and refined carbohydrates are compounded by physical inactivity. Elevated sodium content in processed foods and condiments contribute to the estimated 8.7 g/d (3.5 g/d sodium) salt intake of the average American (Table 8). Studies of dietary modulation, specifically the Dietary Approaches to Stop Hypertension (DASH), demonstrated significant BP reduction with reduced salt intake *(25,26)*. These effects are amplified by other lifestyle modifications (Table 9). The Treatment of Mild Hypertension Study (TOMHS) confirmed that lifestyle modification is synergistic with antihypertensive therapy to achieve BP reduction and reduce CV risk *(27)*. Alternatively, the Trial of Preventing Hypertension (TROPHY), started in 1999, is an ongoing 4-yr multicenter trial of untreated prehypertensive patients randomized to

Table 7
Laboratory Tests Appropriate for Newly Diagnosed Hypertensive Patients

Assessing risk	Screening for common asymptomatic diseases
Fasting lipid profile	Complete blood count
Fasting serum glucose	Serum calcium
Serum creatinine	
Urinalysis (both macroscopic and microscopic)	
12-lead electrocardiogram	

Establishing cause	Guiding therapy
Serum potassium	Lipid profile
Serum creatinine	Fasting serum glucose
Urinalysis (both macroscopic and microscopic)	Serum creatinine
Thyroid-stimulating hormone	

Adapted from ref. *27a*.

Table 8
Foods With High Sodium Content

Potato chips	Bouillon
Pretzels	Ham
Salted crackers	Sausages
Biscuits	Frankfurters
Pancakes	Smoked meats or fish
Fast foods	Sardines
Olives	Tomato juice (canned)
Pickles	Frozen lima beans
Sauerkraut	Frozen peas
Soy sauce	Canned spinach
Catsup	Canned carrots
Some cheeses	Pastries/cakes from self-rising flour mixes
Commercially prepared soups	

placebo and fixed-dose candesartan. This trial is examining whether development of stage I hypertension can be intercepted with early pharmacological intervention *(28)*.

INITIATION AND SELECTION OF DRUG THERAPY

Although comprehensive data on the effectiveness of new drug classes is now available, recommendations continue to focus on BP reduction rather than specific drug selection. The Antihypertensive and Lipid-Lowering Treatment to Prevent Heart Attack (ALLHAT) trial demonstrated that diuretics are equivalent to calcium channel blockers (CCBs) and angiotensin-converting enzyme (ACE) inhibitors in preventing CV complications of hypertension. Unless compelling indications are present warranting a specific drug therapy, JNC 7 advocates low-cost thiazide-type diuretics as the initial basis of antihypertensive therapy, because they have been thoroughly studied for decades.

Table 9
Effects of Lifestyle Modification on Blood Pressure[a]

Type	Description	Blood pressure effect
Weight reduction	Target body mass index 18.5–24.9	5–20 mmHg decrease for every 10 kg of weight loss
Dietary Approaches to the Stop Hypertension eating plan	Diet rich in fruits, vegetables, and low-fat dairy products, with reduced total and saturated fats	8–14 mmHg reduction
Dietary sodium restriction	Reduce dietary sodium intake to less than 100 mmol/d (2.4 g sodium or 6 g of sodium chloride)	2–8 mmHg reduction
Physical activity	Regular aerobic exercise at least 30 min/d most days of the week	4–9 mmHg reduction
Moderation of alcohol consumption	Limit consumption to no more than 2 drink equivalents for most men and 1 drink equivalent for women or lighter weight individuals (1 equivalent = 12 oz. beer, 5 oz. wine, or 1.5 oz. spirits)	2–4 mmHg reduction

[a]Adapted from Joint National Committee on the Detection, Evaluation, and Treatment of High Blood Pressure 7 (14).

The treatment algorithm of JNC 7 illustrates goal-directed therapy (Fig. 1). Application of this process should occur at each patient encounter. The question of ideal strategy when the initial choice fails to attain goal BP has been a long-standing debate: should additional agents be added ("stepped-care") or should the first agent be stopped in favor of another class of agents ("sequential monotherapy")? JNC 5 allowed both approaches but JNC 6 and 7 strongly favor stepped-care unless therapeutic unresponsiveness or side effects are noted with the first choice. For patients with stage 2 hypertension, initial two-drug combination therapy including a thiazide-type diuretic is advised because trials have shown that multidrug therapy is frequently required to achieve the goal (13,29,30). However, until the Avoiding CV Events Through Combination Therapy in Patients Living with Systolic Hypertension (ACCOMPLISH) trial is completed in 5 to 7 yr, we will not have the necessary evidence to help us select the optimal combination of currently available drugs (31).

In addition to the CV risk benefit of achieving target BP, intensive treatment in high-risk hypertensive patients can save many more lives. The Valsartan Antihypertensive Long-term Use Evolution (VALVE) study showed fewer endpoints with early intensive BP reduction. The amlodipine (CCB) group achieved a 4.0/2.1 mmHg greater difference in BP reduction after 1 mo compared with the valsartan (angiotensin receptor blocker [ARB]) group. The groups averaged a 13.9/7.2 mmHg (amlodipine) and 11.3/5.3 mmHg (valsartan) reduction in the first 6 mo, however, the differences in BP reduction were less (1.5/1.3 mmHg) at the end of the study. The 63% excess strokes in the valsartan group occurred in the first 6 mo, and 76% within the first year, likely a consequence of early intensive BP reduction with amlodipine (32). Vigilance is appropriate for those at risk for orthostatic hypotension, such as patients with diabetes, autonomic dysfunction, and older patients.

Monthly follow-up is recommended until the BP goal is reached. Visit frequency may be increased for those with stage 2 hypertension or comorbidities that necessitate caution. Serum studies of electrolytes and renal function should be monitored within a few weeks of initiation of either diuretics or angiotensin antagonists and one to two times per year thereafter (33). Likewise, management of comorbid conditions should impact laboratory analysis (e.g., lipid evaluation, diabetes monitoring, markers of inflammation, or evaluation of microalbuminuria or proteinuria).

COMPELLING INDICATIONS FOR MEDICATION SELECTION

Ischemic Heart Disease

Because ischemic heart disease is the most common target-organ effect of hypertension, BBs, or long-acting CCBs are the first drug choices for this risk group. Additionally, ACE-Is may also be used in patients with acute coronary syndromes, however, BB and aldosterone antagonists have also been shown to benefit after myocardial infarction (29,30,34). The Heart Outcomes Prevention Evaluation (HOPE) study examined patients with increased CV risk with preserved systolic left ventricular function. A 22% reduction of composite CV endpoints was found with ramipril (ACE-I) vs placebo (35). Whether benefit is ascribable to intrinsic properties of ACE-I that go beyond BP reduction has been debated.

The Comparison of Amlodipine vs Enalapril to Limit Occurrences of Thrombosis (CAMELOT) study, evaluating a three-arm protocol of enalapril vs amlodipine vs

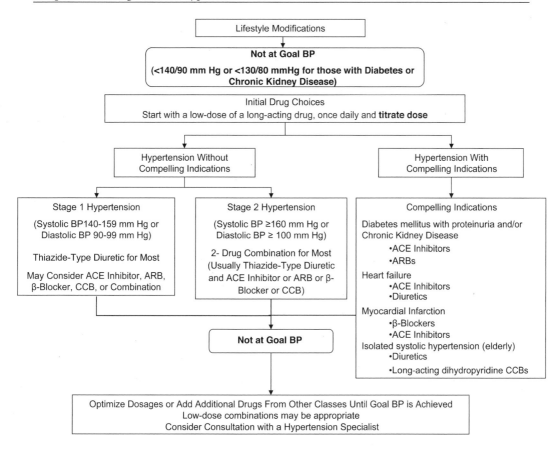

Fig. 1. Algorithm for the treatment of hypertension. (Adapted from ref. *14.*) BP, blood pressure; ACE, angiotensin-converting enzyme; ARB, angiotensin receptor blocker; CCB, calcium channel blocker.

placebo in nearly 2000 normotensive patients with coronary artery disease, showed cardioprotective effects in treated patients after 2 yr. Patients randomized to amlodipine had a 5/3 mmHg reduction from a baseline BP of 129/77 mmHg, similar to the 5/2 mmHg reduction achieved with enalapril, however, only the amlodipine group experienced a 31% reduction in CV events. This suggested that ACE-I may not have protective effects beyond BP reduction, as suggested by the HOPE study *(36).*

Congestive Heart Failure

For patients with CHF, either systolic or diastolic left ventricular dysfunction, medical regimens including ACE-Is or ARBs, selective BBs, and nonselective BBs are recommended *(37–42).* Additionally, diuretics and aldosterone antagonists have been shown to be beneficial, especially for symptomatic CHF *(43,44).* Although the Prospective Randomized Amlodipine Survival Evaluation (PRAISE) study showed better outcomes in patients with nonischemic cardiomyopathy for amlodipine vs placebo, there was no increased morbidity or mortality among patients with severe CHF. Nonetheless, CCBs are not the mainstay of treatment for patients with CHF *(45).*

Diabetes Mellitus

Until 1996, published data had not yet addressed treatment of hypertensive type 2 diabetic patients. Only the Captopril trial by Lewis et al. in 1993 evaluated treatment for type 1 diabetic patients *(46)*. Insight into management of diabetic hypertensive patients proceeds from two sources: trials enrolling diabetic hypertensive patients, and subgroup analyses of larger studies in which a proportion of subjects had diabetes. Multiple drug classes were evaluated, including diuretics, BBs, ACE-Is, ARBs, and CCBs, all reducing CV risk with BP reduction.

The UKPDS 38 was the first trial in diabetic patients with hypertension that examined BP and glycemic control in 1148 diabetic hypertensive patients. Investigators tracked both microvascular and macrovascular complications of diabetes, as well as CV and all-cause mortality. Subjects were followed for a mean of 8.4 yr and multiple drugs were required to attain target BP. Diabetic complications were 24% fewer ($p = 0.0046$), diabetes-related deaths were 32% fewer ($p = 0.019$), strokes were 44% fewer ($p < 0.013$), and myocardial infarctions were 21% fewer (p was nonsignificant) in the group with BP that was controlled more tightly. Tight blood glucose control was associated with only a 12% reduction in diabetic complications, underscoring the importance of BP regulation in diabetic patients, although optimization of both BP and glucose are clearly essential *(47)*.

Substudies of diabetic populations within large randomized trials demonstrated accentuated risk reduction in treated diabetic hypertensive patients relative to nondiabetic subjects. In the HOT trial, 1501 diabetic patients among 18,790 HOT volunteers had a 51% reduction in CV mortality, demonstrated in the group randomized to the lowest DBP goal (<80 mmHg). No other subgroup had benefit, although none showed harm from aggressive therapy *(48)*. In HOPE, ACE-Is were proven effective in diabetic patients. There was a 22% relative risk reduction in CV events for the 3577 diabetic patients of the 9297 patients enrolled *(49)*.

Two studies published in 2001 examined the efficacy of ARBs in diabetic patients with nephropathy and further examined benefits of specific drugs vs the degree of BP control achieved. The Irbesartan Type II Diabetic Nephropathy Trial (IDNT; irbesartan), and the Reduction of End Points in Non-Insulin Dependent Diabetes Mellitus with Angiotensin II Antagonist Losartan (RENAAL) trial (losartan), demonstrated specific renal protective benefits of angiotensin II blockade in delaying the progression of renal dysfunction to end-stage renal disease. In both studies, there was equally good BP control in the ARB-treatment arm vs the non-ARB-treatment arm. Investigators concluded that the 20 to 30% risk reduction in renal endpoints was attributable to the inherent properties of ARBs rather than to the degree of BP control achieved *(50,51)*.

The ALLHAT study represents the largest diabetic patient subgroup analysis in any clinical hypertension trial. There were 13,101 diabetic patients, an additional 1399 volunteers with impaired fasting glucose, and 17,012 normoglycemic patients. ALLHAT randomized subjects to three different first-line agents: diuretics, CCBs, or ACE-Is. A fourth group received a peripheral α-adrenergic blocker, doxazosin, as initial therapy, but that arm of the trial was stopped early. Results from ALLHAT showed no evidence of superiority in patients initially treated with the newer agents in any of the three glycemic subgroups or in the overall trial. No significant increase in fasting glucose was noted in patients previously classified as diabetic *(52)*, however, there were differences in the incidence of new diabetes in the volunteers randomized to each class of drugs. Only 8.1%

of those randomized to lisinopril developed new diabetes compared with 9.8% receiving amlodipine and 11.6% receiving chlorthalidone *(30)*. The significance of these findings is unclear because the diabetic subgroup of ALLHAT that started therapy with chlorthalidone did as well or better than those randomized to begin treatment with the other drugs *(53)*.

Recent evaluation of glucose and BP control with the use of BB was investigated in the Glycemic Effects in Diabetes Mellitus: Carvedilol-Metoprolol Comparison in Hypertensive (GEMINI) study. In addition to either ACE-I or ARB, subjects were randomized to a selective (metoprolol tartate) or nonselective (carvedilol) BB. Although using surrogate metabolic outcomes, carvedilol proved superior because it stabilized hemoglobin A_{1C} and improved insulin resistance. Carvedilol slowed development of microalbuminuria with comparable BP control, benefits that may relate to carvedilol's α- and β-blocking properties, allowing greater peripheral blood flow and glucose disposal *(54)*.

Chronic Kidney Disease

Patients with CKD are another at-risk group that has shown promise when tighter BP control is applied. Multiple trials show that lower BP preserves renal function, motivating stricter guidelines for patients with CKD of less than 130/80 mmHg *(47,48,55)*. As stated in the previous section, both ACE-Is and ARBs exhibit renoprotective effects beyond simple BP control.

Cerebrovascular Disease

Patients with history of cerebrovascular disease similarly benefit from BP control. Results from the Perindopril Protection Against Recurrent Stroke Study (PROGESS) demonstrated that the combination of ACE-I and diuretic reduced the risk of stroke and major vessel events in hypertensive patients compared with ACE-I alone *(56,57)*.

RESISTANT HYPERTENSION

Defined as a failure to reach optimal BP despite using full doses of an appropriate three-drug regimen including a diuretic *(14)*, resistant hypertension is becoming more prevalent, particularly as stricter targets are recommended. Evaluation of a resistant hypertensive includes assessment of six domains:

1. Specific identifiable disorder (secondary hypertension).
2. Inappropriate or inadequate medical treatment by the clinician.
3. Patient nonadherence to the prescribed regimen.
4. Older patients with systolic hypertension who are unresponsive to appropriate therapy.
5. Exogenous substances that raise BP or interfere with antihypertensive agents.
6. Obesity and metabolic syndrome *(58)*.

If the BP goal still cannot be achieved, it may be useful to consult with a hypertension specialist *(59)*.

BARRIERS TO SUCCESS

The best strategy to achieve BP targets remains undefined. Solving this problem requires identifying the source and determining aggravating factors. That goals are dif-

ficult to achieve should not discourage the practitioner from striving for excellence. Clinical trials show that current goals are achievable indeed.

Guideline targets have shifted only slightly in the last decade. The goal of less than 140/90 mmHg advocated by JNC 5 continues in JNC 7. More intensive goals of less than 130/85 mmHg for diabetic patients were advocated in the 1993 guidelines, with only slight modification to less than 130/80 mmHg in 2003. Data from clinical practice lags behind these recommendations. Improvement is noted in recent surveys, reflecting a time delay between guideline publication and physician implementation. Control in diabetic patients still remains suboptimal.

Clinical inertia may explain the physician's recognition of a problem without acting on it. In this case, clinic inertia is manifested as a failure to initiate or intensify therapy during patient encounters *(60)*. Hypertension, especially in diabetic patients, represents an asymptomatic modifiable CV risk factor in which abnormalities are solely numerical in the presymptomatic phase of the disease. Therefore, opportunities for intervention are clear and frequent. Therapeutic failures cannot be attributed to lack of feasibility, as contradicted by clinical trial experience. Clinical inertia remains a principal force in lack of goal achievement *(61)*.

Hypertension is generally an asymptomatic disease for which patients have no complaints or requests for intervention. In addition to addressing other symptomatic complaints, the physician is obliged to approach high BP at every encounter in light of the great benefit associated with its control. Likewise, the physician is responsible for translating enthusiasm in the treatment of chronic asymptomatic diseases. Because BP is checked at each encounter, it should be discussed at each encounter. What message do physicians send if the problem of an unrealized goal is not addressed?

In examining barriers to diabetes care, El-Kebbi et al. identified provider's self-reported reasons for not advancing therapy in uncontrolled diabetic patients. Perception of patient improvement was noted in a 34% of responses, with lack of adherence with diet or medications cited in 26% and acute intervening illness in 8%. Patient refusal for more intensive care, side effects, or lack of a specific reason played only a minor role *(62)*. Goal-oriented management should acknowledge but not allow these issues to become barriers to good CV health. Although medication nonadherence may confound an office BP reading, it should not preclude intensive follow-up with a plan of titration. Signs of improvement should be a mechanism of encouragement that treatment is working. If the goal is achieved and maintained with drug therapy, the patient should be informed that medication reduction may be possible after evidence of further lifestyle modification.

Physicians need to identify competing substances that will impede the path to the goal. Illicit adrenergic substances, dietary supplements, and over-the-counter medications counteract treatment and exacerbate already existing hypertension *(63)*. Most patients are unaware of potential interactions and will not speak of their use unless directly questioned. If the substance is recommended for treatment of another clinical condition, its use should be monitored and discontinued as soon as possible. It is estimated that one out of every five patients who take prescription medication are also using herbs or high-dose dietary supplements. Because herbal supplements are not classified as drugs, Food and Drug Administration testing and quality control standards may not apply *(64)*. Physicians should remain nonjudgmental and sensitive to patients' views, and inform the patients of potential untoward effects of these substances, especially drug interactions.

GOAL-ORIENTED MANAGEMENT

Although evidence validates the intensive recommendations of JNC 7, it remains to be seen whether these goals can be achieved. Although favorable outcomes from trials are encouraging, methods must be devised to translate trial conclusions into practice if disappointing rates of BP control are to improve. Although a dichotomized goal (above or below a prespecified target) is clearly artificial and not physiological, we think that it is easier in a busy practice to implement a specific numerical goal. This approach will also make it easier to assess performance and it sets a clear basis for quality comparison among different health care providers and delivery systems.

The choice of an appropriate goal is also a key issue. A goal that cannot be reached is too severe and, thus, unachievable, but a goal that is too easily reached will not optimize outcomes in high-risk subjects. Results from the Controlled Onset Verapamil Investigation of Cardiovascular End Points (CONVINCE) and ALLHAT studies have shown that excellent control rates are available in clinical trials in which study coordinators maintain fidelity to protocols that demand forced titration or the addition of a new drug or drugs if the goal BP is not reached.

In a study of 437 consecutive patients seen at a University hypertension specialty clinic, goal-oriented management was evaluated for treatment efficacy. Similar to forced titration algorithms in clinical trials, goal-oriented management requires stepping up therapy until the goal is achieved. No specific drug-treatment algorithm was mandated and physicians were free to choose any lifestyle or drug combination they wished. Results paralleled evidence from large clinical trials, because 59% of patients achieved the SBP goal of less than 140 mmHg and the DBP goal of less than 90 mmHg, with 86% of patients having DBP less than 90 mmHg, similar to CONVINCE and ALLHAT. As in HOT and CONVINCE, in which 30 and 32% of participants received monotherapy at 3 yr, respectively, greater than two-thirds of patients required two or more medications *(65)*. In diabetic patients, 52% achieved a BP less than 140/90 mmHg, but only 22% of diabetic patients reached the previous JNC 6 target of less than 130/85 mmHg, and a dismal 15% reached the American Diabetes Association, National Kidney Foundation, and JNC 7 target of less than 130/80 mmHg *(66)*.

A similar study was published in Spain, examining 4049 difficult-to-control subjects in 47 hospital-based hypertension clinics. Using similar methods, the overall goal BP (<140/90 mmHg) in patients with uncomplicated hypertension was reached in 42% of patients, with the DBP goal reached in 70% of patients and the SBP goal reached in 47% of patients. However, only 36.7% of diabetic patients reached the goal of less than 140 mmHg for SBP and also less than 90 mmHg for DBP. Similarly, only 13.2% reached goals of less than 130/85 mmHg and fewer (10.5%) had BPs of less than 130/80 mmHg *(67)*.

Further studies have analyzed guideline adherence and goal achievement in the managed care setting. A retrospective analysis of 502 patients in three primary care clinics operated by a commercial Managed Care Organization looked at target achievement based on Health Plan Employer Data and Information Set and JNC 6 guideline criteria for patients with uncomplicated hypertension and diabetic patients. Subjects had full health insurance, including prescription coverage. The goal of BP of at most 140/90 mmHg was attained by 74% of patients, with 46% of the 148 diabetic patients having BPs of less than 130/85 mmHg *(68)*.

We doubt that specific algorithms are applicable or appropriate in the general practice setting. The pathophysiology of hypertension in individual patients varies widely, and response to single agents or combinations may be patient specific. Access, cultural, language, and economic factors introduce further variation. Physicians must choose the regimen they view as best for each patient. Indeed, JNC 7 and other contemporary guidelines grant considerable flexibility to clinicians in allowing choice based on judgment regarding how an individual patient will respond, what other diseases or risk factors are present, and what economic factors exist.

The issue of second-step therapy is more complex. Ideally, a second agent should have a mechanism of action different from the first. Although there are eight different pharmacological classes, physiologically, there are three mechanisms of action that can serve as therapeutic targets: stroke volume (best affected by thiazide diuretics, loop diuretics, and aldosterone antagonists), heart rate (BB and nondihydropyridine CCBs), and vascular resistance (dihydropyridine CCBs, renin–angiotensin blockade agents [ACE-I or ARB], α-adrenergic blockers, and direct vasodilators). Within each medication, there may be shared physiological effects. For example, thiazide diuretics exhibit direct volume effects in addition to smooth muscle-based vasodilatory attributes. The BB class exhibits both heart rate and anti-renin properties. Certain BBs, such as carvedilol and labetalol, possess α-adrenergic blocking influences. ACE-I and ARBs modulate salt and water balance through aldosterone blockade as well as direct reduction of vascular resistance.

If BP still resists control after these three physiological elements are addressed, centrally acting agents, such as clonidine, methyldopa, and reserpine can be introduced, however, doses may be limited by excessive sedation or depression. Although direct vasodilators are effective, concomitant BB and loop diuretics are necessary to offset reflex tachycardia and fluid retention, respectively. Unconventional combinations within the same physiological class have proved effective in resistant cases. Examples include the addition of aldosterone inhibitors (spironolactone) to thiazide diuretics, ACE-I, or ARBs, concurrent use of ACE-I with ARBs, or combination of dihydropyridine with nondihydropyridine calcium antagonists (69–72).

Whereas a forced titration algorithm specifies which drug to add when a patient is not at the goal BP (appropriate for a clinical trial), a goal-oriented algorithm advocates vigorous drug titration using available and well-tolerated agents, regardless of initial drug therapy or lifestyle approach. The rational use of second, third, or fourth agents, as described in the previous paragraphs, will typically allow control even for the most difficult hypertensive patients (59).

SUMMARY

JNC 7 has taken an aggressive approach to assessment of the hypertensive patient, together with subsequent recommendations for aggressive treatment not only in patients with sustained systolic and or diastolic hypertension, but also in selected patients identified with high-normal BP. When possible, sound, evidence-based data from randomized, controlled trials was used in making therapeutic recommendations.

The disparity between hypertension control efforts is a major concern, because only one in four hypertensive individuals in the United States are currently controlled to below target BP levels (140/90 mmHg). Efforts are being made to change physicians' attitudes

toward treatment that led to this significant shortfall in control. We must translate the evidence in support of aggressive treatment to lower BP into an action plan that will encourage all providers to take a more vigorous role in their treatment strategies. Current guidelines for lower treatment goals are soundly grounded in research data. Recently reported clinical trials fully support these treatment recommendations. Treating BP to at least normal levels would seem appropriate for most patients as we hope to reduce CV risk in this new millennium.

REFERENCES

1. Veterans Administration Cooperative Study Group on Antihypertensive Agents. Effects of treatment on morbidity in hypertension. Results in patients with diastolic BP averaging 115 through 129 mmHg. JAMA 1967;202:1028–1034.
2. Veterans Administration Cooperative Study Group on Antihypertensive Agents. Effects of treatment on morbidity in hypertension. II. Results in patients with diastolic blood pressure averaging 90 through 114 mmHg. JAMA 1970;213:1143–1152.
3. Moser, M. Evolution of the treatment of hypertension from the 1940s to JNC V. Am J Hypertens 1997;10(part 2):2S–8S.
4. National High Blood Pressure Education Program. Report to the Hypertension Information and Education Advisory Committee. Task Force I Data Base. Recommendations for a national high blood pressure program database for effective antihypertensive therapy. DHEW Publication No. (NIH) 75-593, September 1, 1973.
5. Kannel WB, Gordon T, Schwartz MJ. Systolic versus diastolic blood pressure and risk of coronary heart disease. The Framingham study. Am J Cardiol 1971;27:335–346.
6. Report of the Joint National Committee on Detection, Evaluation and Treatment of High Blood Pressure (JNC IV). Arch Intern Med 1988;148:1023–1038.
7. Hulley SB, Furberg CD, Gurland B, et al. Systolic Hypertension in the Elderly Program (SHEP): antihypertensive efficacy of chlorthalidone. Am J Cardiol 198;56:913–920.
8. Systolic Hypertension in the Elderly Program Cooperative Research Group. Prevention of stroke by antihypertensive drug treatment in older persons with isolated systolic hypertension. Final results of the systolic hypertension in the elderly program (SHEP). JAMA 1991;265:3255–3264.
9. Hypertension Detection and Follow-up Program Cooperative Group. Five-year findings of the Hypertension Detection and Follow-Up Program (HDFP). Reduction in mortality of persons with high blood pressure, including mild hypertension. JAMA 1979;242:2562–2571.
10. Working Group on Hypertension in Diabetes. Statement on hypertension in diabetes mellitus: final report. Arch Intern Med 1987;147:830–842.
11. Laasko M. Benefits of strict glucose and blood pressure control in type 2 diabetes: lessons from the UK Prospective Diabetes Study. Circulation 1999;99:461–462.
12. UK Prospective Diabetes Study Group. Tight blood pressure control and risk of macrovascular and microvascular complications in type 2 diabetes: UKPDS 38. BMJ 1998;317:703–713.
13. Hansson L, Zanchetti A, Carruthers SG, et al. Effects of intensive blood pressure lowering and low-dose aspirin in patients with hypertension: principal results of the Hypertension Optimal Treatment (HOT) randomized trial. Lancet 1998;351:1755–1762.
14. Chobanian AV, Bakris GL, Black HR, et al. and the National High Blood Pressure Education Program Coordinating Committee. The Seventh Report of the Joint National Committee on the Prevention, Detection, Evaluation, and Treatment of High Blood Pressure. JAMA 2003;289:2560–2572.
15. Lewington S, Clarke R, Qizilbash N, Peto R, Collins R. Age-specific relevance of usual blood pressure to vascular mortality: a meta-analysis of individual data for one million adults in 61 prospective studies. Lancet 2002;360:1903–1913.
16. Must A, Spadano J, Coakley E, Field A, Colditz G, Dietz W. The disease burden associated with overweight and obesity. JAMA 1999;282:1523–1529.
17. Ford ES, Giles WH, Dietz WH. Prevalence of the metabolic syndrome among US adults—findings from the Third National Health and Nutrition Examination Survey. JAMA 2002;287:356–359.
18. Gregg EW, Cheng YJ, Cadwell BI, et al. Secular trends in cardiovascular disease risk factors according to body mass index in US adults. JAMA 2005;293:1868–1874.

19. Kannel WB. Risk stratification in hypertension: new insights from the Framingham Study. Am J Hypertens 2000;13:3S–10S.

20. Vasan RS, Beiser A, Seshadri S, et al. Residual lifetime risk for developing hypertension in middle-aged women and men: the Framingham Heart Study. JAMA 2002;287:1003–1010.

21. Perloff D, Grim C, Flack J, et al. Human blood pressure determination by sphygmomanometry. Circulation 1993;88:2460–2470.

22. Staessen JA, Fagard R, Thijs L, et al. Randomised double-blind comparison of placebo and active treatment for older patients with isolated systolic hypertension. The Systolic Hypertension–Europe (Syst-Eur) Trial Investigators. Lancet 1997;350:757–764.

23. Julius S, Mejia A, Jones K, et al. White coat versus sustained borderline hypertension in Tecumseh, Michigan. Hypertension 1990;16:617–623.

24. Pickering TG. A new role for ambulatory blood pressure monitoring? JAMA 1997;278:1110.

25. Obarzanek E, Proschan MA, Vollmer WM, et al. Individual blood pressure responses to changes in salt intake: results from the DASH-Sodium Trial. Hypertension 2003;42:459–467.

26. Sacks FM, Svetkey LP, Vollmer WM, et al. for the DASH-Sodium Collaboration Research Group. Effects on blood pressure of reduced dietary sodium and the dietary approaches to stop hypertension (DASH) diet. N Engl J Med 2001;344:3–10.

27. Neaton JD, Grimm RH, Prineas RJ, et al. Treatment of Mild Hypertension Study (TOMHS). JAMA 1993;270:713–724.

27a. Elliot WJ, Black HR. Hypertension. In: Wong NE, ed. Preventive Cardiology: A Practical Approach, 2nd ed. New York: McGraw-Hill, 2005, p. 169.

28. Julius S, Nesbitt S, Egan B, et al. for the TROPHY study group. Trial of Preventing Hypertension: design and 2-year progress report. Hypertension 2004;44:146–151.

29. Black HR, Elliott WJ, Grandits G, et al. CONVINCE Research Group. Principal results of the Controlled Onset Verapamil Investigation of Cardiovascular End Points (CONVINCE) trial. JAMA 2003;289:2073–2082.

30. The ALLHAT Officers and Coordinators for the ALLHAT Collaborative Group. Major outcomes in high-risk hypertensive patients randomized to angiotensin converting enzyme inhibitor or calcium channel blocker vs diuretic. The Antihypertensive and Lipid-Lowering Treatment to Prevent Heart Attack Trial (ALLHAT). JAMA 2002;288:1981–1997.

31. Jamerson KA. The first hypertension trial comparing the effects of two fixed-dose combination therapy regimens on cardiovascular events: Avoiding Cardiovascular Events Through Combination Therapy in Patients Living with Systolic Hypertension (ACCOMPLISH). J Clin Hypertens 2003;5(4 Suppl 3):29–35.

32. Julius S, Kjeldsen SE, Weber M, et al. for the VALUE trial group. Outcomes in hypertensive patients a high cardiovascular risk treated with regimens based on valsartan or amlodipine: the VALUE randomized trial. Lancet 2004;3663:2022–2031.

33. Bakris GL, Weir MR, on behalf of the Study of Hypertension and Efficacy of Lotrel in Diabetes (SHIELD) investigators. Achieving goal blood pressure in patients with type 2 diabetes: conventional versus fixed-dose combination approaches. J Clin Hypertens 2003;5:201–210.

34. Pitt B, Remme W, Zannad F, et al. Eplerenone, a selective aldosterone blocker, in patients with left ventricular dysfunction after myocardial infarction. N Engl J Med 2003;348:1309–1321.

35. The Heart Outcomes Prevention Evaluation Study Investigators. Effects of an angiotensin converting-enzyme inhibitor, ramipril, on cardiovascular events in high-risk patients. N Engl J Med 2000;342:145–153.

36. Nissen SE, Tuzcu EM, Libby P, et al. for the CAMELOT Investigators. Effect of antihypertensive agents on cardiovascular events in patients with coronary disease and normal blood pressure The CAMELOT Study: a randomized controlled trial. JAMA 2004;292:2217–2226.

37. Tepper D. Frontiers in congestive heart failure: effect of Metoprolol CR/XL in chronic heart failure: metoprolol CR/XL Randomised Intervention Trial in Congestive Heart Failure (MERIT-HF). Congest Heart Fail 1999;5:184–185.

38. The SOLVD Investigators. Effect of enalapril on survival in patients with reduced left ventricular ejection fractions and congestive heart failure. N Engl J Med 1991;325:293–302.

39. Cohn JN, Tognoni G. A randomized trial of the angiotensin-receptor blocker valsartan in chronic heart failure. N Engl J Med 2001;345:1667–1675.

40. Packer M, Coats AJ, Fowler MB, et al. Effect of carvedilol on survival in severe chronic heart failure. N Engl J Med 2001;344:1651–1658.

41. Poole-Wilson PA, Swedberg K, Cleland JG, et al. Carvedilol or Metoprolol European Trial Investigators. Comparison of carvedilol and metoprolol on clinical outcomes in patients with chronic heart failure in the Carvedilol or Metoprolol European Trial (COMET): randomised controlled trial. Lancet 2003;362:7–13.
42. Pfeffer MA, Swedberg K, Granger CB, et al. CHARM Investigators and Committees. Effects of candesartan on mortality and morbidity in patients with chronic heart failure: the CHARM-Overall programme. Lancet 2003;362:759–766.
43. Pitt B, Zannad F, Remme WJ, et al. The effect of spironolactone on morbidity and mortality in patients with severe heart failure. Randomized Aldactone Evaluation Study Investigators. N Engl J Med 1999;341:709–717.
44. Hunt SA, Baker DW, Chin MH, et al. ACC/AHA guidelines for the evaluation and management of chronic heart failure in the adult: executive summary. A report of the American College of Cardiology/American Heart Association Task Force on Practice Guidelines (Committee to revise the 1995 Guidelines for the Evaluation and Management of Heart Failure). J Am Coll Cardiol 2001;38:2101–2113.
45. Packer M, O'Connor CM, Ghali JK, et al. Effect of amlodipine on morbidity and mortality in severe chronic heart failure. Prospective Randomized Amlodipine Survival Evaluation Study Group. N Engl J Med 1996;335:1107–1114.
46. Lewis EJ, Hunsicker LG, Bain RP, Rohde RD for the Collaborative Study Group. The effect of angiotensin-converting-enzyme inhibition on diabetic nephropathy. N Engl J Med 1993;329:1456–1462.
47. UK Prospective Diabetes Study Group. Tight blood pressure control and risk of macrovascular and microvascular complications in type 2 diabetes: UKPDS 38. BMJ 1998;317:703–713.
48. Hansson L, Zanchetti A, Carruthers SG, et al. Effects of intensive blood pressure lowering and low-dose aspirin in patients with hypertension: principal results of the Hypertension Optimal Treatment (HOT) randomized trial. Lancet 1998;351:1755–1762.
49. Yusuf S, Sleight P, Pogue J, Bosch J, Davies R, Dagenais G. Effects of an angiotensin-converting-enzyme inhibitor, ramipril, on cardiovascular events in high-risk patients. The Heart Outcomes Prevention Evaluation Study Investigators. N Engl J Med 2000;342:145–153.
50. Lewis EJ, Hunsicker LG, Clarke WR, et al. Renoprotective effect of the angiotensin receptor antagonist irbesartan in patients with nephropathy due to type 2 diabetes. N Engl J Med 2001;345:851–860.
51. Brenner BM, Cooper ME, de Zeeuw D, et al, for the Reduction of End Points in Non–Insulin-Dependent Diabetes Mellitus with the Angiotensin II Antagonist Losartan (RENAAL) Study Investigators. Effects of losartan on renal and cardiovascular outcomes in patients with type 2 diabetes and nephropathy. N Engl J Med 2001;345:861–869.
52. Whelton PK, Barzilay J, Cushman WC, et al. for the ALLHAT Collaborative Research Group. Clinical Outcomes in ALLHAT antihypertensives trial participants with type 2 diabetes, impaired fasting glucose, and normoglycemia. Ann Intern Med 2005;165:1401–1409.
53. Singer GM, Setaro JF. The ALLHAT (The Antihypertensive and Lipid-Lowering to Prevent Heart Attack Trial) Study: implications for resistant hypertension. J Clin Hypertens 2004;7:31–32.
54. Bakris GL, Fonseca V, Katholi RE, et al. for the GEMINI Investigators. Metabolic effects of carvedilol vs metoprolol in patients with type 2 diabetes mellitus and hypertension. A randomized controlled trial. JAMA 2004;292:2227–2236.
55. Lazarus JM, Bourgoignie JJ, Buckalew VM, et al. Achievement and safety of a low blood pressure goal in chronic renal disease. The Modification of Diet in Renal Disease Study Group. Hypertension 1997;29:641–650.
56. PROGRESS Collaborative Group. Randomised trial of a perindopril-based blood-pressure-lowering regimen among 6,105 individuals with previous stroke or transient ischaemic attack. Lancet 2001;358:1033–1041.
57. PROGRESS Collaborative Group. Effects of a perindopril-based blood pressure lowering regimen on cardiac outcomes among patients with cerebrovascular disease. Eur Heart J 2003;24:475–484.
58. Setaro JF. Resistant hypertension. In: Black HR, Elliott WP, eds. Clinical Hypertension: A Companion to Braunwald's Heart Disease, 1st edition. Philadelphia, Elsevier, 2006, in press.
59. Garg JP, Elliott WJ, Folker A, Izhar M, Black HR and RUSH University Hypertension Service. Resistant hypertension revisited: a comparison of two university-based cohorts. Am J Hypertens 2005;18:619–626.
60. Phillips LS, Branch WT Jr, Cook CB, et al. Clinical inertia. Ann Intern Med 2001;135:825–834.
61. Berlowitz DR, Ash AS, Hickey EC, et al. Inadequate management of blood pressure in a hypertensive population. N Engl J Med 1998;339:1957–1963.

62. El-Kebbi IM, Ziemer DC, Gallina DL, Dunbar V, Phillips LS. Diabetes in urban African-Americans. XV. Identification of barriers to provider adherence to management protocols. Diabetes Care 1999;22:1617–1620.
63. Setaro JF, Black HR. Refractory hypertension. N Engl J Med 1992;327:543–547.
64. Valli G, Giardina EV. Benefits, adverse effects and drug interactions of herbal therapies with cardiovascular effects. J Am Coll Cardiol 2002;39:1083–1095.
65. Singer GM, Izhar M, Black HR. Goal-oriented management of hypertension: translating clinical trial results into practice. Hypertension 2002;40:464–469.
66. Singer GM, Izhar M, Black HR. Guidelines of hypertension: are quality assurance measures on target? Hypertension 2004;43:198–202.
67. Banegas JR, Segura J, Ruilope LM, et al. on behalf of the CLUE Study Group Investigators. Blood pressure control and physician management of hypertension in hospital hypertension units in Spain. Hypertension 2004;43:1338–1344.
68. Romain TM, Patel RT, Heaberlin AM, Zarowitz BJ. Assessment of factors influencing blood pressure control in a managed care population. Pharmacotherapy 2003;23:1060–1070.
69. Saseen JJ, Carter BL, Brown TE, Elliott WJ, Black HR. Comparison of nifedipine alone and with diltiazem or verapamil in hypertension. Hypertension 1996;28:109–114.
70. Nishizaka MK, Zaman MA, Calhoun DA. Efficacy of low-dose spironolactone in subjects with resistant hypertension. Am J Hypertens 2003;16:925–930.
71. Nakao N, Yoshimura A, Morita H, Takada M, Kayano T, Ideura T. Combination treatment of angiotensin II receptor blocker and angiotensin-converting enzyme inhibitor in non-diabetic renal disease (COOPERATE): a randomized controlled trial. Lancet 2003;361:117–124.
72. Mogensen CE, Neldam S, Tikkanen I, et al. Randomised controlled trial of dual blockade of rennin-angiotensin system in patients with hypertension, microalbuminuria, and non-insulin dependent diabetes: the Candesartan and Lisinopril Microalbuminuria (CALM) Study. Br Med J 2000;321:1440–1444.

7

Diabetes Mellitus, Hyperinsulinemia, and Coronary Artery Disease

Byron J. Hoogwerf, MD

CONTENTS

INTRODUCTION

Diabetes mellitus (DM) is associated with an increased risk for coronary heart disease (CHD), less favorable outcomes from intervention procedures, and CHD-related mortality *(1–56)* (Table 1). Hyperglycemia by itself likely contributes to this risk, however, DM—especially type 2 DM—and impaired glucose tolerance are associated with a number of other CHD risk factors. These risk factors include dyslipidemia, hypertension, central obesity, albuminuria, a procoagulant state, and markers of inflammation *(10,26–28,45,57–88)*. These risk factors are associated with insulin resistance and have also been described as the "metabolic syndrome" for coronary artery disease (CAD). There are accumulating data to suggest that these abnormalities may be associated with endothelial cell dysfunction. In addition to these risk factors, the concepts of protein glycation, as well as oxidized lipoproteins as possible mechanisms for CHD have been proposed *(89–92)*.

From: *Contemporary Cardiology: Preventive Cardiology:*
Insights Into the Prevention and Treatment of Cardiovascular Disease, Second Edition
Edited by: J. M. Foody © Humana Press Inc., Totowa, NJ

Table 1
Summary of Relationships Between DM and CHD Risk

CHD risk in DM
    Two- to fivefold increased risk for CHD
    Two- to fivefold increased risk for CHD death
    Increased risk for morbidity and mortality after MI
    Increased risk for adverse outcomes after PTCA/stent/CABG
Clustering of CHD risk factors in DM
    Traditional risk factors
        Dyslipidemia
            Increased triglycerides
            Decreased HDL-C
            Small, dense LDL
        Hypertension
        Central obesity
    Nontraditional risk factors
        Hyperinsulinemia
        Procoagulant profile
            Increased platelet aggregation
            Increased PAI-1
            Increased fibrinogen
        Proteinuria
        Glycation of proteins
        Oxidation of lipoproteins
        Inflammation

DM, diabetes mellitus; CHD, coronary heart disease; MI, myocardial infarciton; PTCA, percutaneous transluminal coronary angioplasty; CABG; coronary artery bypass graft; HDL-C, high-density lipoprotein cholesterol; LDL, low-density lipoprotein; PAI, plasminogen activator inhibitor.

Accumulating intervention trial data suggests that intervention on these CHD risk factors may reduce the risk for CHD in patients with diabetes. Perhaps the most robust data on CHD risk reduction is now related to lipid-lowering therapy. Favorable reduction in risk has been reported from analysis of patients with diabetes in several intervention trials, as well as the reports of studies whose study populations included only subjects with diabetes Collaborative Atorvastatin Diabetes Study (CARDS) or large cohorts with diabetes (Heart Protection Study, Anglo-Scandinavian Cardiac Outcomes Trial (AS-COT) Lipid-Lowering Arm (LLA) *(93–121)*. Observational data and intervention trials have shown a relationship between the level of hyperglycemia and atherosclerotic disease risk *(38,122)*. CHD risk reduction from management of hypertension *(123–138)* and use of anti-platelet regimens *(110,120,139,140)* can be inferred from other studies in patients with diabetes. Finally, independent effects of angiotensin-converting enzyme (ACE) inhibitor therapy and lack of benefit from vitamin E in patients with diabetes have been reported *(141–148)*.

This chapter summarizes the observational studies showing the relationship between glucose and CHD risk, the intervention trial data assessing reduction in glucose, lipids, and blood pressure on CHD risk, review of treatment strategies for these common risk variables, a summary of outcomes after myocardial infarction (MI) and intervention therapy in patients with diabetes, and a summary of diabetes prevention studies.

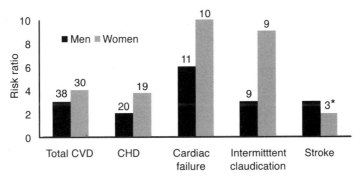

p < 0.001 for all values except *p < 0.05.

Fig. 1. Framingham Heart Study 30-yr follow-up: Age-adjusted annual risk of vascular disease endpoints in patients with diabetes (ages 35–64 yr). From ref. *149*.

RELATIONSHIP OF GLUCOSE TOLERANCE AND CHD

Diabetes Mellitus

DM is associated with a doubling of CHD risk *(1–56,149)*. In women, the risk may increase as much fivefold. Several prospective observational studies have confirmed these risk relationships. The Framingham Study has demonstrated an overall doubling of CHD risks in men and shown that, in women with diabetes, CHD risk is comparable to that of age-matched male counterparts (Fig. 1). Furthermore, this study showed that, in the presence of other CHD risk factors (smoking, hypercholesterolemia, hypertension, left ventricular hypertrophy), diabetes still contributes to CHD risk *(15,16,100)*. The Multiple Risk Factor Intervention Trial has evaluated more than 300,000 subjects. The presence of diabetes in these men tripled the risk for subsequent CHD events and CHD deaths *(48,49)*. This relationship held true even when there was adjustment for other CHD risk factors.

Several observational cohort studies have looked at the relationship between baseline glycemic control and atherosclerotic risk. The Wisconsin Epidemiologic Study of Diabetic Retinopathy study used baseline hemoglobin (Hb)A_{1C} as a predictor of subsequent CHD events in the three diabetes subgroups ($\leq$30 yr old, taking insulin; >30 yr old, taking insulin; and $\leq$30 yr old, not taking insulin). Each of these subgroups carries a progressive increase in CHD events across quartiles of baseline HbA_{1C} *(38)*. Scandinavian studies have demonstrated that higher mean glucose values in patients with diabetes may predict the risk for stroke or cause mortality *(29,109)*. More recently, the meta-analysis reported by Selvin *(150)* and the European Prospective Investigation into Cancer (EPIC) Norfolk study confirm these observations *(27)*. The EPIC Norfolk analyses of 10,232 patients showed that a 1% increase in HbA_{1C} levels was associated with a 20 to 30% increase in cardiovascular events and all-cause mortality in men and women 45 to 79 yr of age. This relation was independent of diabetes status. Therefore, the *presence* of hyperglycemia as well as the *degree* of hyperglycemia and the presence of other CHD risk factors are associated with an increased risk for CHD events in patients with diabetes.

Impaired Glucose Tolerance

Impaired glucose tolerance has been defined either in terms of fasting glucose values of at most 126 mg/dL, (previously, <140 mg/dL and >110 mg/dL). Other definitions also included a 30- to 90-min plasma glucose value higher than 200 mg/dL with a blood glucose value of between 140 and 200 mg/dL 2 h after a 75-g glucose challenge. Subjects with impaired glucose tolerance are also at increased risk for CHD. A number of studies have now demonstrated that impaired glucose tolerance is associated with central (or visceral) obesity, hypertension, and dyslipidemia. The dyslipidemia is further characterized as one in which there is an elevation of total triglyceride level, a reduction in high-density lipoprotein (HDL)-cholesterol (C) level, and increased concentrations of small, dense low-density lipoprotein (LDL)-C *(10,80,103,151)*. Clustering of such risk factors may be greater in women *(85)*.

Normal Glucose Concentration

Recent data suggest that CHD risk may be associated with increasing glucose concentrations *(4,14,73,152)* even in the normal range (≤110 mg/dL). These studies have not uniformly adjusted for the other, more traditional, CHD risk factors. However, a large cross-sectional study that adjusted for traditional and nontraditional risk factors still demonstrated increased CHD risk with increasing glucose concentrations in the nondiabetic range *(88)*. Some of these data sets suggest that there is an increased risk for clustering of other CHD risk factors with high-normal glucose concentrations.

CHD RISK FACTORS ASSOCIATED WITH GLUCOSE INTOLERANCE

Traditional

DYSLIPIDEMIA

The dyslipidemia of diabetes has been characterized in a number of studies. Typically, patients with diabetes have higher mean triglyceride concentrations, lower HDL-C concentrations, and LDL-C concentrations that are comparable to a nondiabetic population (Fig. 2). However, the LDL composition is altered, with higher concentrations of small, dense LDL. This is the more atherogenic moiety and may be more susceptible to oxidation (*see* Glycation and Glycoxidation of Proteins section). Increased triglyceride concentrations may be the result of increased production of the very low-density lipoprotein (VLDL; perhaps related to the hyperglycemia) as well as diminished clearance of triglyceride concentrations. Hydrolysis of triglycerides via capillary lipoprotein lipase may be impaired. Lipoprotein lipase is an insulin-sensitive enzyme. Therefore, either insulinopenia or insulin resistance contribute to diminished clearance of triglycerides.

HYPERTENSION

Patients with both type 1 and type 2 diabetes have an increased risk for hypertension. In type 1 diabetes, hypertension is almost always associated with evidence of diabetic nephropathy (in the early stages, with evidence of microalbuminuria). Hypertension in type 2 diabetes occurs independently of clinical evidence of diabetic nephropathy. The mechanism for hypertension is not entirely established. Some evidence suggests that hyperinsulinemia may be associated with salt retention or increased sympathetic tone. Both mechanisms have been invoked as contributors to hypertension associated with diabetes.

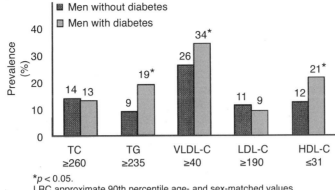

Fig. 2. Frequency of abnormal lipid levels in men with and without type 2 diabetes. (Adapted from ref. *178*.)

OBESITY

Increased body weight has been associated with diabetes for several decades. Several observational studies have demonstrated that central obesity or an increased waist-to-hip ratio (more recently simply a waist circumference) is associated with an increased risk for diabetes as well as associated CHD risk factors. Such obesity is associated with hyperinsulinemia and insulin resistance. Studies of central obesity have shown that visceral fat (more than subcutaneous fat in the abdominal) is associated with diabetes, hyperinsulinemia, and the other risk factors for CHD. The mechanism by which obesity may contribute to CHD risk is uncertain. Visceral fat may increase delivery of free fatty acids to the liver. There are reports that visceral fat may be a release of cytokines, which contribute to endothelial cell dysfunction.

SMOKING *(153)*

Smoking has long been known to be a risk for CAD. There are now data to suggest that smoking increases the risk for insulin resistance in type 2 DM and impaired glucose tolerance. The mechanism by which this occurs is not yet established.

Nontraditional CHD Risk Factors

There are a series of risk factors that may be associated with diabetes and impaired glucose tolerance that, in turn, may be associated with an increased risk of CAD.

HYPERINSULINEMIA

Hyperinsulinemia, especially when associated with central obesity, is associated with increased CHD risk in several observational studies *(12,43,58,59,61,62,64,65,73,75,79–81,83)*. In many of these studies, hyperinsulinemia is associated with traditional risk factors. Hyperinsulinemia seemed to be additive to risks associated with lipid abnormalities, including increased LDL-C and lipoprotein B. Hyperinsulinemia is associated with increased plasminogen activator inhibitor (PAI)-1. Insulin is also associated with tissue growth, suggesting that it may contribute to such things as smooth muscle proliferation that may be important in the atherosclerotic process. However, it is not yet clear whether insulin (or perhaps proinsulin) is itself atherogenic or whether this increased risk for CHD is a result of the other factors.

Exogenous Hyperinsulinemia

Patients with diabetes who are taking insulin are also at increased risk for CHD events. Insulin has been proposed as the culprit. However, these studies cannot consistently take into account the duration of diabetes. Because one-third to one-half of people in the United States who have diabetes are unaware of the diagnosis, adjusting for the duration of the disease is difficult. Furthermore, the accumulating evidence that type 2 diabetes is characterized not only by insulin resistance, but by declining β-cell function, suggests that all patients with type 2 diabetes have had the disease for a sufficiently long time to exhibit β-cell failure.

Proteinuria/Albuminuria

There is increasing attention to proteinuria, renal failure, and the associated dyslipidemia as risk factors for CAD in patients with diabetes *(66,71,108,122)*. Whether proteinuria again simply marks for duration of diabetes or reflects loss of vascular integrity in general (both microvascular and macrovascular disease) is not that clear. In the face of proteinuria, the rate of progression to end-stage renal disease can be slowed by aggressive blood pressure management, especially with the use of ACE inhibitors, as well as improved glycemic control. Because both of these interventions may have beneficial effect on CHD risks, whether reduction in proteinuria has independent benefit on CHD risk is not yet established.

Increased Procoagulant State

DM is associated with an increased risk for atherothrombosis, probably as a result of increased platelet aggregation, increased fibrinogen, and elevated PAI-1 levels *(60,111)*. How much these variables affect the risk for initial CHD events, the increased risk for recurrent MI (after the first MI), and worse outcomes after revascularization procedures is not yet established.

Glycation and Glycoxidation of Proteins *(58,89–92)*

Oxidized lipoproteins have several features that suggest that they may increase the risk for the development of atherosclerotic plaque, including increased foam cell formation, cytotoxicity to endothelial cells, and increased smooth muscle formation. Two features of diabetes may increase the risk for oxidation. Glycated lipoproteins seem to have increased susceptibility to oxidation, leading to the term "glycoxidation." In addition, small, dense LDL is also more susceptible to oxidation. Therefore, both hyperglycemia and the presence of increased concentrations of small, dense LDL suggest that if lipoprotein oxidation is important in the atherosclerotic process, it may contribute to the increased risks seen in patients with diabetes.

Inflammation

Multiple observational studies have now demonstrated that inflammation plays a role in CHD risk. The most commonly used marker of inflammation is the ultrasensitive or highly sensitive assay for C-reactive protein (CRP). These studies show an association of elevated CRP with DM, especially when associated with features of the metabolic syndrome *(74,77–78)*. The accumulating data on the importance of metabolically active (or visceral fat) and its role in CHD risk may be partially explained by the fact that visceral fat produces cytokines, such as interleukin-6 and tumor necrosis factor-α, which, in turn, may be associated with increased concentrations of highly sensitive CRP.

INTERVENTION TRIALS OF CHD RISK REDUCTION IN DM
Glycemic Control

Five major randomized trials looking at glycemic control and complications in type 2 DM have been reported. The Japanese study of Ohkkubo et al. was designed to look at microvascular complications *(154)*. The four intervention trials designed to address relationships between glycemic control and CHD risk reduction deserve comment. The University Group Diabetes Program was the first major, randomized clinical trial designed to compare the effects of placebo and four different treatments (tolbutamide, phenformin, variable dose insulin, and standard or fixed-dose insulin) on CHD risk reduction *(155)*. The study reported increased CHD risk associated with tolbutamide use, but no other favorable or adverse outcomes. In retrospect, the University Group Diabetes Program probably was underpowered to test the CHD hypothesis. Furthermore, the well-known results were confounded by the observation that the tolbutamide group had an increased number of coronary events and mortality. The trial could not demonstrate any reduction in CHD risks with the insulin therapies. Conversely, it did not show any adverse effect of insulin therapy. The Veterans Administration (VA) trial was a pilot study that assessed intensive glucose control in 75 diabetic men compared with a conventional control in a similar group. Although an incremental difference in HbA_{1C} of 2% was met (this was the intent of the pilot), the trial could not show clear differences between treatment groups for coronary events *(57,156)*. Although a greater number of events were reported in the intensively controlled group, when adjusted for pre-existing coronary disease, there were no statistically significant differences. A larger VA trial is now in progress. The Diabetes Mellitus Insulin Glucose Infusion in Acute Myocardial Infarction (DIGAMI) study evaluated the effects of insulin therapy in patients with DM who had a recent MI. Patients were randomized to intensified glucose control both in the immediate postinfarction state and for a period after the infarction (compared with a conventional post-MI approach). The risk for subsequent MIs was reduced in the more intensively treated group *(157)*. Whether this was the result of more intensive follow-up, glucose lowering, or insulin use in the postinfarct period could not be answered by this study. In an effort to resolve this issue, the DIGAMI 2 study was convened using three treatment strategies in 1253 subjects: group 1, acute insulin–glucose infusion followed by insulin-based long-term glucose control; group 2, insulin–glucose infusion followed by standard glucose control; and group 3, routine metabolic management according to local practice *(158)*. HbA_{1C} levels were not different among groups at the end of trial. Although there were trends toward reduction in mortality, the study reported a negative outcome with no differences in mortality or atherosclerosis related morbidity among the three groups at the end of 2.1 yr (median duration of follow-up). The study had originally planned to recruit 3000 subjects, therefore, part of the explanation for this negative outcome may be related to inadequate power to address the research question.

Finally, the United Kingdom Prospective Diabetes Study reported a 16% reduction in risk for atherosclerotic events in patients who were more intensively treated *(122,136–138)*. This difference did not quite achieve statistical significance by conventional standards ($p = 0.052$). There were no clear differences among the oral agent and insulin treatment arms (with the exception of what may be an aberration in events associated with metformin and glyburide combination use).

A very large National Institutes of Health trial called Action to Control Cardiovascular Risk in Diabetes (ACCORD; $n = 10{,}251$) is designed to address the question of whether

glycemic control will reduce the risk for coronary disease events. This study is currently underway in 75 centers in the United States and Canada (www.accordtrial.org). This trial is designed to randomize type 2 patients with diabetes to two different HbA$_{1C}$ targets and determine whether the differences in glycemic control reduce the risk for CHD. Results should be available in 2008 to 2009.

Lipid-Lowering Trials (Table 2)

STATIN THERAPY TRIALS

Since the mid-1990s, most of the cholesterol-lowering trials have included some diabetic subjects, and the results of one placebo-controlled trial in study populations comprised entirely of diabetic subjects are now available. The first LDL-C-lowering trial to demonstrate a reduction in all-cause mortality (in addition to a reduction in coronary events) was the Scandinavian Simvastatin Study of Survival. Among the 4444 participants in this trial, there were 202 patients with known DM at the time of the trial *(105,113)*. The benefits of cholesterol lowering were comparable between diabetic subjects and their nondiabetic counterparts, however, even in the statin-treated diabetic subjects, the risk for cardiovascular events was greater than in subjects without diabetes.

In the Cholesterol and Recurrent Events trial, there were 586 patients with a clinical diagnosis of DM and 3573 subjects without DM *(100)*. Baseline and in-trial LDL-C concentrations were comparable between the diabetic and nondiabetic subjects. In this trial, the reduction in risk for diabetic subjects was 23% and the reduction in risk was 25% for nondiabetic subjects. The Heart Protection Study was a study of more than 20,000 subjects randomized to 40 mg simvastatin vs placebo. This study had 5963 subjects with DM *(106)*. In the intention-to-treat analyses, the reduction in risk for CHD events was 24% for the trial as a whole. In patients with diabetes collectively, the results were comparable. In patients with diabetes without previous vascular disease (*N* = 2912), the primary prevention of CHD was 33%. The ASCOT-LLA study also had a large diabetic cohort (*N* = 2532) *(117,118)*. In this cohort of hypertensive diabetic subjects, there was a 23% reduction in the composite cardiovascular events. In several other trials, the beneficial effects of LDL-C lowering were comparable in the diabetic subjects and nondiabetic subjects *(121)*. In many of these trials, the number of diabetic subjects was too small for the favorable reduction in atherosclerotic disease events to be statistically significant.

There is a single trial in which lipid-lowering therapy in diabetic subjects did not favor the statin therapy. The Pravastatin in elderly individuals at risk of vascular disease trial was comprised of 5804 men and women, aged 70 to 82 yr, and treated with pravastatin for 3 yr *(120)*. There were 623 patients with clinically diagnosed diabetes. There was a 19% reduction in CHD events when all participants were analyzed. In the diabetic subjects, the risk ratio for the pravastatin group compared with placebo was 1.27 (95% confidence interval [CI], 0.90–180).

Recently a cholesterol-lowering trial (statin vs placebo) was completed that was performed in cohorts of patients with DM (Fig. 3). CARDS was comprised of 2838 patients with DM *(93)*. Patients were randomized to 10 mg atorvastatin daily (vs placebo) and followed for a mean of 3.9 yr. The risk for cardiovascular events was reduced by 37%, the risk for acute coronary disease events was reduced by 36%, and the risk for stroke was reduced by 48%.

FIBRATE THERAPY TRIALS

Gemfibrozil, a fibric acid derivative, has been studied and compared with placebo in two major cholesterol-lowering trials *(98,109,114)*. Fibrates do not have much effect in

Table 2
Coronary Heart Disease Events for Subjects With Type 2 DM in Randomized, Double-Blind, Lipid-Lowering Trials

Primary Prevention Studies

Study	Treatment	Control (n/n)	Intervention (n/n)	RR (95% CI)	ARR (95% CI)	NNT
AFCAPS/TexCAPS	Lovastatin (± resin) vs placebo	6/71	4/84	0.56 (0.17–1.92)	0.04 (−0.04 to 0.12)	27.1
ALLHAT-LLT	Pravastatin vs usual care	Not reported	Not reported	0.89 (0.71–1.10)	Not reported	Not reported
HHS	Gemfibrozil vs placebo	8/76	2/59	0.32 (0.07–1.46)	0.07 (−0.01 to 0.15)	14.0
HPS	Gemfibrozil vs placebo	367/1976	276/2006	0.74 (0.64–0.85)	0.05 (0.03 to 0.07)	20.8
PROSPER	Pravastatin vs placebo	28/205	32/191	1.23 (0.77–1.95)	−0.03 (−0.10 to 0.04)	−32.3
ASCOT-LLA	Atorvastatin vs placebo	46/1274	38/1258	0.84 (0.55–1.29)	0.01 (−0.01 to 0.02)	169.5
Pooled[b]		—	—	0.78 (0.67–0.89)	0.03 (0.01 to 0.04)	34.5[c]

Secondary prevention studies

Study	Treatment	Control (n/n)	Intervention (n/n)	RR (95% CI)	ARR (95% CI)	NNT
4S	Simvastatin vs placebo	44/97	24/105	0.50 (0.33–0.76)	0.23 (0.10 to 0.35)	4.4
CARE	Pravastatin vs placebo	112/304	81/282	0.78 (0.62–0.99)	0.08 (0.01 to 0.16)	12.3
HPS	Simvastatin vs placebo	381/1009	325/972	0.89 (0.79–1.00)	0.04 (0.00 to 0.09)	23.1
LIPID	Pravastatin vs placebo	88/386	76/396	0.84 (0.64–1.11)	0.04 (−0.02 to 0.09)	27.7
LIPS	Fluvastatin vs placebo	31/82	26/120	0.53 (0.29–0.97)	0.16 (0.03 to 0.29)	6.2
Post-CABG	40–80 mg lovastatin (± resin) vs 2.5–5 mg lovastatin (± resin)	14/53	9/63	0.53 (0.18–1.60)	0.12 (−0.03 to 0.27)	8.2
PROSPER[d]	Pravastatin vs placebo	31/115	38/112	1.26 (0.85–1.87)	−0.07 (−0.19 to 0.05)	NA
VA-HIT	Gemfibrozil vs placebo	116/318	88/309	0.76 (0.57–1.01)	0.08 (0.01 to 0.15)	12.5
Pooled[c]		—	—	0.76 (0.59–0.93)	0.07 (0.03 to 0.12)	13.8[e]

Adapted from ref. 171.

[a]Meta-analysis; caused by no heterogeneity between primary prevention studies ($p = 0.18$); fixed-effects model used.
[b]Number needed to treat for benefit is for 4.3 yr.
[c]Meta-analysis; caused by substantial between-study heterogeneity ($p = 0.026$); random-effects model used.
[d]Number needed to treat for benefit is for 4.9 yr.

n/n, number with events/number in treatment arm; NNT, number needed to treat; AFCAPS/TEXCAPS, Air Force/Texas Coronary Atherosclerosis Prevention Study; LLT, lipid-lowering treatment; HHS, Helsinki Heart Study; HPS, Heart Protection Study; PROSPER, Pravastatin in elderly individuals at risk of vascular disease; 4S, Scandinavian Simvastatin Study of Survival; CARE, Cholesterol and Recurrent Events; LIPID, Long-Term Intervention with Pravastatin in Ischaemic Disease; LIPS, Lescol® Intervention Prevention Study.

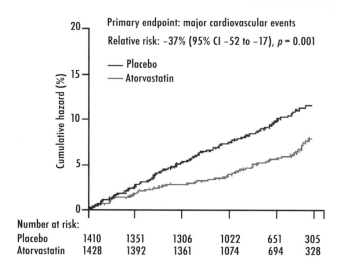

Fig. 3. Reduction in major cardiovascular events in diabetic subjects treated with atorvastatin vs placebo. (Adapted from ref. *92*.)

reducing LDL-C, but they lower triglycerides and raise HDL-C levels. Diabetic and nondiabetic subjects taking fibrates in these trials had fewer coronary events and strokes compared with those subjects taking placebo. This benefit was not associated with reduced LDL concentrations. There were 135 patients with diabetes in the Helsinki Heart Study. Although the relative risk (RR) reduction in the patients with diabetes was greater than in the trial as a whole (RR = 0.32; 95% CI, 0.07–1.46), the small numbers precluded statistically significant differences. In the VA-HDL Intervention Trial (HIT) study, comprised of 2351 men, there were 627 diabetic subjects. There was a 24% risk reduction in both diabetic and nondiabetic subjects.

SUMMARY OF STATIN/FIBRATE TRIALS IN DIABETIC SUBJECTS

Statins (usually compared with placebo) have been used in most of the intervention studies, and the major lipid effect has been a reduction in LDL-C. Patients with diabetes in the statin trials generally had more heart disease than their nondiabetic counterparts. Whereas diabetic subjects had comparable (or even greater) *relative* benefits, the patients with diabetes taking statins still have a greater risk for heart disease than their nondiabetic counterparts. A summary of trials published during the past 20 yr has recently been published (Table 1) *(121)* (this summary was published before CARDS and the subgroup analysis from ASCOT-LLA). Based on all of these studies, statins are now considered standard therapy for CHD risk reduction in most patients with DM. Of note is the observation that LDL-C lowering not only is associated with a reduced risk for heart disease, but also a reduced risk for stroke.

Most of the effects of fibrates are to reduce triglycerides and raise HDL-C levels. They have little effect on LDL-C. In the Helsinki Heart Study, patients were recruited because they had elevated non-HDL-C levels. However, the subjects who received the greatest benefit were those who had elevated VLDL-C (triglyceride-carrying moiety) concentrations. In the VA-HIT study, triglycerides were reduced by approx 30%, and HDL-C levels were increased by approx 7%. The investigators interpreted the increase in HDL-C levels as being responsible for the favorable outcomes in this study.

The Fenofibrate Intervention and Event Lowering in Diabetes (FIELD) study, a randomized, placebo-controlled trial, compared fenofibrate with placebo in 9795 subjects aged 50–75 yr with type 2 diabetes mellitus (159). There was an 11% reduction $(p = 0.16)$ in the primary outcome of coronary heart disease death and non-fatal MI and a 24% reduction $(p = 0.010)$ in non-fatal MI. These results were confounded by high rates of statin drop in, especially in the placebo arm.

Although both statins and fibrates are commonly used to treat cholesterol and triglyceride abnormalities in patients with DM, the ACCORD trial will refine our understanding of lipid-altering therapy in patients with diabetes. This trial will address the question of whether a combination of a statin plus a fibrate will improve the results seen with either agent used alone. The ACCORD study includes 10,251 patients with diabetes; among whom, approx 5518 are enrolled in the lipid arm. In the lipid arm, all subjects will be treated with a statin and then randomized to fenofibrate or a placebo. Until the results of the ACCORD trial are available, statins will continue to be the mainstay of therapy. Fibrates may be used either alone or in combination in selected patients with diabetes.

HYPERTENSION

Several trials of blood pressure lowering have shown a reduction in CHD events in patients with and without DM $(123–132,143–148)$. Most of the studies on coronary vascular disease as well as stroke have been performed in type 2 patients with diabetes. This section reviews selected studies showing general effects of blood pressure lowering on atherosclerotic disease events, as well as the observations with selected classes of antihypertensive agents. There seems to be accumulating data that short-acting calcium channel blockers should be avoided in both patients with and without DM. This subject will not be further discussed in this chapter.

The largest body of reported data in patients with diabetes is regarding the use of ACE inhibitors, long-acting calcium channel blockers, and diuretics, with accumulating data on the angiotensin receptor blockers (ARBs). With the exception of Antihypertensive and Lipid-Lowering Treatment to Prevent Heart Attack Trial (ALLHAT), there are limited comparisons with single agents in each class within a single trial. Blood pressure levels at entry have also been somewhat variable for both systolic and diastolic blood pressure. Most of the trials use a reduction of 20 mmHg for either systolic or diastolic blood pressure or both. There are also widely varying endpoints, including combined or individual endpoints that include all-cause mortality, fatal or nonfatal MI, and strokes. Selected trials have used other endpoints, including hospitalization for angina. In some of the trials, cardiovascular endpoints were secondary endpoints and the analyses in patients with diabetes were often performed after trial completion. Nevertheless, the following general conclusions can be drawn. There is atherosclerotic risk reduction in the range of 20 to 55% with blood pressure lowering in patients with diabetes (these risk reductions are comparable to what can be achieved with aggressive lipid lowering). In general, there is greater risk reduction in stroke than there is for CHD in these studies.

Several studies have looked at ACE inhibitor therapy in diabetic subjects. The Appropriate Blood Pressure Control in Diabetes (ABCD) trial had a change in creatinine clearance as its primary endpoint, with fatal and nonfatal MI as a secondary endpoint (129). It compared 235 diabetic subjects taking Enalapril with 235 diabetic subjects taking Nisoldipine. There were both normotensive and hypertensive patients in this study. In the report of 470 hypertensive, type 2 patients with diabetes, there was comparable blood

pressure lowering in the two treatment groups. There was an increased risk for fatal and nonfatal MI with nisoldipine (adjusted risk ratio [ARR] of 7, with a 95% CI of 2.3–21.4), as well as nonfatal MIs (ARR, 5.9) and cerebrovascular accidents (ARR, 2.2; CI that bounded unity of 0.7 to 7.1). The fact that other blood pressure treatment was not controlled may also be a confounding variable because there was a high discontinuation rate in both groups. Furthermore, the authors acknowledged that they could not "distinguish among a deleterious effect of Nisoldipine, protective effect of Enalapril and a combination of both as the reason for the difference…" The Fosinopril vs Amlodipine Cardiovascular Events Randomized Trial in Patients with Hypertension and noninsulin-dependent DM trial looked at 380 hypertensive patients (160). The primary outcome was changes in lipid levels. Cardiovascular events were a secondary outcome. Target blood pressures were 140/90 (or >20 mmHg blood pressure drop if initial blood pressures are >160/110). This trial demonstrated that a greater number of patients in both groups achieved diastolic blood pressure targets than achieve systolic blood pressure targets. Furthermore, amlodipine was added to more than 30% of the Fosinopril group. Fosinopril was added to more than 26% of the amlodipine group. Overall event rates were less with Fosinopril than with amlodipine. A beneficial effect of other agents, including calcium channel blockers, is available from other hypertensive trials. Most notable is the Hypertension Optimal Treatment Trial with 18,790 patients aged 50 to 80 yr (130). Target blood pressures include diastolic pressures of less than 90 in one group, to at most 85 in a second group, and to at most 80 in a third group. There were approx 500 patients with type 2 diabetes in each arm (total of 1501). Compared with the diastolic blood pressure target group of less than 90, the patients with diabetes with a diastolic blood pressure target of less than 80 had a 51% decrease in major cardiovascular events (aspirin use in this trial also demonstrated a reduction in atherosclerotic vascular events). The Systolic Hypertension in Europe (Syst-Eur) (135) trial used nitrendipine to lower blood pressure. It included 492 patients with diabetes (4203 patients did not have diabetes). The blood pressure target was a 20-mmHg reduction of systolic blood pressure. In the patients with diabetes with blood pressure reduction, there was a reduction in mortality by 55% and decreases in cardiovascular events of 26% and in strokes of 38%. The potential beneficial effects of low-dose thiazides have been demonstrated in a number of studies. The Systolic Hypertension in the Elderly Program trial (134) was really the first to show significant benefit in patients with diabetes. The Systolic Hypertension in the Elderly Program trial did not demonstrate a statistically significant reduction in mortality; however, the reported reduction was 26%. There was a reduction in cardiovascular events of 34% and in coronary events of 56%. Stroke reduction was also not statistically significant, at 22%. The use of β-blockers has been incorporated in a number of trials. The beneficial effects of both ACE inhibitors and β-blockers were demonstrated in the United Kingdom Prospective Diabetes Study (37). Furthermore, there seems to be additive effects of blood pressure lowering to HbA_{1C} reduction in this trial. Greater incremental effects of blood pressure on risk reduction may be seen in patients with higher HbA_{1C} levels, and, similarly, greater effects of HbA_{1C} reduction may be seen in patients with higher blood pressure.

The largest blood pressure trial ever undertaken (and one that included a large number of diabetic subjects) was ALLHAT (124,125). In 2000, the ALLHAT investigators discontinued the doxazosin arm because of increased risk for heart failure compared with chlorthalidone. The remaining ALLHAT participants were comprised of 33,357 subjects aged older than 55 yr who had hypertension and at least one other CHD risk factor. They were randomized to receive chlorthalidone (n = 15,255), amlodipine (n = 9048) or

lisinopril (n = 9054). The primary outcome was combined fatal CHD or nonfatal MI; secondary outcomes were all-cause mortality, stroke, combined CHD (primary outcome, coronary revascularization, or angina with hospitalization), and combined cardiovascular disease (combined CHD, stroke, treated angina without hospitalization, heart failure, and peripheral arterial disease). After a mean follow-up of 4.9 yr, there were no significant differences among the groups for the primary outcomes and most of the secondary outcomes; heart failure was lower in the chlorthalidone group than the other two groups (ALLHAT). More than 35% of the ALLHAT participants had DM; outcomes in the diabetic subjects were not different than those demonstrated in all of the participants. Of note was the observed new-onset DM in subjects who did not have DM at the beginning of the study. The highest percentage of DM was associated with chlorthalidone use (11.6%) compared with amlodipine (9.8%) and lisinopril (8.1%). Although this increase in the risk for diabetes did not affect the outcomes, this observation is consistent with other studies, including the Heart Outcomes Prevention Evaluation (HOPE) trial, that showed a reduced risk for new-onset diabetes with ACE inhibitor treatment (*see* Prevention of DM section).

Two studies with large diabetic cohorts evaluated the effects of ACE inhibitors vs other therapy and demonstrated that such interference with the renin–angiotensin–aldosterone system may have benefits that extend beyond the blood pressure reduction. The HOPE study demonstrated that use of the ACE inhibitor, ramipril, at a dose of 10 mg daily was associated with a 22% reduction in MI and a 37% reduction in cardiac death in patients with diabetes *(143–148)*. These results were similar to the reduction in risk reported in the whole HOPE study population of patients either with CHD or at high risk for CHD. The differences in blood pressure explain approx 25% of the CHD effect and slightly more of the stroke effect. Similar results were reported in the European Trial on Reduction of Cardiac Events with Perindopril in Stable Coronary Artery Disease (EUROPA) trial, using perindopril vs placebo *(141)*. The EUROPA study reported a 20% reduction in events with perindopril use, of which approx 15% of the effect was attributable to blood pressure reduction, and a similar reduction (19%) was observed in the diabetic subset. The Prevention of Events with ACE Inhibition (PEACE) trial had a similar design, but did not demonstrate differences with the use of trandolapril *(161)*. This lack of difference may be a result of several factors, including the fact that the PEACE cohort was at lower risk than the study populations of HOPE and EUROPA, and was more aggressively treated with statins and antiplatelet agents. There are fewer data in studies using ARBs. The Losartan Intervention for Endpoint Reduction in Hypertension (LIFE) compared losartan with atenolol in 9193 hypertensive subjects with left ventricular hypertrophy *(128)* (data on diabetic subjects have not been published separately). For a comparable blood pressure reduction, there was a 13% (p = 0.021) lower event rate in the losartan group; most of this difference was a reduction in strokes.

OTHER ATHEROSCLEROTIC RISK FACTORS RELATED TO DM

Hyperinsulinemia

Hyperinsulinemia, and the commonly associated insulin resistance, has been associated with increased risk for CHD. Hyperinsulinemia is often associated with known or suspected risk factors for atherosclerotic vascular disease, such as central obesity, DM, dyslipidemia (high triglyceride levels, low HDL-C levels, and small, dense LDL-C), hypertension, and increased PAI-1 activity. This association had been demonstrated in

studies of clinical CHD as well as angiographic studies of the carotid arteries. It is not yet clear whether insulin, or perhaps proinsulin, is atherogenic, or whether the risk for atherosclerosis is because hyperinsulinemia is associated with the well-established risk factors noted previously.

The role by which hyperinsulinemia or "hyperproinsulinemia" may increase the risk for CHD is not yet established. Furthermore, whether it contributes to the risk similarly in various arterial systems (coronary, cerebral, or peripheral) is also not yet established. Many studies have looked at clinical outcomes and, more recently, angiographic outcomes have been investigated using such methodologies as angiography of native vessels, saphenous vein graft conduits, and ultrasound of the carotid arteries.

Several observational studies have looked at insulin concentration as a predictor of CHD risk. As early as 1968, Tzargournis et al. reported an association of hyperinsulinemia and hypertriglyceridemia in young men with CHD (83). This observation has been confirmed in several subsequent studies that also show an association of hyperinsulinemia with one or more of the following: central obesity, low HDL-C levels, hypertension, and impaired glucose tolerance. Prospective observational studies have also shown that increased insulin concentrations were associated with an increased risk for future CHD events and CHD related mortality. Insulin levels obtained 1-h after oral glucose challenge were associated with increased CHD incidence and mortality in the 3390 participants of the Busselton (Australia) study (52). RR for the top quintile of insulin concentrations (compared with the bottom four quintiles) was 1.67 for CHD events at 6 yr and 1.66 for CHD death at 12 yr. In the Paris Prospective Study, the highest quintiles of fasting insulin and insulin concentrations 2 h after a 75-g oral glucose challenge ($n =$ 7029) were associated with a more than twofold increase in CHD risk compared with the lower quintiles (12). In the Quebec Cardiovascular Study (61) of 2103 men, insulin concentration predicted CHD events (along with several lipid abnormalities, including apolipoprotein B, LDL-C, and HDL-C); insulin concentration amplified the adverse effects of low HDL-C, elevated triglycerides, and elevated apolipoprotein B levels.

In the last decade, several studies have looked at the relationship between insulin concentrations and other measures of vascular disease. The Atherosclerosis Risk in Communities Study (45) used several measures of arterial stiffness in carotid arteries and reported that insulin concentrations were associated with measures reflecting increased stiffness in univariate analyses performed in nondiabetic subjects. In multivariate analyses, serum insulin remained a significant predictor in white men and women, but not in black examinees. In addition, insulin showed a synergistic effect with glucose and triglycerides in this study. Kekäläinen et al. could not show a relationship between insulin concentration or insulin sensitivity in the progression of atherosclerosis as measured by serial ultrasounds in femoral arteries in 118 subjects (26). Agewall et al. used carotid ultrasound to look at intima media thickness and plaque status in 25 men with cardiovascular risk factors and 23 matched controls without such risk factors (58). Insulin sensitivity was determined by hyperinsulinemic, euglycemic clamp techniques. Lower insulin sensitivity was associated with intima media thickness (even when adjusted for body weight). However, these authors reported no relationship of insulin sensitivity to plaque status. Laakso et al. reported that men with either femoral or carotid (or both) atherosclerosis as determined by ultrasonography had lower glucose disposal rates (insulin resistance) during hyperinsulinemic clamp studies compared with controls without ultrasound evidence of disease (70). However, mean fasting insulin and C-peptide concentrations were similar.

Dysfibrinolysis and Atherosclerosis

There are several lines of evidence to suggest that patients with diabetes may be at increased risks for atherothrombosis as a result of increased platelet aggregation, elevated PAI levels and perhaps altered endothelial cell function. Nevertheless, there are few randomized controlled trials that assess the benefits of interventions to reduce the risk for thrombogenic in patients with diabetes. One such study was the Early Treatment Diabetic Retinopathy Study *(140)*. The purpose of this study was to assess whether 650 mg aspirin daily vs placebo would reduce the risk for progression of diabetic retinopathy. Although there was no benefit in this primary endpoint, there was a reduction in life table cumulative event rates for fatal or nonfatal MI (RR = 0.83; CI, 0.66–1.04; p = 0.04) in patients with diabetes. This study was an important consideration in the position statement from the American Diabetes Association in recommending aspirin for patients with DM.

GLUCOSE-LOWERING AGENTS

Overview

In type 1 DM, insulin use is necessary for adequate glycemic control. Similarly, with increasing duration of type 2 DM, the use of insulin is often necessary for adequate glycemic control. It is beyond the scope of this chapter to discuss the spectrum of insulins and insulin regimens in diabetes. The oral agents to lower glucose deserve summary comments, however. These agents fall into several general mechanistic classes: insulin secretagogues (sulfonylureas, meglitinide, and nateglinide); reduction in hepatic glucose production (metformin); insulin sensitizers (thiazolidinediones); gut-related delay in glucose absorption (carbohydrase inhibitors); and incretins (exenatide). The mechanisms that increase glucose in type 2 diabetes include abnormalities of insulin production, increased hepatic glucose production, and insulin resistances, as well as exaggerated postprandial hyperglycemia. As such, agents that work by different mechanism have additive effects on glucose control. However, the limited ability to characterize the main biochemical abnormality in any single patient limits the ability to select a single agent that will have the greatest efficacy in a single patient. The general efficacy, contraindications and side effects of each class of agents is discussed briefly.

Sulfonylureas

At maximal doses, mean glucose-lowering effects are in the range of 30 to 60 mg/dL (HbA$_{1C}$ change of 1–2%). The incremental reduction may be greater with more marked hyperglycemia. In addition to glucose-lowering effects, there are data for these agents (as well as other sulfonylureas) to indicate that they may have a beneficial effect on the dyslipidemia associated with diabetes by lowering triglycerides. In some cases, this may be associated with an increase in HDL-C concentrations.

Hypoglycemia may occur with any of the sulfonylureas, however, severe hypoglycemia is infrequent. Weight gain is common with sulfonylureas. Sulfonylureas are cleared by both hepatic and renal routes (depending on the agent). In patients with elevated serum creatinine concentrations, sulfonylurea dosing schedules should be reduced, and increased attention should be given to increased risk for hypoglycemia.

Meglitinide (Repaglinide), Neteglinide (Starlix)

These agents are oral glucose-lowering agents that work by stimulating prandial insulin and reducing postprandial glucose. They are rapidly absorbed and have short meta-

bolic half-lifes. Therefore, they must be taken with meals. The overall efficacy is modest, with reductions in HbA$_{1C}$ in the range of 0.5 to 1.5%. Among the insulin secretagogue medications, these agents have the advantage of being acceptable for use in patients who have renal compromise. There is relatively little risk for hypoglycemia, especially compared with the sulfonylureas. Extensive data on the beneficial effects on lipid profiles are not available.

Metformin

The efficacy of metformin is comparable to that of the sulfonylureas and comparison data with glyburide have been reported. Mean reduction in HbA$_{1C}$ is between 1 and 2% in many studies. In addition, there is a small reduction in total cholesterol, total triglycerides, and LDL-C. Several studies also report weight reduction in conjunction with metformin use.

A small percentage of people develop a metallic taste with metformin use. This is usually transient. Starting with a low dose and increasing doses as tolerated can ameliorate the metallic taste. Approximately 5% of patients may develop diarrhea of sufficient degree to preclude metformin use. Finally, with selected patients who have risk for hypoxemia (e.g., with congestive heart failure), liver disease, or renal compromise, there may be an increased risk for lactic acidosis. Some clinicians also suggest that metformin should not be used in the elderly.

Thiazolidinediones (Pioglitazone and Rosiglitazone)

Thiazolidinediones are insulin sensitizers, which require insulin (endogenous or exogenous) to work effectively. As monotherapy, they are similar to sulfonylureas and metformin, with HbA$_{1C}$ reductions in the approx 0.5 to 1.5% range. There are some data that suggest that use of thiazolidinediones may be associated with improved insulin secretory capacity (although they are not primarily an insulin secretagogue). These data suggest that with improved insulin sensitivity there is improved β-cell response, with entraining of endogenous insulin to nutrient stimulation. The glucose-lowering efficacy of troglitazone (removed from the market because of hepatoxicity), pioglitazone, and rosiglitazone are comparable. There is an evolving understanding of the potential benefits (and differences) among thiazolidinediones on lipid profiles. These include changes in LDL-C size from a small, dense LDL to a larger LDL that may be less atherogenic and less susceptible to oxidation. Head-to-head comparisons of lipid-related effects have been reported in abstract form, but not yet been reported in the reviewed literature.

Finally, there is some data to suggest that because of the interaction with a peroxisome proliferator-activated receptor-γ receptor, there may be a beneficial affect on CHD risk factor reduction. There are favorable effects on inflammatory markers and there is evidence that there is a reduction in measures of carotid intimal medial thickness with thiazolidinedione use (162,163). Weight gain and peripheral edema are common side effects of thiazolidinedione use. Whether this weight gain is associated with increased risk for atherosclerotic disease is unknown. Furthermore, fluid retention is common. Thiazolidinedione use is generally considered to be contraindicated in heart failure, although the retrospective study of Tang suggests that peripheral edema does not correlate well with other measures of heart failure (164). Cautious use in patients at risk for heart failure is currently prudent.

Carbohydrase Inhibitors

The efficacy of the carbohydrate inhibitors (acarbose and miglitol) is modest in mean glycemic reduction. In many trials, the reduction in HbA_{1C} is approx 0.5 to 1%. However, postmarketing data suggest that with marked hyperglycemia the actual reduction in HbA_{1C} may be somewhat greater than that reported from phase 3 trials. There is a beneficial affect on lipid profiles. The agents do not predispose to weight gain and may ameliorate some of the weight gain associated with sulfonylurea use. The gastrointestinal side effects of the carbohydrase inhibitors are significant in both frequency and intensity. This has limited their use in the clinical arena in the United States.

Incretins (Exenatide)

Additional glucose-lowering agents have recently been approved, but are not yet clinically available. These are gut peptides that stimulate insulin secretion and suppress glucagon production. The early versions are analogs of glucagon-like peptide-1 an injectable compound that reduces HbA_{1C} by approx 1% *(165,166)*. Native glucagon-like peptide-1 is degraded by an enzyme called dipeptidyl-dipeptidase IV, and oral DPP-IV inhibitors are under investigation. Nausea is a common side effect. Weight loss with these agents is also common.

LIPID MANAGEMENT IN PATIENTS WITH DIABETES

Diabetes is a significant risk factor in risk assessment strategies. Consequently, aggressive lipid-lowering strategies have been recommended for patients with diabetes *(167)* (Table 3). In the most recent National Cholesterol Education Program guidelines, DM was considered to be a CHD risk equivalent, and LDL-C targets were set at 100 mg/dL *(46)* (Table 4). In the recent revision to these guidelines, very high-risk patients, such as those with diabetes and established CHD should be considered to have an LDL-C target of 70 mg/dL *(167)*. When LDL-C targets have been achieved, but triglyceride (and VLDL-C) concentrations are elevated, then the non-HDL target is set at 30 mg/dL above the LDL-C goal. Intervention trial and general clinical experience indicate that use of statins or fibric acid derivatives in patients with diabetes are efficacious and safe. Furthermore, these agents have no known adverse effect on glucose tolerance. Bile acid sequestrants may be somewhat more difficult to use in patients with diabetes who are more likely to be hypertensive or require oral agents to manage glucose levels. This "polypharmacy" and the potential of the bile acid sequestrants to interfere with absorption of other agents limit their use in some patients with diabetes. Increased triglyceride levels with bile acid sequestrant use are also a problem in some patients with diabetes. More recently, ezetimibe is being used as an alternative to the bile acid sequestrants. Ezetimibe has a modest LDL-C-lowering effect either as monotherapy or in combination with statins, and a modest triglyceride-lowering effect. The concerns regarding interference with absorption of other medications is not a concern with ezetimibe. Niacin may increase insulin resistance and adversely affect glycemic control. Its use is generally limited to patients with diabetes with satisfactory glycemic control.

MANAGEMENT OF HYPERTENSION IN PATIENTS WITH DIABETES

The beneficial effects of blood pressure lowering are now well-established in both nondiabetic and patients with diabetes. Studies show that reductions in systolic blood

Table 3
Order of Priorities for Treatment of Diabetic Dyslipidemia in Adults

I. LDL cholesterol lowering
   Lifestyle interventions
   Preferred
      HMG-CoA reductase inhibitor (statin)
   Others
      Bile acid-binding resin (resin), cholesterol absorption inhibitor, fenofibrate or niacin
II. HDL cholesterol raising
   Lifestyle interventions
   Nicotinic acid or fibrates
III. Triglyceride lowering
   Lifestyle interventions
   Glycemic control
   Fibric acid derivative (gemfibrozil, fenofibrate)
   Niacin
   High-dose statins (in those who also have high LDL cholesterol)
IV. Combined hyperlipidemia
   First choice
      Improved glycemic control plus high-dose statin
   Second choice
      Improved glycemic control plus statin plus fibric acid derivative
   Third choice
      Improved glycemic control plus statin plus nicotinic acid

Adapted from ref. 9.

pressure will result in substantial reductions in atherosclerotic risk. Furthermore, beneficial effects have been show in patients with diabetes with ACE inhibitors, long-acting calcium channel blockers, β-blockers, and diuretics. The absence of extensive head-to-head comparisons limits the capability to determine which class of agents may have the greatest benefit. The ALLHAT study data suggests that there are no significant differences in outcomes between diuretics, calcium channel blockers, and ACE inhibitors in terms of outcomes. However, the greater risk for new-onset diabetes is highest with diuretics and lowest with ACE inhibitors, raising concerns regarding how this may confound long-term follow-up results. Because of the accumulating data that ACE blockade of the renin–angiotensin–aldosterone system with ACE inhibitors or ARBs may have some advantage in protecting renal function in patients with diabetes, these classes of agents should generally be considered as the first line agents. Potential adverse effects of β-blockers and diuretics on glycemic control and dyslipidemia need to be balanced by their indications in the face of CHD risk management. Such considerations usually favor their use with the usual clinical indications.

Smoking Risk in Patients With Diabetes

Smoking clearly increases the risk for CHD risk in patients with diabetes. The American Diabetes Association has formally endorsed the importance of smoking cessation in patients with diabetes (153).

Table 4

ATP III LDL-C Goals and Cutpoints for Therapeutic Lifestyle Changes (TLC) and Drug Therapy in Different Risk Categories and Proposed Modifications Based on Recent Clinical Trial Evidence

Risk category	LDL-C goal	Initiate TLC	Consider drug therapy[k]
High risk: CHD[c] or CHD risk equivalents[d] (10-yr risk >20%)	<100 mg/dL (optional goal: <70 mg/dL)[j]	≥100 mg/dL[b]	≥100 mg/dL (<100 mg/dL; consider drug options)[k]
Moderately high risk: 2+ risk factors[i] (10-yr risk 10% ot 20%)	<130 mg/dL[h]	≥130 mg/dL[b]	≥130 mg/dL (100–120 mg/dL; consider drug options)[f]
Moderate risk: 2+ risk factors[i] (10-yr risk <10%)[e]	<130 mg/dL	≥130 mg/dL	≥160 mg/dL
Lower risk: 0–1 risk factor[a]	<160 mg/dL	≥160 mg/dL	≥190 mg/dL (160–189 mg/dL; LDL-lowering drug optional)

[a]Almost all people with zero or one risk factor have a 10-yr risk <10%, and 10-yr risk assessment in people with zero or one risk factor is thus not necessary.

[b]Any person at high risk or moderately high risk who has lifestyle-related factors (e.g., obesity, physical inactively, elevated triglyceride, low HDL-C, or metabolic syndrome) is a candidate for therapeutic lifestyle changes to modify these risk factors regardless of LDL-C level.

[c]CHD includes history of myocardial infarction, unstable angina, stable angina, coronary artery procedures (angioplasty or bypass surgery), or evidence of clinically significant myocardial ischemia.

[d]CHD risk equivalents include clinical manifestations of noncoronary forms of atherosclerotic disease (peripheral arterial disease, abdominal aortic aneurysm, and carotid artery disease [transient ischemic attacks or stroke of carotid origin or >50% obstruction of a carotid artery]), diabetes, and 2+ risk factors with 10-yr risk for hard CHD >20%.

[e]Electronic 10-yr risk calculations are available at www.nhlbi.nih.gov/guidelines/cholesterol.

[f]For moderately high-risk persons, when LDL-C level is 100 to 129 mg/dL, at baseline or on lifestyle therapy, initiation of an LDL-lowering drug to achieve an LDL-C lever <100 mg/dL to a therapeutic option on the basis of available clinical trial results.

[g]If baseline LDL-C is <100 mg/dL, institution of an LDL-lowering drug is a therapeutic option on the basis of available clinical trial results. If a high-risk person has high triglycerides or low HDL-C, combining a fibrate or nicotinic acid with an LDL-lowering drug can be considered.

[h]Optional LDL-C goal <100 mg/dL.

[i]Risk factors include cigarette smoking, hypertension (BP ≥ +40/90 mmHg or an antihypertensive medication), low HDL cholesterol (<40 mg/dL), family history of premature CHD (CHD in male first-degree relative <55 yr of age; CHD in female first-degree relative <65 yr of age), and age (men ≥45 yr; women ≥55 yr).

[j]Very high risk favors the optional LDL-C goal of <70 mg/dL, and in patients with high triglycerides, non-HDL-C <100 mg/dL.

[k]When LDL-lowering drug therapy is employed, it is advised that intensity of therapy be sufficient to achieve at least a 30 to 40% reduction in LDL-C levels. From ref. 47, see also refs. 46, 67, and 180–182.

131

Acute Coronary Syndromes in Patients With Diabetes

In addition to an increased risk for CHD, many studies have shown that patients with diabetes have a worse outcome after an MI both in terms of morbidity and mortality *(4,11)* (Fig. 4). Many of these studies report that women with diabetes are at a much greater risk for an adverse outcome than their nondiabetic counter parts. Furthermore, the increased number of CHD risk factors in patients with diabetes and more diffuse disease seem to be contributing risk factors. Khot et al. analyzed the prevalence of CHD risk factors in 122,458 patients from 14 randomized clinical trials of CHD patients who had been enrolled because of ST-elevation MI ($n = 76,716$), unstable angina/non-ST-elevation MI ($n = 35,527$), or undergoing percutaneous coronary intervention (PCI) ($n = 10,215$) *(28)*. The purpose of the study was to determine the percentage of patients who had conventional risk factors, including smoking, dyslipidemia, hypertension, and DM. Diabetes was present in 23.2% of women and 15.3% of men.

Acute management of an acute coronary syndrome is similar in diabetic and nondiabetic patients. The outcomes of thrombolytic therapy may be less favorable in patients with diabetes *(18,21,34,55)*. The early, compelling data suggesting that intensive glycemic control in the period surrounding the MI may improve outcomes in DIGAMI has been tempered by the absence of similarly dramatic results from DIGAMI-2 *(115,116)*.

Vascular Interventions in Patients With Diabetes

The results of surgical intervention, such as coronary artery bypass procedures and angioplasty, generally have less favorable long-term outcomes in patients with diabetes, with evidence of earlier graft closure and increased mortality compared with nondiabetic patients undergoing such procedures. The mechanisms for more these adverse outcomes may be related to the increased number of CHD risk factors, including an increased procoagulant risk. Limited data on the effects of aggressive risk factor management suggest that aggressive cholesterol lowering may slow the rate of progression of disease in saphenous vein graft conduits *(107)*. The Bypass Angioplasty Revascularization Investigation trial was designed to compare coronary artery bypass graft (CABG) vs percutaneous transluminal coronary angioplasty (PTCA) *(8)*. This trial did not show a difference in outcomes in all patients in the study. The subgroup with diabetes had a more favorable outcome with CABG. The changing intervention technologies for both CABG and PTCA/stent procedures, and more aggressive use of antiplatelet therapy limit the ability to apply the Bypass Angioplasty Revascularization Investigation results to current clinical practice. However, a propensity analysis of patients studied at the Cleveland Clinic suggest favorable mortality with CABG vs PTCA intervention *(7)*. Brener reported on 6033 consecutive patients who had coronary vascular interventions (PCI, $n = 872$; CABG, $n = 5161$) to compare mortality rates using propensity analyses. Mortality rates were higher at 1 yr for PCI than CABG (5 vs 4%) and at 5 yrs (16 vs 14%). Thirty percent of the patients undergoing PCI and 40% of the patients undergoing CABG had DM. The mortality difference with PCI was demonstrated in patients with diabetes (21 vs 17%). Furthermore, diabetes was one of the independent predictors of mortality.

PREVENTION OF DM

Several studies have been performed that evaluated lifestyle and pharmacological ways to reduce the risk for new onset of DM, usually in patients who were at high risk

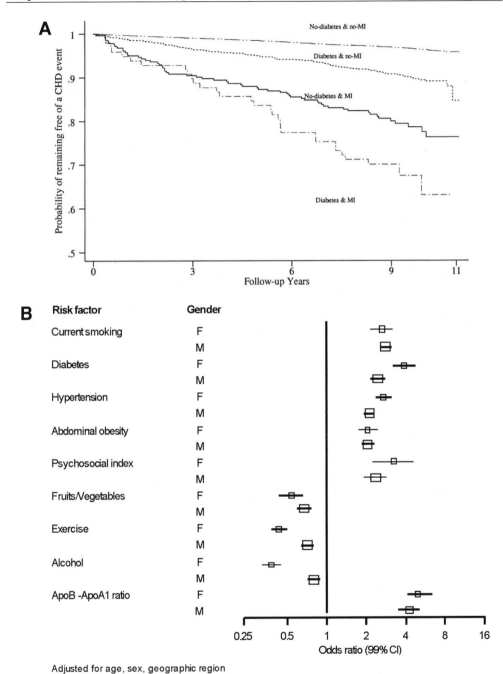

Fig. 4. (**A**) Coronary heart disease events in diabetic subjects compared with nondiabetic subjects in the ARIC study. (From ref. *30*.) (**B**) Risk factors associated with MI in the INTERHEART study (*n* = 26,916) (From ref. *30*.)

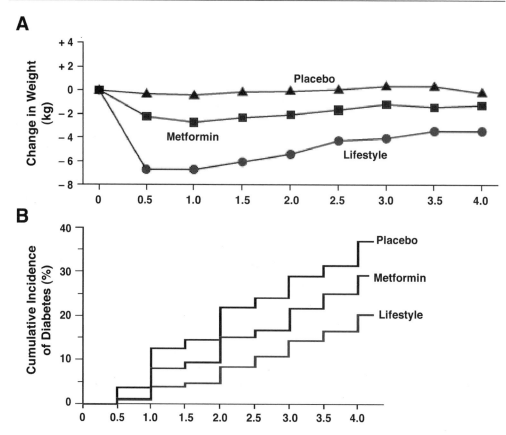

Fig. 5. Diabetes Prevention Trial (adapted from ref. *168*). (**A**) Change in body weight for each study group. (**B**) Incidence of DM for each study group. The diagnosis of diabetes was based on the criteria of the American Diabetes Association *(179)*. The incidence of diabetes differed significantly among the three groups ($p < 0.001$ for each comparison).

to develop DM *(168–170)*. In addition, post hoc analyses of trials (convened to evaluate the effects of various interventions on atherosclerotic vascular disease risk) have assessed the effects of the intervention on the reduction in risk for new-onset DM.

The Diabetes Prevention Program (DPP) in more than 3000 subjects followed for a mean of 2.8 yr studied the effects of intensive lifestyle modification (vs standard lifestyle), and metformin on the risk to develop DM in subjects with impaired glucose tolerance *(99)*. In the DPP, an achieved weight reduction of 4% from baseline and 150 min/wk of exercise was associated with a 58% reduction in the risk to develop DM (Fig. 5). Metformin had a more modest effect, with a 31% reduction in risk. The effects of intensive lifestyle changes were greater in subjects older than 60 yr of age, whereas metformin had very little effect in this age group. The DPP had a troglitazone arm that was discontinued when troglitazone was removed from the market because of increased risk for hepatotoxicity *(171)*. The results of the troglitazone arm showed a favorable effect of troglitazone during its use, but the effect seems to have been lost with discontinuation. Similarly, the smaller (*n* = 522) Finish Diabetes Prevention study showed favorable effects of intensive life style on the reduced risk to develop DM *(172)*. The Study to Prevent (STOP)-NIDDM trial compared the carbohydrase inhibitor, acarbose, to placebo

in 1368 randomized subjects (with 341 dropouts) and showed a 25% reduction in new-onset DM *(173)*. Furthermore, this study showed a 49% RR reduction in cardiovascular events and a 34% RR reduction in new onset of hypertension *(169)*—this observation was supported by the meta-analyses of seven acarbose trials *(174)*.

The Troglitazon in the Prevention of Diabetes (TRIPOD) study was designed to assess whether the thiazolidinedione, troglitazone, would reduce the risk for new-onset DM in women with a history of gestational DM, who were at high risk to develop type 2 DM *(169)*. The annual rate of new-onset diabetes in the placebo group was 12.1% compared with 5.4% in the troglitazone (thiazolidinedione)-treated group. When troglitazone was taken off the market, the study was forced to stop. Of interest was the observation that the reduction in risk for new-onset DM in the troglitazone group seemed to be durable, with persistence of a reduced incidence of new-onset diabetes for the next 8 mo *(165)*.

Post hoc analyses from several trials have evaluated the effects of various antihypertensive agents on the risk to develop DM *(175)*. In the HOPE trial, new-onset DM was more than 30% reduced in the ramipril group vs the placebo group at the end of the trial, as well as after the extended follow-up of an additional 2.6 yr *(176)*. Enalapril has also been associated with reduced risk for new-onset DM in Studies of Left Ventricular Dysfunciton (SOLVD) *(177)*. The LIFE trial showed a reduced risk of new-onset diabetes with an ARB (losartan) compared with the β-blocker atenolol *(128)*. It is not clear whether this is a favorable effect of the ARB or an adverse effect of the β-blocker. In ALLHAT, the lowest risk for new-onset diabetes was associated with lisinopril and the highest risk was associated with the diuretic, whereas the calcium channel blocker arm had an intermediate risk *(125)*. Finally, the preliminary results of ASCOT also reported a 30% reduction in new-onset DM in the perindopril/amlodipine arm compared with the atenolol/bendroflumethiazide-K arm. As with the LIFE study, this result may be caused by a favorable effect of ACE inhibitors (or calcium channel blockers) or an adverse effect of diuretics/β-blockers *(117)*. There are diabetes prevention trials underway that are using thiazolidinediones (Diabetes Reduction Assessment With Ramipril and Rosiglitazone Medication [DREAM], Actos Now for Prevention of Diabetes [ACTNOW]), ACE inhibitors (DREAM), and ARBs (Nateglinide and Valsartan in Impaired Glucose Tolerance Outcomes Research [NAVIGATOR]). The results of these studies will help to clarify the observations from the post hoc analyses of potential medication effects on the risk for new-onset DM.

SUMMARY

Patients with diabetes are at increased risk for CHD, and have an associated increased morbidity and mortality from CHD compared with their nondiabetic counterparts. Patients with diabetes often have a greater number of traditional risk factors, such as hypertension, dyslipidemia, and obesity, as well as a relatively higher procoagulant state (increased fibrinogen, increased PAI-1, and increased platelet aggregation). Hyperglycemia is associated with a modest increase in risk for the development of CHD and for adverse outcomes after an MI. Aggressive risk factor management, especially lipid lowering, has comparable or greater benefit in patients with diabetes compared with patients without DM (Table 3). Management of acute coronary syndromes and indications for surgical interventions are essentially the same in diabetic and nondiabetic patients, although long-term outcomes are still worse in patients with diabetes.

REFERENCES

1. Abbott RD, Donahue RP, Kannel WB, Wilson PW. The impact of diabetes on survival following myocardial infarction in men vs. women. The Framingham Study. JAMA 1988;260:3456–3460.
2. Anderson, KM, Wilson PWF, Odell PM, Kannel WB. An updated coronary risk profile: a statement for health professionals. Circ 1991;83:356–362.
3. American Diabetes Association. Dyslipidemia management in adults with diabetes. American Diabetes Association: Clinical Practice Recommendations. 2004;27(Suppl 1):S68–S71.
4. Aronson D, Rayfield EJ, Chesebro JH. Mechanisms determining course and outcome of diabetic patients who have had acute myocardial infarction [review]. Ann Intern Med 1997;126:296–306.
5. Behar S. Boyko V. Reicher-Reiss H. Goldbourt U. Ten-year survival after acute myocardial infarction: comparison of patients with and without diabetes. SPRINT Study Group. Secondary Prevention Reinfarction Israeli Nifedipine Trial. Am Heart J 1997;133:290–296.
6. Bjønholt JV, Erikssen G, Aaser E, et al. Fasting blood glucose: an underestimated risk factor for cardiovascular death: Results from a 22-year follow-up of healthy nondiabetic men: Diabetes Care 1999;22:45–49.
7. Brener SJ, Lytle BW, Casserly IP, et al. Percutaneous revascularization in patients with multivessel coronary disease and high-risk features. Circulation 2004;109:2290–2295.
8. Chaitman BR, Rosen AD, Williams DO, et al. Myocardial infarction and cardiac mortality in the Bypass Angioplasty Revascularization Investigation (BARI) randomized trial. Circulation 1997;96:2162–2170.
9. Coutinho M, Gerstein HC, Wang Y, Yusuf, S. The relationship between glucose and incident cardiovascular events: a metaregression analysis of published data from 20 studies in 95,783 individuals followed for 12.4 years. Diabetes Care 1999;22:233–240.
10. DeFronzo RA, Ferrannini E. A multifaceted syndrome responsible for NIDDM obesity, hypertension, dyslipidemia, and atherosclerotic cardiovascular disease. Insulin resistance [review]. Diabetes Care 1991;14:173–194.
11. Donahue RP, Goldberg RJ, Chen Z, Gore JM, Alpert JS. The influence of sex and diabetes mellitus on survival following acute myocardial infarction: a community-wide perspective. J Clin Epidemiol 1993;46:245–252.
12. Eschwège E, Richard JL, Thibult N, et al. Coronary heart disease mortality in relation with diabetes, blood glucose and plasma insulin levels: the Paris Prospective Study, ten years later. Horm Metab Res 1985;(Suppl 15):41–46.
13. Fava S, Aquilina O, Azzopardi J, Agius Muscat H, Fenech FF. The prognostic value of blood glucose in diabetic patients with acute myocardial infarction. Diabet Med 1996;13:80–83.
14. Fietsam R, Bassett J, Glover JL. Comparisons of coronary artery surgery in diabetic patients. The American Surgeon 1991;57:551–557.
15. Garcia MJ, McNamara PM, Gordon T, Kannell WB. Morbidity and mortality in diabetics in the Framingham population. Sixteen year follow-up study. Diabetes 1974;23:105–111.
16. Gerstein HC, Pais P, Pogue J, Yusuf S. Relationship of glucose and insulin levels to the risk of myocardial infarction: a case-control study. J Am Coll Cardiol 1999;33:612–619.
17. Gowda MS, Vacek JL, Hallas D. One-year outcomes of diabetic versus nondiabetic patients with non-Q-wave acute myocardial infarction treated with percutaneous transluminal coronary angioplasty. Am J Cardiol 81(9):1998;1067–1071.
18. Granger CB, Califf RM, Young S, et al. Outcome of patients with diabetes mellitus and acute myocardial infarction treated with thrombolytic agents. The Thrombolysis and Angioplasty in Myocardial Infarction (TAMI) Study Group. J Am Coll Cardiol 1993;21:920–925.
19. Herlitz J, Bang A, Karlson BW. Mortality, place and mode of death and reinfarction during a period of 5 years after acute myocardial infarction in diabetic and non-diabetic patients. Cardiology 1996;87:423–428.
20. Jacoby RM, Nesto RW. Acute myocardial infarction in the diabetic patient: pathophysiology, clinical course and prognosis [review]. J Am Coll Cardiol 1992;20:736–744.
21. Jelesoff NE, Feinglos M, Granger CB, Califf RM. Outcomes of diabetic patients following acute myocardial infarction: a review of the major thrombolytic trials [review]. Coron Artery Dis 1996;7:732–743.
22. Johnson WE, Pedraza PM, Kayser KL. Coronary artery surgery in diabetics: 281 consecutive patients followed four to seven years. Am Heart J 1982;104:824–829.
23. Kannel WB, D'Agostino RB, Wilson PW, Belanger AG, Gagnon DR. Diabetes, fibrinogen, and risk of cardiovascular disease: the Framingham experience. Am Heart J 1990;120:672–676.
24. Kannel WB. Lipids, diabetes, and coronary artery disease: insights from the Framingham Study. Am Heart J 1985;110:1100–1107.

25. Karlson BW, Herlitz J, Hjalmarson A. Prognosis of acute myocardial infarction in diabetic and non-diabetic patients. Diabet Med 1993;10:449–454.
26. Kekäläinen P, Sarlund H, Farin P, Kaukanen E, Yang X, Laakso M. Femoral atherosclerosis in middle-aged subjects: association with cardiovascular risk factors and insulin resistance. Am J Epid 1996;144:742–748.
27. Khaw KT, Wareham N, Bingham S, et al. Association of hemoglobin A1c with cardiovascular disease and mortality in adults: the European Prospective Investigation into Cancer in Norfolk. Ann Intern Med 2004;141:413–420.
28. Khot UM, Khot MB, Bajer CT, et al. Prevalence of conventional risk factors in patients with coronary heart disease. JAMA 2003;290:898–904.
29. Kuusisto J, Mykkänen L, Pyörälä K, Laakso M. NIDDM and its metabolic control predict coronary heart disease in elderly subjects. Diabetes 1994;43:960–967.
30. Lee CD, Folsom AR, Pankow JS, Brancati FL. for the Atherosclerosis Risk in Communities (ARIC) Study Investigators Cardiovascular events in diabetic and nondiabetic adults with or without history of myocardial infarction. Circulation 2004;109;855–860.
31. Lehto S, Ronnemaa T, Haffner SM, Pyörälä K, Kallio V, Laakso M. Dyslipidemia and hyperglycemia predict coronary heart disease events in middle-aged patients with NIDDM. Diabetes 1997;46:1354–1359.
32. Lundberg V, Stegmayr B, Asplund K, Eliasson M, Huhtasaari F. Diabetes as a risk factor for myocardial infarction: population and gender perspectives. J Intern Med 1997;241:485–492.
33. Lytle B, Loop FD, Cosgrove DM, et al. Long-term (5–12 years) serial studies of internal mammary artery and saphenous vein coronary bypass grafts. J Thorac Cardiovasc Surg 1985;80:258–278.
34. Mak KH, Moliterno DJ, Granger CB, et al. Influence of diabetes mellitus on clinical outcome in the thrombolytic era of acute myocardial infarction. GUSTO-I Investigators. Global Utilization of Strep-tokinase and Tissue Plasminogen Activator for Occluded Coronary Arteries. J Am Coll Cardiol 1997;30:171–179.
35. Melchior T, Kober L, Madsen CR, et al. Accelerating impact of diabetes mellitus on mortality in the years following an acute myocardial infarction. TRACE Study Group. Trandolapril Cardiac Evaluation. Eur Heart J 1999;20:973–978.
36. Miettinen H, Lehto S, Salomaa V, et al. Impact of diabetes on mortality after the first myocardial infarction. The FINMONICA Myocardial Infarction Register Study Group Diabetes Care. 1998;21:69–75.
37. Morris JJ, Smith LR, Jones RH, et al. Influence of diabetes and mammary artery grafting on survival after coronary bypass. Circulation 1991;84(Suppl III):III-275–III-284.
38. Moss SE, Klein R, Klein BE, Meuer SM. The association of glycemia and cause-specific mortality in a diabetic population. Arch Int Med 1994;154:2473–2479.
39. Niles NW, McGrath PD, Malenka, et al. Survival of patients with diabetes and multivessel coronary artery disease after surgical or percutaneous coronary revascularization: results of a large regional prospective study: Northern New England Cardiovascular Disease Study Group. J Am Coll Cardiol 2001;37:1008–1015.
40. O'Sullivan JJ, Conroy RM, Robinson K, Hickey N, Mulcahy R. In-hospital prognosis of patients with fasting hyperglycemia after first myocardial infarction. Diabetes Care 1991;14:758–760.
41. Panzram G. Mortality and survival in type 2 (non-insulin dependent) diabetes mellitus. Diabetologia 1987;30:123–131.
42. Prasad B, Stone GW, Stuckey TD, et al. Impact of diabetes mellitus on myocardial perfusion after primary angioplasty in patients with acute myocardial infarction. J Am Coll Cardiol 2005;45:508–514.
43. Pyörälä K. Relationship of glucose intolerance and plasma insulin to the incidence of coronary heart disease: results from 2 population studies in Finland. Diabetes Care 1972;2:131–141.
44. Risum Ø, Abdelnoor M, Svennevig JL, et al. Diabetes mellitus and morbidity and mortality risks after coronary artery bypass surgery. Scand J Thor Cardiovasc Surg 1996;30:71–75.
45. Saloma V, Riley W, Kark JD, Nardo C, Folsom A. Non-insulin dependent diabetes mellitus and fasting glucose and insulin concentrations are associated with arterial stiffness indexes: The Atherosclerosis Risk in Communities (ARIC) Study. Circulation 1995;91:1432–1443.
46. Saltiel AR, Olefsky JM. Thiazolidinediones in the treatment of insulin resistance and type II diabetes mellitus. Diabetes1996;45:1661–1669.
47. Silva JA, Nunez E, White CJ, et al. Predictors of stent thrombosis after primary stenting for acute myocardial infarction. Catheter Cardiovasc Interv 1999;47:415–422.
48. Stamler R, Stamler J. Asymptomatic hyperglycemia and coronary heart disease. J Chron Dis 1979;32:683–691.

49. Stamler J, Vaccaro I, Neaton JD, Wentworth D. Diabetes, other risk factors, and 12-yr cardiovascular mortality for men screened in the Multiple Risk Factor Intervention Trial. Diabetes Care 1993;16:434–444.
50. Stone PH, Muller JE, Hartwell T, et al. The effect of diabetes mellitus on prognosis and serial left ventricular function after acute myocardial infarction: contribution of both coronary disease and diastolic left ventricular dysfunction to the adverse prognosis. The MILIS Study Group. J Am Coll Cardiol 1989;14:49–57.
51. Walter DP, Gatling W, Houston AC, Mullee MA, Julious SA, Hill RD. Mortality in diabetic subjects: an eleven-year follow-up of a community-based population. Diabet Med 1994;11:968–973.
52. Welborn TA, Wearne K. Coronary heart disease incidence and cardiovascular mortality in Busselton with reference to glucose and insulin concentrations. Diabetes Care 1979;2:154–160.
53. Wilson PWF, D'Agostino RB, Levy D, Belanger AM, Silbershatz H, Kannel WB. Prediction of coronary heart disease using risk factor categories. Circulation 1998;97:1837–1847.
54. Wong ND, Cupples LA, Ostfeld AM, Levy D, Kannel WB. Risk factors for long-term coronary prognosis after initial myocardial infarction: the Framingham Study. Am J Epidemiol 1989;130:469–480.
55. Woodfield SL, Lundergan CF, Reiner JS, et al. Angiographic findings and outcome in diabetic patients treated with thrombolytic therapy for acute myocardial infarction: the GUSTO-I experience J Am Coll Cardiol 1996;28:1661–1669.
56. Yusuf S, Hawken S, Ounpuu S, et al. for the INTERHEART Study Investigators. Effect of potentially modifiable risk factors associated with myocardial infarction in 52 countries (the INTERHEART study): case-control study. Lancet 2004;364:937–952.
57. Abraira C, Colwell J, Nuttall F. Veterans Affairs cooperative study on glycemic control and complications in type II diabetes (VACSDM): results of the feasibility trial. Diabetes Care 1995;18:1113–1123.
58. Agewall S, Fagerberg B, Atvall S, Wendelhage I, Urbanavicius V, Wikstrand J. Carotid artery wall intima-media thickness is associated with insulin-mediated glucose disposal in men at high and low coronary risk. Stroke 1995;26:956–960.
59. Bonora E, Targier G, Zenere MB, et al. Relationship between fasting insulin and cardiovascular risk factors in already present in young men: the Verona Young Men Atherosclerosis Risk Factors Study. Eur J Clin Invest 1997;27:248–254.
60. Davi G, Violi F, Giammarresi C, et al. Increased plasminogen activator inhibitor antigen levels in diabetic patients with stable angina. Blood Coagul Fibrinolysis 1991;2:41–45.
61. Deprès J-P, Lamarche B, Mauriège P, et al. Hyperinsulinaemia as an independent risk factor for ischaemic heart disease. New Engl J Med 1996;334:952–957.
62. Ducimetière P, Eschwège E, Papoz L, Richard JL, Claude JR, Rooselin GE. Relationship of plasma insulin levels to the incidence of myocardial infarction and coronary heart disease mortality in a middle-aged population. Diabetologia 1980;19:205–210.
63. Folsom AR, Szklo M, Stevens J, Liao F, Smith R, Eckfeldt JH. A prospective study of coronary heart disease in relation to fasting insulin, glucose, and diabetes. The Atherosclerosis Risk in Communities (ARIC) Study. Diabetes Care 1997;20:935–942.
64. Fontbonne A, Charles MA, Thilbult N, et al. Hyperinsulinemia as a predictor of coronary heart disease mortality in a healthy population: the Paris Prospective Study, 15 year follow-up. Diabetologia 1991;34:356–361.
65. Haffner SM, Mykkänen L, Stern MP, Valdez RA, Heisserman JA, Bowsher RR. Relationship of pro-insulin and insulin to cardiovascular risk factors in nondiabetic subjects. Diabetes 1993;42:1297–1302.
66. Hanninen J, Takala J, Keinanen-Kiukaanniemi S. Albuminuria and other risk factors for mortality in patients with non-insulin-dependent diabetes mellitus aged under 65 years: a population-based prospective 5-year study. Diabetes Res Clin Pract 1999;43:121–126.
67. Kaplan NM. Upper-body obesity, glucose intolerance, hypertriglyceridemia, and hypertension. The deadly quartet [review]. Arch Intern Med 1989;149:1514–1520.
68. Kwaan HC. Changes in blood coagulation, platelet function, and plasminogen-plasmin system in diabetes [review]. Diabetes 1992;41(suppl 2)32–35.
69. Laakso M, Barrett-Connor E. Asymptomatic hyperglycemia is associated with lipid and lipoprotein changes favoring atherosclerosis. Arteriosclerosis 1989;9:665–672.
70. Laakso M, Sarlund H, Salonen R, et al. Asymptomatic atherosclerosis and insulin resistance. Arterioscler Thromb 1991;11:1068–1076.
71. Marso SP, Ellis SG, Tuzcu M, et al. The importance of proteinuria as a determinant of mortality following percutaneous coronary revascularization in diabetics. J Am Coll Cardiol 1999;33:1269–1277.

72. Matsuda T, Morishita E, Jokaji H, et al. Mechanism on disorders of coagulation and fibrinolysis in diabetes. Diabetes 1996;45(Suppl 3):S109–S110.

73. Perry IJ, Wannamethee SG, Whincup PH, Shaper AG, Walker MK, Alberti KGMM. Serum insulin and incident coronary heart disease in middle-aged British men. Am J Epidemiol 1996;144:224–234.

74. Pradhan AD, Manson JE, Rifai N, Buring JE, Ridker PM. C-reactive protein, interleukin 6 and risk of developing type 2 diabetes mellitus. JAMA 2001;286:327–334.

75. Pyörälä K, Savolainen E, Kaukola S, Haapakoski J. Plasma insulin as coronary heart disease risk factor: relationship to other risk factors and predictive value during 9¬ -year follow-up of the Helsinki Policemen Study population. Acta Med Scand 1985;(Suppl)701:38–52.

76. Rantala AO, Paivansalo M, Kauma H, et al. Hyperinsulinemia and carotid atherosclerosis in hypertensive and control subjects. Diabetes Care 1998;21:1188–1193.

77. Ridker PM, Wilson PWF, Grundy S. Should C-reactive protein be added to metabolic syndrome and to assessment of global cardiovascular risk? [Review] Circulation 2004;109:2818–2825.

78. Ridker PM, Brown NJ, Vaughan DE, Harrison DG, Jehta JL. Established and emerging plasma biomarkers in the prediction of first atherothrombotic events. Circulation 2004;109(Suppl IV):IV-6–IV-19.

79. Rönnemaa T, Laakso L, Pyörälä K, Kallio V, Puuka P. High fasting plasma insulin is an indicator of coronary heart disease in non-insulin-dependent diabetic patients and nondiabetic subjects. Arterioscler Thromb 1991;11:80–90.

80. Sowers JR. Insulin resistance, hyperinsulinemia, dyslipidemia, hypertension, and accelerated atherosclerosis [review]. J Clin Pharmacol 1992;32:529–535.

81. Stout, RA. Insulin and atheroma: 20-yr perspective. Diabetes Care 1990;13;631–654.

82. Tuttle KR, Phulman ME, Cooney SK, Short R. Urinary albumin and insulin as predictors of coronary artery disease: an angiographic study. Am J Kid Dis 1999;34:918–925.

83. Tzargournis M, Chiles JM, Ryan JM, Skillman TG. Interrelationships of hyperinsulinism and hypertriglyceridemia in young patients with coronary heart disease. Circulation 1968;38:1156–1163.

84. Wick G, Schett G, Amberger A, Kleindienst R, Xu Q. Is atherosclerosis an immunologically mediated disease? Immunol Today 1995;16:27–33.

85. Winegard DL, Barrett-Connor E, Criqui M, Suarez L. Clustering of heart disease risk factors in diabetic compared to non-diabetic adults. Am J Epidemiol 1983;117:19–26.

86. Winocour PD. Platelet abnormalities in diabetes mellitus. Diabetes 1992;41(Suppl 2):26–32.

87. Yudkin JS, Denver AE, Mohamed AV, et al. The relationships of concentrations of insulin and proinsulin-like molecules with coronary heart disease prevalence and incidence: a study of two ethnic groups. Diabetes Care 1997;20:1093–1100.

88. Hoogwerf BJ, Sprecher DL, Pearce GL, et al. Blood glucose concentrations ‚â§125 mg/dL and coronary heart disease risk. Am J Cardiol 2002;89:596–599.

89. Brownlee M, Cerami A, Vlassara H. Advanced glycosylation end products in tissue and the biochemical basis of diabetic complications. N Engl J Med 1988;318:1315–1321.

90. Chisolm GM, Irwin KC, Penn MC. Lipoprotein oxidation and lipoprotein-induced cell injury in diabetes. Diabetes 1992;41(Suppl 2):61–66.

91. Lyons T. Lipoprotein glycation and its metabolic consequences. Diabetes 1992;(Suppl 2):67–73.

92. Steinberg D, Parthasarathy S, Carew TE, Khoo JC, Witztum JL. Beyond cholesterol: modifications of low-density lipoprotein that increase its atherogenicity [review]. N Engl J Med 1989;320:915–924.

93. Calhoun HM, Betteridge J, Durrington PM, et al. on behalf of the CARDS investigators. Primary prevention of cardiovascular disease with atorvastatin in type 2 diabetes in the Collaborative Atorvastatin Diabetes Study (CARDS): multicentre randomized placebo-controlled trial. Lancet 2004;364:685–696.

94. Campeau L, Hunninghake DB, Knatterud G, et al. for the Post CABG Study. Aggressive cholesterol lowering delays saphenous vein graft atherosclerosis in women, in the elderly and in patients with associated risk factors: NHLBI Post CABG Clinical Trial. Circulation 1999;99:3241–3247.

95. Downs JR, Clearfield M, Weis S, et al. Primary prevention of acute coronary events with lovastatin in men and women with average cholesterol levels: results of AFCAPS/TexCAPS. Air Force/Texas Coronary Atherosclerosis Prevention Study. JAMA 1998;279:1615–1622.

96. Expert Panel of Detection, Evaluation, and Treatment of High Blood Cholesterol in Adults. National Cholesterol Education Program. National Cholesterol Education Program. Executive summary of the Third Report of the National Cholesterol Education Program (NCEP) Expert Panel on Detection, Evaluation and Treatment of High Blood Cholesterol in adults (Adult Treatment Panel III). JAMA 2001;283:2486–2497.

97. Grundy SM, Cleeman JL, Merz CN, et al. for the Coordinating Committee of the National Cholesterol Education Program. Arterioscler Thromb Vasc Biol 2004;24:e149–161.
98. Frick MH, Elo O, Haapa K, et al. Helsinki Heart Study: primary-prevention trial with gemfibrozil in middle-aged men with dyslipidemia. Safety of treatment, changes in risk factors, and incidence of coronary heart disease. N Engl J Med 1987;317:1237–1245.
99. Friedrich CA, Rader DJ. Management of lipid disorders. Rheum Dis Clin North Am 1999;25:507–520.
100. Goldberg RB, Mellies MJ, Sacks FM, et al. The Care Investigators. Cardiovascular events and their reduction with pravastatin in diabetic and glucose intolerant myocardial infarction survivors with average cholesterol levels: subgroup analyses in the cholesterol and recurrent events (CARE) trial. Circulation 1998;98:2513–2519.
101. Grundy SM, Balady GJ, Criqui MH, et al. Primary prevention of coronary heart disease: guidelines from Framingham. A statement for healthcare professionals from the American Heart Association's Task Force on Risk Reduction. Circulation 1998;97:1876–1887.
102. Grundy, SM. Integrating risk assessment with intervention. Primary Prevention of Coronary Heart Disease Circ 1999;100:988–998.
103. Grundy SM, Cleeman JI, Merz CN, et al. Implications of recent clinical trials for the National Cholesterol Education Program Adult Treatment Panel III guidelines. Circulation 2004;110:227–239.
104. Haffner SM. Management of dyslipidemia in adults with diabetes: technical review. Diabetes Care 1998;21:160–178.
105. Haffner SM, Alexander CM, Cook TJ, et al. for the Scandinavian Simvastatin Survival Study Group. Reduced coronary events in simvastatin-treated patients with coronary heart disease and diabetes or impaired glucose levels: subgroup analyses in the Scandinavian Simvastatin Survival Study. Arch Intern Med 1999;159:2661–2628.
106. Heart Protection Study Collaborative Group. MRC/BHF Heart Protection Study of cholesterol-lowering with simvastatin in 5963 people with diabetes; a randomized placebo-controlled trial. Lancet 2003;361:2005–2015.
107. Hoogwerf, BJ, Waness A, Cressman M, et al. for the Post CABG Trial Investigators. Effects of aggressive cholesterol lowering on clinical and angiographic outcomes in patients with diabetes mellitus: post CABG trial. Diabetes 1999;48:1289–1294.
108. Kasiske B. Hyperlipidemia in patients with chronic renal disease. Am J Kidney Dis 1998;32:S142–S156.
109. Koskinen P, Manttari M, Manninen V, Huttunen JK, Heinonen OP, Frick MH. Coronary heart disease incidence in NIDDM patients in the Helsinki Heart Study. Diabetes Care 1992;15:820–825.
110. The Long-Term Intervention with Pravastatin in Ischaemic Disease (LIPID) Study Group. Prevention of cardiovascular events and death with pravastatin in patients with coronary heart disease and a broad range of initial cholesterol levels. N Engl J Med 1998;339:1349–1357.
111. American Diabetes Association. Aspirin therapy in diabetes. American Diabetes Association: clinical practice recommendations. Diabetes Care 2004;27(Suppl 1):S73–S74.
112. The Post Coronary Artery Bypass Graft Trial Investigators. The effect of aggressive lowering of low density lipoprotein cholesterol levels and low dose anticoagulation on obstructive changes in saphenous-vein coronary-artery bypass grafts [published erratum appears in N Engl J Med 1997;337:1859]. N Engl J Med 1997;336:153–162.
113. Pyörälä K, Pedersen TR, Kjekshus J, Faergeman O, Olsson AG, Thorgeirsson G. Cholesterol lowering with simvastatin improves prognosis of diabetic patients with coronary heart disease. A subgroup analysis of the Scandinavian Simvastatin Survival Study (4S) [published erratum appears in Diabetes Care 1997;20:1048]. Diabetes Care 1997;20:614–620.
114. Rubins HB, Robins SJ, Collins D, et al. for the Veterans Affairs High-Density Lipoprotein Cholesterol Intervention Trial Study Group. Gemfibrozil for the secondary prevention of coronary heart disease in men with low levels of high-density lipoprotein cholesterol. N Engl J Med 1999;341:410–418.
115. Sacks FM, Pfeffer MA, Moye LA, et al. The effect of pravastatin on coronary events after myocardial infarction in patients with average cholesterol levels. Cholesterol and Recurrent Events Trial Investigators. N Engl J Med 1996;335:1001–1009.
116. Scandinavian Simvastatin Survival Study (4S). Randomized trial of cholesterol lowering in 4444 patients with coronary heart disease: the Scandinavian Simvastatin Survival Study (4S). Lancet 1994;344:1383–1389.
117. Sever PS, Dahlof B, Poulter NR, et al. Prevention of coronary and stroke events with atorvastatin in hypertensive patients who have average or lowering-than-average cholesterol concentrations, in the Anglo-Scandinavian Cardiac Outcomes Trial—Lipid Lowering Arm (ASCOT-LLA): a multicentre randomized controlled trial. Lancet 2003;361:1149–1158.

118. Sever PS, Poulter NR, Dahlof B, et al. for the ASCOT investigators. Reduction in cardiovascular events with atorvastatin in 2,532 patients with type 2 diabetes: Anglo-Scandinavian Cardiac Outcomes Trial—Lipid-lowering arm (ASCOT-LLA). Diabetes Care 2005;28:1151–1157.
119. Shepherd J, Cobbe M, Ford I, et al. for the West of Scotland Coronary Prevention Study Group. Prevention of coronary heart disease with pravastatin in men with hypercholesterolemia. N Engl J Med 1995;333:1301–1307.
120. Shepherd J, Blauw GJ, Murphy MB, et al. Pravastatin in elderly individuals at risk of vascular disease (PROSPER): a randomized controlled trial. Lancet 2002;360:162–130.
121. Vijan S, Hayward RA. Pharmacologic lipid-lowering therapy in type 2 diabetes mellitus: background paper for the American College of Physicians. Ann Intern Med 2004;140:644–649.
122. Turner R, Cull C, Holman R for the United Kingdom Prospective Diabetes Study Group. United Kingdom Prospective Diabetes Study 17: a 9-year update of a randomized controlled trial on the effect of improved metabolic control on complications in non-insulin-dependent diabetes mellitus. Ann Int Med 1996;124:136–145.
123. Alderman MH, Cohen H, Roque R, Madhavan S. Effect of long-acting and short-acting calcium antagonists on cardiovascular outcomes in hypertensive patients. Lancet 1997;349:594–598.
124. The ALLHAT Officers and Coordinators for the ALLHAT Collaborative Research Group. Major cardiovascular events in hypertensive patients randomized to doxazosin vs chlorthalidone: the Antihypertensive and Lipid-Lowering Treatment to Prevent Heart Attack Trial (ALLHAT). JAMA 2000;283:1967–1975.
125. The ALLHAT Officers and Coordinators for the ALLHAT Collaborative Research Group. Major outcomes in high-risk hypertensive patients randomized to angiotensin-converting enzyme inhibitor or calcium channel blocker vs diuretic: the Antihypertensive and Lipid-Lowering Treatment to Prevent Heart Attack Trial (ALLHAT). JAMA 2002;288:2981–2997.
126. Borhani NO, Mercuri M, Borhani PA, et al. Final outcome results of the multicenter isradipine diuretic atherosclerosis study. JAMA 1996;276:785–791.
127. Curb JD, Pressel SL, Cutler JA, et al. Effect of diuretic-based antihypertensive treatment on cardiovascular disease risk in older diabetic patients with isolated systolic hypertension. JAMA 1996;276:1886–1892.
128. Dahlöf B, Devereux RB, Kjeldsen SE for the LIFE Study Group. Cardiovascular morbidity and mortality in the Losartan Intervention for Endpoint reduction in hypertension study (LIFE): a randomized trial against atenolol. Lancet 2002;359:995–1003.
129. Estacio RO, Jeffers BW, Hiatt WR, Biggerstaff SL, Gifford, N, Schrier RX. The effect of nisoldipine as compared with enalapril on cardiovascular outcomes in patients with non-insulin-dependent diabetes and hypertension. N Engl J Med 1998;338:645–652.
130. Hansson L, Znachetti A Carruthers SG, et al. Effect of intensive blood-pressure lowering and low-dose aspirin in patients with hypertension: principal results of the Hypertension Optimal Treatment (HOT) randomized trial. Lancet 1998;351:1755–1762.
131. Jonas M, Reicher-Reiss H, Boyko V, et al. Usefulness of beta-blocker therapy in patients with non-insulin-dependent diabetes mellitus and coronary artery disease. Bezafibrate Infarction Prevention (BIP) Study Group. Am J Cardiol 1996;77:1273–1277.
132. Joint National Committee (JNC-VII). The seventh report of the Joint National Committee on prevention, detection, evaluation and treatment of high blood pressure. JAMA 2003;289:2560–2572.
133. Psaty BM, Heckbert SR, Koepsell TD, et al. The risk of myocardial infarction associated with antihypertensive drug therapies. JAMA 1995;274:620–625.
134. SHEP Cooperative Research Group. Prevention of stroke by antihypertensive drug treatment in older persons with isolated systolic hypertension: final results of the Systolic Hypertension in the Elderly Program (SHEP). JAMA 1991;265:3255–3264.
135. Tuomilehto J, Rastenyte D, Birkenhager WH, et al. Effects of calcium-channel blockade in older patients with diabetes and systolic hypertension. Systolic Hypertension in Europe Trial Investigators. New Engl J Med 1999;340:677–684.
136. UK Prospective Diabetes Study (UKPDS) Group. Intensive blood-glucose control with sulphonylureas or insulin compared with conventional treatment and risk of complications in patients with type 2 diabetes (UKPDS 33) Lancet 1998;352:837–853.
137. UK Prospective Diabetes Study (UKPDS) Group. Effect of intensive blood-glucose control with metformin on complications in overweight patients with type 2 diabetes (UKPDS 34). Lancet 1998;352:854–865.
138. UK Prospective Diabetes Study (UKPDS) Group. Tight blood pressure control and risk of macrovascular and microvascular complications in type 2 diabetes: (UKPDS 38). BMJ 1998;317(7160): 703–713.

139. Colwell JA. Aspirin therapy in diabetes [technical review]. Diabetes Care 1997;20:1767–1771.
140. ETDRS Study Group. Aspirin effects on mortality and morbidity in patients with diabetes mellitus—Early Treatment Diabetic Retinopathy Study Report—14. JAMA 1992;268:1292–1300.
141. Fox KM, European Trial on Reduction of Cardiac Events with Perindopril in Stable Coronary Artery Disease Investigators. Efficacy of perindopril in reduction of cardiovascular events among patients with stable coronary artery disease: randomized, double-blind, placebo-controlled trial (the EUROPA study). Lancet 2003;362:782–788.
142. Bosch J, Lonn E, Pogue J, Arnold JM, Dagenais GR, Yusuf S, HOPE/HOPE-TOO Study Investigators. Long-term effects of ramipril on cardiovascular events and on diabetes: results of the HOPE study extension. Circulation 2005;112:1339–1346.
143. The HOPE Study Investigators. The HOPE (Heart Outcomes Prevention Evaluation) Study: the design of a large, simple randomized trial of an angiotensin-converting enzyme inhibitor (ramipril) and vitamin E in patients at high risk of cardiovascular events. Can J Cardiol 1996;12:127–137.
144. The Heart Outcomes Prevention Evaluation Study Investigators. Effects of an angiotensin-converting-enzyme inhibitor, ramipril, on death from cardiovascular causes, myocardial infarction, and stroke in high-risk patients. N Engl J Med 2000;342:145–153.
145. The Heart Outcomes Prevention Evaluation Study Investigators. Vitamin E supplementation and cardiovascular events in high-risk patients. N Engl J Med 2000;342:154–160.
146. The Heart Outcomes Prevention Evaluation Study Investigators. The MICRO-HOPE Study: rationale and design of a large study to evaluate the renal and cardiovascular effects of an ACE inhibitor and vitamin E in high-risk patients with diabetes. Diabetes Care 1996;19:1225–1228.
147. The Heart Outcomes Prevention Evaluation Study Investigators. Effects of ramipril on cardiovascular and microvascular outcomes in people with diabetes mellitus: results of the HOPE and MICRO-HOPE study. Lancet 2000;355:253–259.
148. The HOPE and HOPE-TOO Trial Investigators. Effects of long-term vitamin E supplementation on cardiovascular events and cancer: a randomized controlled trial. JAMA 2005;293:1138–1147.
149. Wilson PWF, Kannel WB. Epidemiology of hyperglycemia and atherosclerosis. In: Ruderman N, Williamson J, Brownlee M, eds. Hyperglycemia, Diabetes and Vascular Disease. Oxford University Press, New York, 1992.
150. Selvin E, Marinopoulos S, Berkenblit G, et al. Meta-analysis: glycosylated hemoglobin and cardiovascular disease in diabetes mellitus. Ann Intern Med 2004;141:421–431.
151. Reaven GM. Role of insulin resistance in human disease. Diabetes 1988;37:1495–1507.
152. Chiasson JL, Josse RG, Hunt JA, et al. The efficacy of acarbose in the treatment of patients with non-insulin-dependent diabetes mellitus. Ann Int Med 1994;121:928–935.
153. American Diabetes Association. Smoking and Diabetes. American Diabetes Association: clinical practice recommendations. Diabetes Care 2004;27(Suppl 1):S74–S75.
154. Ohkkubo Y, Kishikawa H, Araki E, et al. Intensive insulin therapy prevents the progression of diabetic microvascular complications in Japanese patients with non-insulin-dependent diabetes mellitus: a randomized prospective 6-year study. Diabetes Res Clin Pract 1995;28:103–117.
155. Knatterud GL, Klimt CR, Goldner MG, et al. The University Group Diabetes Program: effects of hypoglycemic agents on vascular complications in patients with adult-onset diabetes, VIII. Evaluation of insulin therapy: final report. Diabetes 1982;31(Suppl 15):1–79.
156. Abraira C, Emanuele N, Colwell J, et al. Glycemic control and complications in type II diabetes: design of the feasibility trial. Diabetes Care 1995;15:1560–1571.
157. Malmberg K, Ryden L, Efendic S, et al. Randomized trial of insulin-glucose infusion followed by subcutaneous insulin treatment in diabetic patients with acute myocardial infarction (DIGAMI study): effects on mortality at 1 year. J Am Coll Cardiol 1995;26:57–65.
158. Malmberg KL, Ryden L, Wedel H, et al. for the DIGAMI 2 Investigators Intense metabolic control by means of insulin in patients with diabetes mellitus and acute myocardial infarction (DIGAMI 2): effects on mortality and morbidity. Eur Heart J 2005;26:650–661.
159. The Field Study Investigators. Effects of long-term fenofibrate therapy on cardiovacul events in 9795 people with type 2 diabetes mellitus (the FIELD study): randomised controlled trial. Lancet 2005;366:1849–1861.
160. Tatti P, Pahor M, Byrington RP, et al. outcome results of the fosinopril versus amlodipine cardiovascular events randomized trial (FACET) in patients iwth hypertension and NIDDM. Diabetes Care 1998;21:597–603.

161. Braunwald E, Domanski MJ, Fowler SE, et al. for the PEACE Trial Investigators. Angiotensin-converting-enzyme inhibition in stable coronary artery disease. N Engl J Med 2004;351:2058–2068.

162. Koshiyama H, Shimono D, Kuwamura N, Minamikawa J, Nakamura Y. Inhibitory effect of pioglitazone on carotid arterial wall thickness in type 2 diabetes. J Clin Endo Metab 2001;86:3452–3456.

163. Sidhu JS, Kaposzta Z, Markus HS, Kaski JC. Effect of rosiglitazone on common carotid intima-mediated thickness progression in coronary artery disease patients without diabetes mellitus. Arterioscler Thromb Vasc Biol 2004;24:930–934.

164. Tang HWH, Francis GS, Hoogwerf B, Young JB. Fluid retention following initiation of thiazolidinedione therapy in patients with established chronic heart failure. J Am Coll Cardiol 2003;41: 1394–1398.

165. Kendall DM, Riddle MC, Rosenstock J, et al. Effects of exenatide (exendin-4) on glycemic control over 30 weeks in patients with type 2 diabetes treated with metformin and a sulfonylurea. Diabetes Care 2005;28:1083–1091.

166. DeFronzo FA, Ratner RE, Han J, et al. Effects of exenatide (exendin-4) on glycemic control and weight over 30 weeks in metformin-treated patients with type 2 diabetes. Diabetes Care 2005;28:1092–1106.

167. Huang J, Hoogwerf BJ. Cholesterol guidelines update: more aggressive therapy for high risk patients. Cleve Clin J Med 2005;72:253–262.

168. Buchanan TA, Xiang AH, Peters RK, et al. Preservation of pancreatic beta-cell function and prevention of type 2 diabetes by pharmacological treatment of insulin resistance in high-risk Hispanic women. Diabetes 2002;51:2796–2803.

169. Chiasson JL, Josse RF, Gomis R, et al. for the STOP-NIDDM Trial Research Group. Acarbose treatment and the risk of cardiovascular disease and hypertension inpatients with impaired glucose tolerance: the STOP-NIDDM trial. JAMA 2003;290:486–494.

170. Knowler WC, Barrett-Connor E, Fowler SE, et al. for the Diabetes Prevention Program Research Group. Reduction in the incidence of type2 diabetes with lifestyle intervention or metformin. N Engl J Med 2002;346:393–403.

171. Knowler WC, Hamman RF, Edelstein SL for the Diabetes Prevention Program Research Group. Prevention of type 2 diabetes with troglitazone in the Diabetes Prevention Program. Diabetes 2005;54:1150–1156.

172. Tuomilehto J, Lindstom J, Eriksson JF, et al. for the Finnish Diabetes Prevention Study Group. Prevention of type diabetes mellitus by changes in lifestyle among subjects with impaired glucose tolerance. N Engl J Med 2001;344:1343–1350.

173. Chiasson JL, Josse RG, Gomis R, for the STOP-NIDDM Trial Research Group. Acarbose for prevention of type 2 diabetes mellitus: the STOP-NIDDM randomized trial. Lancet 2002;359:2072–2077.

174. Hanefeld M, Cagatary M, Petrowitsch T, et al. Acarbose reduces the risk for myocardial infarction in type 2 diabetic patients: meta-analysis of seven long-term studies. Eur Heart J 2004;24:10–16.

175. Pepine CJ, Cooper-DeHoff RM. Cardiovascular therapies and risk for development of diabetes (Viewpoint). J Am Coll Cardiol 2004;44:509–512.

176. Yusuf S, Gerstein H, Hoogwerf B, et al. for the HOPE Study Investigators: ramipril and the development of diabetes JAMA 2001;286:1882–1889.

177. Vermes E, Cucharme A, Bourassa MG, et al. for Studies of Left Ventricular Dysfunction. Enalapril reduces the incidence of diabetes in patients with chronic heart failure: insight from the Studies of Left Ventricular Dysfunction (SOLVD). Circulation 2003;107:1291–1296.

178. Garg A, Grundy SM. Management of dyslipidemia in NIDDM. [Review] [103 refs] Diabetes Care 1990;13:153–169.

179. The Expert Committee on the Diagnosis and Classification of Diabetes Mellitus. Report of the expert committee on the diagnosis and classification of diabetes mellitus. Diabetes Care 1997;20:1183–1197.

180. Expert Panel on Detection, Evaluation, and Treatment of High Blood Cholesterol in Adults. Executive summary of the third report of the National Cholesterol Educaiton Program (NCEP) expert panel on the detection, evaluation, and treatment of high blood cholesterol in adults (Adult Treatment Panel III). JAMA 2001;285:2486–2497.

181. National Cholesterol Education Program (NCEP), Expert Panel on Detection, Evaluation, and Treatment of High Blood Cholesterol in Adults (ATP III) Third report of the National Cholesterol Educaiton Program (NCEP) expert panel on the detection, evaluation, and treatment of high blood cholesterol in adults (Adult Treatment Panel III) final report. Circulation 2002;106:3143–3421.

182. Grundy SM, Cleeman JI, Merz CN, et al. Implications of recent clinical trials for the National Cholesterol Education Program Adult Treatment Panel III guidelines. Circulation 2004;110:227–239.

8 Exercise in the Prevention of Coronary Artery Disease

Gordon G. Blackburn, PhD

CONTENTS

INTRODUCTION

Coronary artery disease (CAD) is a chronic, multifactor disease that has powerful contributing genetic components as well as strong lifestyle components that increase the risk for the development and progression of the disease. Risk factors for CAD have been historically divided into nonmodifiable, primary modifiable, and secondary modifiable factors. The primary focus of medicine has been on the treatment of established CAD, and preventive efforts have more aggressively addressed areas in which direct pharmacological intervention is available *(1)* *(see* Table 1). This is especially evident with respect to hypertension, hyperlipidemia, and antiplatelet aggregation therapy.

For centuries, the medical community has supported the role of regular, moderate exercise as means of maintaining health and preventing disease. Scientific data, collected extensively in the last half of the 20th century, has repeatedly validated this concept. Most studies have been underpowered, and no single randomized clinical trial has definitively demonstrated the benefits of exercise in the prevention of CAD. However, the data supporting the benefits of exercise in reducing the risk of development and progression of CAD are so striking that multiple national health care agencies and organizations have issued recent position statements regarding the benefits and recommendations for regular physical activity as a strategy to reduce the risk of CAD. These have included the Centers for Disease Control and Prevention *(2)*, the American Heart Association *(3)*, the National Institutes of Health *(4)*, the Surgeon General *(5)*, and the American College of Sports Medicine *(6)*. The evidence of the association between sedentary living and the development of heart disease is so strong that the American Heart Association moved "sedentary

From: *Contemporary Cardiology: Preventive Cardiology:*
Insights Into the Prevention and Treatment of Cardiovascular Disease, Second Edition
Edited by: J. M. Foody © Humana Press Inc., Totowa, NJ

Table 1
Estimates of Levels of Utilization of Risk Reduction
Measures Patients Surviving an MI in the United States in 1996

Exercise (cardiac rehabilitation)	<10%
Smoking cessation	20%
Estrogen replacement (women)	20%
Cholesterol-lowering diet	20%
Cholesterol-lowering drug	30%
β-blocker therapy	40%
ACE inhibitor therapy	60%
Aspirin therapy	70%

lifestyle" into the primary modifiable" risk category in 1992, stating that "inactivity increases the risk of CAD" and regular exercise can help to control blood lipid abnormalities, control obesity, independently but modestly lower blood pressure in the hypertensive patient, and lower coronary mortality *(7)*. However, despite half a century of recurrent scientific findings outlining the benefits of exercise both for primary and secondary prevention, our society remains remarkably sedentary, and the use of cardiac rehabilitation programs abysmally low. It has been estimated that 20% of the North American population is totally sedentary and 60% have no regular exercise. It has also been estimated that only 20 to 25% of the North American population exercise appropriately to achieve the desired benefits attributed to an active lifestyle.

EXERCISE AND PRIMARY PREVENTION

Modern epidemiological studies investigating the relationship between activity and the development of CAD began with the report by Morris and colleagues *(8)* looking at a large population of civil servants from England. The authors compared CAD rates between sedentary bus drivers and the more active conductors, who at that time walked throughout the double-decker buses collecting fares. Comparisons were also made between active postal workers, who walked, delivering letters, and the more sedentary clerks. In both groups, the active cohort had half of the age-adjusted incidence for myocardial infarction (MI), and the sedentary cohort was at twice the risk for sudden or early death after an MI. Although these studies were later revealed to have significant design flaws that may have accounted for a higher-risk population being hired for the sedentary jobs, it suggested the positive relationship between regular activity and decreased risk of developing heart disease. However, as stated by Oberman *(9)*, "The observed association between inactivity and CAD in the prospective studies could represent several possible hypotheses:

1. Exercise protects against CAD.
2. Exercise indirectly reduces the risk of CAD through changes in other risk factors.
3. Subclinical disease prevents people from exercising vigorously at work or during leisure.
4. People predisposed to CAD prefer sedentary activities.
5. Social, cultural, and other factors determine both activity levels and likelihood of CAD.

Although epidemiological studies cannot definitively determine a cause-and-effect relationship, if the first hypothesis is not true, one would expect to see variation in the

benefits of exercise on the prevention of CAD between studies, the impact of exercise should disappear if other risk factors are not affected by exercise, changes in physical activity levels should not effect CAD risk, there should not be a dose–response effect of exercise on reduction of CAD, and the relationship between physical activity and CAD should vary between cultures and job types.

A homogeneous lifestyle and standard of living with varying levels of occupational activity was studied in men and women living on kibbutzim (collective settlements) in Israel. More than 5000 men and 5000 women were studied to determine the relationship between activity and CAD risk. The population was divided into those who spent less than 80% of their work time seated and those who spent more than 80% of their work time seated. Although the active population had a higher caloric intake of food, there was no difference between cholesterol levels of the groups. The risk of MI was 2.5 times greater for the sedentary man and 1.8 times greater for the sedentary woman. The sedentary kibbutz member was also at greater risk for death from CAD (2.0 times increase for men and 3.0 times increase for women). Controlling for lifestyle and selected risk factors, the protective benefit of physical activity was supported *(10)*.

The protective role of exercise was also supported in a large cohort of longshoremen, in the United States. This longitudinal study objectively measured energy requirements of various job tasks and tracked job assignments for four age cohorts (35–44, 45–54, 55–64, and 65–74 yr at entry into the study in 1951). Tasks were classified into three categories: high (5.2–7.5 kcal/min), intermediate (2.4–5.0 kcal/min), and light (1.5–2.0 kcal/min). Subjects were contacted annually to evaluate job energy requirements and underwent repeated multiphase screening for cigarette smoking, hypertension, history of MI, obesity, abnormal glucose metabolism, and higher cholesterol level during a 21-yr period. All subjects were followed for 22 yr or until age 75 yr, or death. During the follow-up period, fewer than 1% of participants were lost to follow-up.

The age-adjusted coronary death rates were 26.9, 46.3, and 49.0 per 10,000 work-years for those in the heavy, moderate, and light caloric output jobs, respectively. Cigarette smoking, hypertension, and history of a previous MI all added to the risk of a fatal heart attack. However, differences in mortality rates persisted after correction for risk factors for CAD by multiple logistic analyses. To account for a drop in activity level secondary to subclinical disease, men with job transfers within 6 mo of death were excluded from the analysis without affecting the relationship between higher activity level and lower CAD rates *(11–13)*.

If a genetic predisposition exists that excludes individuals prone to CAD from exercise, it could be argued that athletes should be at lower risk for CAD than nonathletes. However, if it is habitual activity that offers a protective effect, then regular daily activity, carried on throughout life should be a key factor in reducing CAD risk. Paffenbarger and colleagues *(14)* studied the relationship between college athleticism and postcollege physical exercise in 16,936 Harvard alumni. The physical exam records of students who entered Harvard between 1916 and 1950 were analyzed along with a questionnaire regarding postcollege physical activity. Physical activity was standardized based on specific activities and estimated weekly caloric expenditures were calculated. During the follow-up period from 1962 to 1972 there were 572 first-time heart attacks, and from 1962 to 1978, there were 1413 total deaths. Student athletic participation did not predict low CAD risk, although habitual postcollege exercise did. A strong, inverse, dose-related correlation was observed between exercise level and death from all causes, cardiovascu-

lar disease (CVD) and respiratory disease, with individuals expending more than 2000 kcal/wk at the lowest risk. In addition, the exercise benefit was independent of other risk factors (smoking, obesity, weight gain, hypertension, and family history). Sedentary alumni (<2000 kcal/wk expended in activity) were at a 49% greater risk for heart attack as compared with the most active alumni.

Summary papers, outlining the risk of sedentary lifestyle and increased risk of developing CAD were published in 1987 and 1990. The article by Powell and colleagues (15) reviewed 43 prospective studies that investigated the relationship between the primary risk for CAD and sedentary lifestyles. The quality of the study designs were evaluated and rated. The authors reported that, for studies with good scientific design, a strong inverse relationship between physical activity and CAD mortality was consistently observed, with the sedentary population being at twice the risk of the active population. In addition, they found the risk of a sedentary lifestyle to be similar to that of other risk factors, such as elevated cholesterol, cigarette smoking, and hypertension. The studies reported in Powell (15) were reevaluated, along with eight more-recent studies using meta-analysis (16), and revealed similar findings regardless of whether activity was performed on the job or during leisure time.

Not only has daily activity been associated with a reduction in CAD risk, but fitness level has also been correlated with lower mortality levels from CAD. Ekelund and colleagues (17) reported on data from the Lipid Research Clinics in which 4276 men between the ages of 30 and 69 yr of age were followed for an average of 8.5 yr. For patients without clinical evidence of CAD and who were not taking cardiovascular drugs, there was approximately a three times greater risk of both cardiovascular and CAD death in the less-fit group, even after adjustment for age and cardiovascular risk factors.

Most studies have focused on the benefits of exercise and fitness in reducing CAD risk in men. Blair and colleagues (18) evaluated the impact of fitness on both all-cause death, CAD death, and cancer death in 10,224 men and 3120 women. All individuals were relatively healthy, with no known CVD at entry into the study. Each individual underwent a physical exam, blood work, and a maximal treadmill exercise test. Based on the results of the exercise test, subjects were assigned to a fitness level, adjusted for age, and based on gender and treadmill time. Subjects were followed for an average of 8 yr, during which time there were 283 deaths in the group. Age-adjusted rates of death were calculated, with a strong inverse relationship observed between fitness level and mortality. In comparison to the most-fit group of men, the least-fit group had a 3.4 times greater risk of all-cause death, and, for women, the risk was 4.7 times greater for the least-fit group. Lower mortality rates from CVD and cancer were also observed for both the most-fit men and women, and the trends remained significant after adjustment for age, smoking, cholesterol, systolic blood pressure, fasting blood glucose level, family history of CAD, and follow-up interval. It was also observed that decline in death rates associated with higher fitness levels was more pronounced in the older individuals.

The benefit of regular activity for the elderly to reduce the risk of primary CVD was further supported by the recent findings from a follow-up study to the Honolulu Heart Program (19), in which 707 nonsmoking retired men between the ages of 61 and 81 yr of age at entry into the study were evaluated for walking habits. The gentlemen were followed for 12 yr, and the primary endpoint evaluated for this study was mortality. At the end of the study period, there were 208 deaths, with a strong inverse relationship observed between distance walked and all-cause death, coronary heart disease deaths,

and cancer deaths. Individuals who walked less than 1 mile per day had a 1.8 times greater risk for all-cause death, a 2.6 times greater risk for coronary heart disease death, and a 2.4 times greater risk for cancer death as compared with those who walked more than 2 miles per day. The inverse relationship between distance walked and mortality remained significant even after adjustment for age, overall activity levels, and other risk factors. These findings suggest that the benefits of activity are dose related and can be beneficial for older men.

Although point estimates of physical fitness have repeatedly demonstrated an increased risk associated with a low fitness level (17,20–23), it can always be argued that genetic factors or subclinical disease limit the fitness level and, therefore, it is that relationship rather that fitness itself that accounts for the relationship with mortality. If changes in fitness over time were associated with changes in CAD risk, the cause-and-effect association between fitness and CAD would be strengthened. To test this hypothesis, Blair and colleagues (24) studied 9777 men who were initially seen for preventive physical exams that included an exercise test. The participants in the study ranged from 20 to 82 yr old at intake. All subjects returned for a second exam and exercise test approx 4.9 yr after the first visit and were followed an average of 5.1 yr after the second exam. Of the 9777 men, 6819 were classified as healthy and 2958 were classified as unhealthy because of previous MI, hypertension, diabetes, cancer, abnormal resting electrocardiogram, or abnormal exercise electrocardiogram. All subjects were followed throughout the study and the relationship between fitness change and mortality was evaluated.

Subjects who maintained a fit level at both exams had the lowest risk of mortality and those who were classified as least fit at both exams had the highest risk of mortality. This was true for all-cause as well as cardiovascular mortality. However, of greater significance is the fact that those who went from the unfit to fit category from the first exam to the second exam had a 44% reduction in all-cause mortality and a 52% reduction in cardiovascular mortality. The improvement in fitness was associated with a reduction in death rates even after adjusting for health status, age, and risk factors.

Longitudinal studies demonstrating an inverse relationship between fitness levels or activity patterns and coronary mortality strengthen the concept of a cause-and-effect relationship, but underlying genetic or early environmental biases cannot be controlled for. However, evaluation of activity and mortality in twin pairs can control for both of these issues. Such a study was conducted by Kujala and colleagues (25). In this study same-sex twin pairs (7925 men and 7977 women) between the ages of 25 and 64 yr were followed for mortality from 1977 to 1994. Leisure-time physical activity level was evaluated by questionnaire in 1975 and again in 1981. Subjects were free of clinical disease at entry into the study and all subjects were able to exercise. Individuals were classified into one of three categories based on reported intensity and total volume of activity. Sedentary individuals reported no leisure time activity, whereas individuals who reported participating in activities at least as strenuous as vigorous walking, for at least 30 min on average per session and at least six times per month, were placed in the conditioning category. All others were placed in the occasional exercise category.

During the 17-yr follow-up period, 1253 subjects died. After adjusting for age and sex, the conditioning exercisers had a 43% reduction in mortality compared with the sedentary group, which is similar to previous non-twin-pair study findings. However, a more detailed analysis of 434 discordant twin deaths (only one of the twin pair died during follow-up), there was a 56% reduction in all-cause death favoring the conditioning

exercisers over the sedentary individual and 34% reduction for the occasional exercisers. The benefits of physical exercise persisted after controlling for age, sex, and other predictors of mortality. Even when genetic and early life familial factors are controlled, a reduction in mortality is associated with chronically higher levels of activity.

EXERCISE AND SECONDARY PREVENTION

The role of exercise in individuals with documented CAD has been investigated extensively since the early 1970s, with consistent findings with respect to safety, improved functional ability, and the relative reduction of both all-cause and cardiac mortality. However, all of the studies have been statistically underpowered with respect to mortality outcomes, limiting the statistical significance and clinical impact of exercise for individuals with CAD. It is estimated that only 11 to 38% of qualifying patients participate in cardiac rehabilitation programs *(26)*.

Functional Capacity Improvement

An excellent summary of exercise trials in CAD patients is presented in the Clinical Practice Guidelines for Cardiac Rehabilitation *(26)*. Fourteen randomized trials from the United States and 21 foreign trials were reviewed. Exercise training was found to improve functional level in patients with catheterization-documented CAD, as well as after MI, coronary artery bypass grafting, and percutaneous transluminal coronary angioplasty. The extent of the improvement varied based on the frequency, intensity, and duration of exercise, as well as the time interval during which training was conducted. It is also important to note that no deterioration in exercise tolerance occurred in any patient who underwent exercise training.

Physical Training and Mortality

Numerous trials have been conducted in the United States and internationally, designed to look at exercise and mortality in a CAD population. However, only one trial focusing on activity had more than 1000 patients entering the exercise arm *(27)*. This pales to the 3837 patients randomized to β-blocker or placebo in the β-Blocker Heart Attack Trial *(28)*. Low patient numbers and few endpoints have limited the statistical significance of studies looking at exercise and CAD mortality.

Kentala reported one of the first randomized, controlled studies looking at exercise and mortality after MI *(29)*. In a 6 to 8 wk event, 152 patients were randomized to either exercise three times per week for 20 min per session or consultation once per week. In a 12-mo follow-up period, there were 11 deaths in each of the groups.

Kallio and colleagues *(30)* reported on the results of a multifactorial intervention program of education, antismoking and dietary advice, discussions regarding psychosocial problems, and a supervised cycle activity program, as compared with the usual care in 375 post-MI patients. The patients were randomized to the intervention group or usual care and followed for 3 yr. The cumulative mortality in the intervention group was 18.6% as compared with 29.4% in the usual care group ($p < 0.02$). This represented a 37% reduction in mortality for the treatment group.

The National Exercise and Heart Disease Project *(31)* was a multicenter study conducted in the United States. A total of 651 post-MI patients (2–36 mo after event) were randomized to either usual care or exercise. The exercise prescription was set to 85% of

the peak heart rate achieved on the entry exercise test. Exercising patients were monitored by electrocardiography for the first 8 wk and then were allowed to exercise in a supervised gym setting for the next 34 mo. The patients performed interval exercise in the lab for 24 min total and 15 min of steady-state aerobic activity in the gym, followed by 25 min of games. Patients were encouraged to exercise three times per week. At the end of the study period, the cumulative mortality rate for the exercise group was 4.6 vs 7.3% for the control group. These differences were not statistically significant, but the exercise group had a 37% reduction in mortality.

A recent report on the 19-yr follow-up of long-term survival of patients in the National Exercise and Heart Disease Project revealed a steady decline in all-cause mortality risk estimates for the exercise group compared with the control subjects. The authors concluded that protective mechanisms associated with exercise may be short lived and suggested that to maintain the benefits of exercise it must be performed on a continuous, regular basis. Of note is the finding that for individuals who increased their functional capacity, regardless of study group, there was a consistent 8 to 14% reduction (per metabolic equivalent [MET]) increase in all-cause mortality at every follow-up period (32).

At the end of the 1980s, two meta-analyses were reported, each analyzing 21 randomized, controlled studies of cardiac rehabilitation and the impact on mortality. The findings of both studies were similar, revealing an approx 20 to 25% relative reduction in mortality, both all-cause and cardiovascular, for the exercise group as compared with the control group after a 3-yr follow-up period (33,34). The benefits in mortality were realized when exercise was started early after the event as well as late, but the benefit improved the longer the activity was maintained. No difference was observed between the exercise group and the control group for nonfatal infarcts at any follow-up period. The consistent, reproducible finding of reduced cardiac and all-cause mortality strongly argues for the increased use of regular activity as a component of any comprehensive risk reduction program.

Safety of Exercise

The benefits of regular, aerobic exercise has been repeatedly documented in both the primary and secondary preventive population. However, any truly effective therapeutic intervention must provide benefit without increasing morbidity or mortality. The most frequently voiced concerns regarding regular aerobic exercise is that it will precipitate or aggravate an orthopedic complication or trigger sudden death.

In a study reported by Panush and colleagues (35), 17 recreational runners, mean age 56 yr, were compared with age-matched, sedentary controls. There was no significant difference reported for problems with degenerative joint disease, osteoarthritis, joint pain, or joint swelling. For individuals with known osteoarthritis, regular, moderate intensity activity, such as walking, increased functional ability and, at the same time, decreased the amount of joint pain in the active participants as compared with the sedentary subjects (36). Overall, the incidence of injury in individuals involved in recreational activity, requiring medical care, has been estimated as low as 5% annually (37).

Regular moderate-intensity exercise is associated with decreased risk of cardiac mortality, and the incidence of sudden death associated with even vigorous exercise is low, at one death in 396,000 jogging hours (38) or one sudden coronary death in 25,000 marathoners per year (39). However, it is important to note that vigorous, high-intensity exercise does increase the risk of MI. Siscovick and colleagues studied 133 men with no

known previous history of CAD, who experienced a primary cardiac arrest during vigorous activity (40). For men with low levels of habitual physical activity, the relative risk of a cardiac arrest during vigorous exercise was 56 times greater than at other times. Even for men who were routinely active, the risk of cardiac arrest was increased five times during vigorous activity. However, the overall risk of cardiac risk (at rest and during vigorous exercise) was reduced by 40% for the routinely active man with respect to the sedentary man, thus supporting the overall benefit of routine exercise and the underlying risk of vigorous physical activity. Similar findings were reported by Mittleman and colleagues (41), who found that there was a 5.9 times greater likelihood of experiencing a MI after vigorous exercise (>6 METs), as compared with the likelihood of experiencing a MI after less vigorous activity or no activity. In addition, they found an inverse dose–response relationship in risk with respect to routine frequency of exercise, ranging from 107 times increased relative risk for individuals who exercised less than once per week, to 2.4 times increased risk for individuals who exercised five or more times per week.

The relative safety of individualized, moderate intensity exercise has also been documented in individuals with known CAD. Based on a survey of 167 cardiac rehabilitation programs, covering 51,303 patients during the first half of the 1980s, VanCamp and Peterson reported only 3 deaths, 21 cardiac arrests, and 8 nonfatal MIs (42). This equates to 1 cardiac arrest per 111,996 patient-hours, one MI per 293,990 patient-hours, and an amazingly infrequent 1 death per 783,972 patient-hours—the latter incidence being lower than that reported for sudden cardiac death associated with jogging for men with no known previous CAD (38). It is also important to note that there was no significant difference in the rates of events between patients who received continuous electrocardiogram monitoring or those who received intermittent monitoring. This suggests that it is the supervision of patients during individualized, moderate activity, rather than the extent of monitoring, that provides the safety during cardiac rehabilitation classes.

Initiating an Activity Program

The benefits of regular exercise are well-documented, and, although the risk associated with exercise is relatively small, it is real. The risk of cardiovascular and orthopedic complications increase both as individual risk of CAD increases and as the intensity of exercise increases. Therefore, it is appropriate that individuals about to embark on a regular activity program undergo some form of screening to minimize exercise-related complications. The extent of the evaluation should be dependent on the age of the individuals, their health status, and the intensity of the exercise they will engage in. The American College of Sports Medicine provides recommendations regarding screening evaluations and testing to guide health care providers involved in the development and administration of exercise prescriptions, outlined in Table 2 (43). It is important to note that for apparently healthy and asymptomatic at risk populations embarking on a moderate-intensity exercise program, a medical examination or exercise testing is not recommended, thus, removing a significant barrier for many individuals and not placing a major burden on the health care system.

Regarding exercise prescriptions, the graded-exercise test is conducted to provide far more information than simply the presence or absence of significant ST segment changes on the electrocardiogram or exertional angina. The MET level and rate-pressure product at onset of ST changes or symptoms, coupled with the heart rate and blood pressure response to exertion, as well as an accurate determination of peak METs or onset/exac-

Table 2
ACSM Recommendations for Medical Examination and Exercise Testing
Prior to Participation and Physician Supervision of Exercise Tests

Medical examination and clinical exercise test recommended before:

	Apparently healthy		Increased risk[a]	Known disease[b]	
	Younger[c]	Older	no symptoms	symptoms	
Moderate exercise (40–60% $VO_{2\ max}$)	No	No	No	Yes	Yes
Vigorous exercise (>60% VO_{2max})	No	Yes	Yes	Yes	Yes

Physician supervision recommended during exercise test:

	Apparently healthy		Increased risk	Known disease	
	Younger[c]	Older	no symptoms	symptoms	
Submaximal testing	No	No	No	Yes	Yes
Maximal testing	No	Yes	Yes	Yes	Yes

[a]Persons with two or more risk factors for CAD.
[b]Persons with known cardiac, pulmonary, or metabolic disease.
[c]<40 yr for men, <50 yr for women.

erbation of arrhythmias are all key variables to be considered and factored into the exercise prescription. It is also important to consider the impact of medications on the exercise response. Although it may be desirable to have β-blockers and nitrates held before diagnostic exercise tests to improve sensitivity, to evaluate typical hemodynamic and chronotropic responses during exertion it is desirable to have patients take all medications as normally prescribed before the graded-exercise test.

Mode of exercise testing and conduct of exercise testing are also key factors to consider if the exercise test is to be used to designing activity guidelines. For most individuals, walking-type activity yields the highest functional capacity and peak heart rate. The same person who undergoes a maximal cycle test is likely to achieve a peak functional capacity of approx 85% of that recorded for the treadmill, with a peak heart rate of 95% of that observed during the maximal walking test. For arm-crank exercise tests, the peak functional capacity falls even further, reaching only 50 to 70% of that measured on the treadmill. Peak heart rate also tends to be lower for arm exercise, as compared with treadmill exercise, reaching only 90% of the latter value *(44)*. These changes in chronotropic response and functional level between modes should be factored in when designing exercise prescriptions to avoid excessive or ineffective intensities. Because of the differences in response between modalities, it is recommended that the primary exercise mode be used as the exercise test modality whenever possible.

Test technique and patient population can also have a significant impact on the estimated functional capacity. Most standard nomograms used to estimate peak functional capacity from time and workload are based on young, healthy individuals who exercised without holding onto the treadmill bars *(45)*. Although these nomograms have been shown to be accurate for healthy, young- to middle-aged populations without orthopedic

limitations and not taking cardiac medications *(46)*, a significant overprediction of functional capacity can occur for the senior, clinical population taking medication *(47,48)*. These overestimations can be exaggerated even more if patients are allowed to hold onto the handrails of the treadmill during exercise tests. Peak functional capacity can be overestimated by up to 31% if patients are allowed to pull or even hold onto the front handrail. To achieve the most accurate estimation of functional capacity and minimize patient risk, it is recommended that patients walk, lightly touching the side handrail for balance during the treadmill exercise test *(49,50)*.

Once the patient has been cleared to begin an exercise, the specific components of the program can be addressed. Every activity session should be composed of a warm-up, a conditioning, and a cool-down period *(43)*.

The warm-up period initiates the exercise session and includes static and range-of-motion stretches as well as low-level aerobic activity at 25 to 40% of the individual's functional ability. These activities are designed to avoid musculoskeletal injury and allow for gradual hemodynamic and physiological adaptation to activity. The warm-up period should last between 5 and 15 min, depending on the orthopedic, metabolic, or cardiovascular restrictions of the exercising population.

The focus of the exercise prescription is the conditioning period. The conditioning period must address six key factors, with the emphasis on each area effected by the overall goal of the activity program: frequency, intensity, mode, duration, rate of progression, and compliance.

FREQUENCY

Recent guidelines regarding activity recommend that for cardiovascular benefit, overall risk reduction, and weight management, exercise be conducted on most days of the week. However, the frequency can vary from only three times per week to multiple sessions per day. The goal of the program, the schedule of the individual, and their current level of fitness all impact on frequency. In general, activity must be performed at least three times per week to gain the desired benefit, no matter what the goal. At lower levels of fitness, it may be necessary to increase the frequency of activity to 5 to 7 d per week to achieve a desirable caloric expenditure per week. For individuals with musculoskeletal or pulmonary limitations to activity or limited flexibility in their schedule, multiple sessions per day may be advisable. As a general rule, exercise for health purposes should be performed between a basal threshold of three times per week out to five times per week.

INTENSITY

Intensity of exercise is perhaps the hardest area to prescribe and monitor. It is also the most poorly understood component of the exercise prescription. It has been recommended that the exercise be performed at a "moderate" intensity. Based on the American College of Sports Medicine criteria, this would correspond to activities equivalent to 40 to 60% of peak oxygen uptake, with 40% appearing to be the threshold level below which no improvement in functional ability occurs. However, few individuals know their peak oxygen uptake and in apparently healthy, asymptomatic patients, the need for an exercise test is not indicated *(43)*.

Exercise intensity can be determined in several ways. One of the most common methods is based on a standard, linear, age-dependent chronotropic response to exercise. This assumes a standard age-dependent peak heart rate and a linear relationship between

oxygen uptake and heart rate. When both heart rate response and functional capacity are expressed as percentage of maximal ability, assuming rest levels to be baseline (i.e., resting heart rate equates to 0% and peak heart rate equates to 100%), the linear relationship can be assumed to be a 1:1 relationship, with the intercept passing through the origin. Therefore, when an individual is exercising at 60% of the heart rate reserve {[(peak heart rate – resting heart rate) × 0.6] + resting heart rate} they are exercising at approx 60% of their functional reserve *(51)*. For healthy individuals not taking cardiac medications, this method can be helpful in determining the appropriate intensity of aerobic activity. Accuracy of pulse palpation is critical to the usefulness of this method, and individuals unfamiliar with this skill are likely to require brief training. For those not interested in, or not capable of, palpating their pulse, the development of accurate heart rate monitors that easily provide constant pulse monitoring provides and alternative method to monitor exercise heart rate responses.

For individuals with documented coronary disease or symptoms in whom an exercise test is recommended before initiating an exercise program, the individual heart rate response to activity and actual peak heart rate can be determined. This provides the health care provider developing the exercise prescription with the information necessary to individualize the target heart rate range for exercise. The prescription is more specific to the patient's responses to activity, especially if the patient took all medications, as normally prescribed, before the exercise test.

Intensity can also be determined based on a more subjective, quantified approach, related to the individual's perception of exercise effort. The Rating of Perceived Exertion (RPE) scales were developed by Borg *(52,53)*. The scales provide numeric values with word anchors that the patient uses to rate the level of exertion they perceive for any given activity. The scales include the older, linear 6- to 20-point scale, based on the relationship between heart rate and perceived exertion and the newer logarithmic scale ranging from 0 to 10. Both scales are widely used and correlate well with the relative level of exertion. At an exercise intensity of 50 to 85% of oxygen uptake, most subjects rate the activity between 12 and 16 ("light" to "hard"). On the 10-point scale, a similar level of exertion would correspond to 3 to 6 ("moderate" to "hard").

The RPE method of guiding exercise intensity can be quickly introduced to an individual and can be easily applied during any type of activity. Although there are certain populations who rate activity disproportionately low or high as compared with the actual relative cost *(54)*, for most individuals, the RPE can effectively guide exercise intensity across a variety of exercise modalities *(55)*.

For individuals undergoing a graded-exercise test, the exercise intensity can be set based on the functional capacity or METs, predicted or measured. The relative exercise intensity range should be at least the threshold level of 40% and can range up to 85% of functional reserve, based on the goal of the program, the interest of the patient, and the patient's ability. The majority of individuals receive optimal return on their effort at intensities between 60 and 75% of functional ability.

To prescribe activities based on METs requires a good understanding of exercise and work physiology so that comparable work levels can be calculated or identified for a variety of modalities. Tables outlining the MET cost of a variety of activities have been published to aid the clinician or exercising individual to identify the cost of activities. One such table is displayed here, dividing activities into three categories based on MET ranges (*see* Table 3).

Table 3
Physical Activities Grouped by MET Ranges

A 3–4 Mets	B 5–6 Mets	C 7–8 Mets
Cycling <8 mph	Cycling 8–10 mph	Cycling 11–12 mph
Cycling, stationary— very light effort	Cycling, stationary— light effort	Cycling, stationary— moderate effort
Dancing, slow pace (aerobic, ballroom)	Dance, moderate pace (folk, square, ballet)	Dancing, quick pace
Rowing, stationary 10 mph	Rowing, stationary 15 mph	Rowing, stationary 20 mph
Tennis, table	Tennis, doubles	Tennis, singles
Walking, level 2–3.5 mph	Walking 3.6–4.5 mph	Walk/job intervals
Water aerobics/walking	Swimming, leisure	Walking upstairs/stair stepper
		Swimming, laps
Bowling	Baseball/softball, nongame	Baseball/softball game
Billiards	Basketball, nongame	Basketball game
Croquet	Cross-country skiing <3 mph	Canoeing, 2–5 mph
Golf, driving range, riding cart	Golf, carrying, pulling clubs	Cross-country skiing, 3–4 mph
Horseback riding, walk	Sailing, small boat	
		Hiking
Horseshoe pitching	Skiing, downhill, beginner, moderate effort	
Shuffle board	Volleyball	Horseback riding, trot
Gardening, light (hand tools, planting)	Gardening, moderate (power tools, dig, rake, hoe)	Hockey, ice and/or field
Grass cutting, riding mower	Grass cutting, push power mower	In-line skating, slow
Housework, general cleaning woodwork	Hunting, small-game, light effort	Racquetball/paddleball, Car washing
		Grass cutting, push handmower
		Hunting, big game (no carcass dragging)
		Wood chopping

MODE

For both primary and secondary preventive care, the mode of activity recommended is one that is aerobic or rhythmical and repetitive in nature and uses large muscle groups and satisfies the necessary intensity requirement. There is no one mode of activity that is best, other than that the best activities are the ones that satisfy the components of the exercise prescription for the individual and are engaged in routinely. Common exercise modalities are included in Table 3.

DURATION

A minimum of 30 min of aerobic activity per day is recommended. Again the goal of the program and the individual's exercise history, functional ability, and schedule will all effect the daily duration. One of the goals of most exercise programs, from a preventive standpoint, is to increase the weekly caloric expenditure, targeting at least 2000 kcal/wk.

It will likely be necessary for sedentary individuals to gradually increase to this level, which can be accomplished by starting at the 30 min/session level and gradually increasing the duration until the target is accomplished. The frequency of activity will also impact weekly caloric expenditure. Assuming a fixed intensity, more-frequent exercise can be conducted for a shorter time at each session and still achieve the same weekly caloric expenditure.

Recently, emphasis has been directed at the potential benefits of multiple, shorter sessions per day. For some individuals, three 20-min sessions per day may be easier to accomplish than a single 60-min session. Certainly, multiple shorter sessions can provide benefit, but the threshold duration for each interval is unclear. Divided intervals of no shorter than 15 min each is recommended.

RATE OF PROGRESSION

As individuals embark on exercise programs, it is important to avoid overly aggressive progression of the exercise program. The rate of progression will depend on the individual's past exercise history, level of conditioning, comorbid conditions, and age. In general, the sedentary, deconditioned, elderly patient with multiple comorbid conditions will require longer to adapt to the activity, and progression, in absolute terms, will be slower. RPE and target heart rate ranges can be helpful in determining individual adaptation and targeting progression.

For the first several months in a program, progression will be somewhat rapid. However, after the first 4 to 6 mo of exercise, progression will slow as the individual enters a maintenance phase *(43)*.

COMPLIANCE

The benefits of appropriate, regular aerobic exercise, both in primary and secondary prevention patients, have been documented previously in this chapter. The key is that the activity be performed over the long term, however. Compliance with cardiac rehabilitation programs, a population that could be expected to be more highly motivated than those without known disease, has a compliance rate of 50 to 75% after 6 mo. To optimize compliance, it is necessary to develop activity plans that mesh with the individual's lifestyle and have a minimum number of barriers. In addition to education regarding the benefits of regular exercise, Oldridge recommends that compliance-enhancing strategies should include reinforcement control, stimulus control, and cognitive/self-control procedures *(56)*.

Each activity session should conclude with the cool-down period. This is essentially the opposite of the warm-up period, allowing the body to gradually transition from the more vigorous conditioning period to rest. During the cool-down period, activity should be gradually tapered down, rather than abruptly terminated. This prevents venous pooling, hypotension, and an abrupt, relative catecholamine surge that can cause arrhythmias. The cool-down period usually lasts from 3 to 10 min.

SUMMARY

Although no single, large, prospective trial has been conducted to decisively demonstrated the benefits of exercise in both the primary and secondary preventive population, the preponderance of the research supports the benefit in reducing future cardiovascular risk. The mechanism or mechanisms through which physical activity reduces this risk of

either developing or dying from CAD are unclear. Regardless of the mechanism, it is apparent that regular, aerobic activity should be addressed and optimized in all CAD preventive strategies. Development of an effective exercise program is likely to require more than a casual recommendation. Patients should be appropriately screened, based on their individual risk of complications associated with exercise, and individualized programs addressing frequency, intensity, mode, duration, and progression should be provided. In addition, as with all lifestyle and risk-reduction strategies, strategies to optimize long-term compliance should be incorporated into the management plan.

REFERENCES

1. Pearson TA, Peters TD. The treatment gap in coronary artery disease and heart failure: community standards and the post-discharge patient. Am J Cardiol 1997;80:45H–52H.
2. Pate RR, Pratt M, Blair SM, et al. Physical activity and public health: a recommendation from the Centers for Disease Control and Prevention and the American College of Sports Medicine. JAMA 1995;273:402–407.
3. Fletcher GF, Balady G, Blair SN, et al. Statement on exercise: benefits and recommendations for physical activity programs for all Americans. A statement for health professionals by the committee on exercise and cardiac rehabilitation of the council on clinical cardiology, American Heart Association. Circulation 1996;94:857–862.
4. NIH Consensus Conference. Physical activity and cardiovascular health. JAMA 1996;276:241–246.
5. Department of Health and Human Services. Physical Activity and Health: a Report for the Surgeon General: U.S. Department of Health and Human Services, Centers for Disease Control and Prevention, National Center for Chronic Disease Prevention and Health Promotion, 1996.
6. Pollock ML, Gaesser GA, Butcher JD, et al. The recommended quantity and quality of exercise for developing and maintaining cardiorespiratory and muscular fitness, and flexibility in health adults. Med Sci Sports Exere 1998;30:975–991.
7. Fletcher AF, Blair SN, Blumenthal J, et al. Statement on exercise: benefits and recommendations for physical activity programs for all Americans. Circulation 1992;86:340–344.
8. Morris JN, Heady JA, Raffle PAB, et al. Coronary heart disease and physical activity of work. Lancet 1953;2:1053–1057, 1111–1120.
9. Oberman A. Exercise and the primary prevention of cardiovascular disease. Am J Cardiol 1985;55:10D–20D.
10. Brunner D, Manelis G, Modan M, Levin S. Physical activity at work and the incidence of myocardial infarction, angina pectoris and death due to ischemic heart diasease: an epidemiological study in Israeli collective settlements (kibbutzim). J Chronic Dis 1974;27:217–233.
11. Paffenbarger RS, Hale WE. Work activity and coronary heart mortality. N Engl J Med 1975;292:545–550.
12. Paffenbarger RS, Hale WE, Brand RJ, Hyde RT. Work-energy level, personal characteristics and fatal heart attack: a birth-cohort effect. Am J Epidemiol 1977;105:200–213.
13. Brand RJ, Paffenbarger RS, Sholtz RI, Kampert JB. Work activity and fatal heart attack studied by multiple logistic risk analysis. Am J Epidemiol 1979;110:52–62.
14. Paffenbarger RS, Hyde RT, Wing AL, Steinmetz CH. A natural history of athleticism and cardiovascular health. JAMA 1984;252:491–405.
15. Powell KE, Thompson PD, Caspersen CJ, Kendrick JS. Physical activity and the incidence of coronary heart disease. Ann Rev Public Health 1987;8:253–287.
16. Berlin JA, Colditz GA. A meta-analysis of physical activity in the prevention of coronary heart disease. Am J Epidemiol 1990;132:612–628.
17. Ekelund LG, Haskell WL, Johnson JL, et al. Physical fitness as a predictor of cardiovascular mortality in asymptomatic North American men. The Lipid Research Clinics Mortality Follow-up Study. N Engl J Med 1988;319:1379–1384.
18. Blair SN, Hohl HW, Paffenbarger RS, et al. Physical fitness and all-cause mortality: a prospective study of healthy men and women. JAMA 1989;262:2395–2401.
19. Hakim AA, Petrovitch H, Burchfiel CM, et al. Effects of walking on mortality among nonsmoking retired med. N Engl J Med 1998;338:94–99.
20. Bruce RA, Hossack KF, DeRouen TA, Hofer V. Enhanced risk assessment for primary coronary heart disease events by maximal exercise testing: 10 years' experience of Seattle Heart Watch. J Am Coll Cardiol 1983;2:565–573.

21. Erikssen J. Physical fitness and coronary heart disease morbidity and mortality: a prospective study in apparently healthy, middle-aged men. Acta Med Scand Suppl 1986;711:189–192.

22. Lie H, Mundal R, Erikssen J. Coronary risk factors and incidence of coronary death in relation to physical fitness: seven year follow-up study of middle-aged and elderly men. Eur Heart J 1985;6:147–157.

23. Sandvik L, Erikssen J, Thaulow E, et al. Physical fitness as a predictor of mortality among healthy, middle-aged Norwegian men. N Engl J Med 1993;328:533–537.

24. Blair SN, Kohl HW, Barlow CE, et al. Changes in physical fitness and all-cause mortality: a prospective study of healthy and unhealthy men. JAMA 1995;273:1093–1098.

25. Kujala UM, Kaprio J, Sarna S, Koskenvuo M. Relationship of leisure-time physical activity and mortality: the Finnish twin cohort. JAMA 1998;279:440–444.

26. Wenger NK, Froelicher ES, Smith LK, et al. Cardiac Rehabilitation. Clinical Practice Guideline No. 17. Rockville, MD: US Department of Health and Human Services, Public Health Service, Agency for Health Care Policy and Research, National Heart, Lung, and Blood Institute, 1995.

27. Lamm G, Denolin H, Dorossiev D, Pisa Z. Rehabilitation and secondary prevention of patients after acute myocardial infarction. Adv Cardiol 1982;31:107–111.

28. Beta Blocker Heart Attack Trial. A randomized trial of propranolol in patients with acute myocardial infarction. I. Mortality results. JAMA 1982;26:247:1707–1714.

29. Kentala E. Physical fitness and feasibility of physical rehabilitation after myocardial infarction in men of working age. Ann Clin Res 1972;4(Suppl 9):1–84.

30. Kallio V, Hamalainen H, Hakkila J, Luurila OJ. Reduction in sudden deaths by a multifactorial intervention programme after acute myocardial infarction. Lancet 1979;2:1091–1094.

31. Shaw LW. Effects of a prescribed supervised exercise program on mortality and cardiovascular morbidity in patients after a myocardial infarction. The National Exercise and Heart Disease Project. Am J Cardiol 1981;48:39–46.

32. Dorn J, Naughton J, Imamura D, Trevisan M. Results of a multicenter randomized clinical trial of exercise and long-term survival in myocardial infarction patients. The National Exercise and Heart Disease Project (NEHDP). Circulation 1999;100:1764–1769.

33. Oldridge NB, Guyatt GH, Fischer ME, Rimm AA. Cardiac rehabilitation after myocardial infarction: combined experience of randomized clinical trials. JAMA 1988;260:945–950.

34. O'Connor GT, Burnig JE, Yusuf S, et al. An overview of randomized trials of rehabilitation with exercise after myocardial infarction. Circulation 1989;80:234–244.

35. Panush RS, Schmidt C, Caldwell JR, et al. Is running associated with degenerative joint disease? JAMA 1986;255:1152–1154.

36. Kovar PA, Allegrante JP, MacKenzie CR, et al. Supervised fitness walking in patients with osteoarthritis of the knee. Ann Intern Med 1992;116:529–534.

37. Blair S, Kohl H, Goodyear N. Rates and risks for running and exercise injuries: studies in three populations. Res Q Exer Sports 1987;58:221–228.

38. Thompson PD, Funk EJ, Carleton RA, Sturner WQ. Incidence of death during jogging in Rhode Island from 1975 through 1980. JAMA 1982;247:2535–2538.

39. Noakes TD. Heart disease in marathon runners: a review. Med Sci Sports Exer 1987;19:187–194.

40. Siskovick DS, Weiss NS, Fletcher, RH, Lasky T. The incidence of primary cardiac arrest during vigorous exercise. N Engl J Med 1994;311:874–877.

41. Mittleman MA, Maclure M, Tofler GH, et al. Triggering of acute myocardial infarction by heavy physical exertion: protection against triggering by regular exertion. N Engl J Med 1993;329:1677–1683.

42. VanCamp SP, Peterson RA. Cardiovascular complications of outpatient cardiac rehabilitation programs. JAMA 1986;256:1160–1163.

43. American College of Sports Medicine. ACSM's Guidelines for Exercise Testing and Prescription. 5th ed. Williams & Wilkins, Baltimore, 1995, p. 373.

44. Blackburn GG. Cardiorespiratory responses to six-week limb-specific exercise conditioning programs. The Pennsylvania State University, 1984.

45. Bruce RA, Kusumi F, Hosmer D. Maximal oxygen intake and nomographic assessment of functional aerobic impairment on cardiovascular disease. Am Heart J 1973;85:546–562.

46. Blackburn G, Harvey S, Wilkoff B. A chronotropic assessment exercise protocol to assess the nedd and efficacy of rate responsive pacing. Med Sci Sports Exer 1988;20:S21.

47. Sullivan M, McKirnan MD. Errors in predicting functional capacity for postmyocardial infarction patients using a modified Bruce protocol. Am Heart J 1984;107:486–492.

48. Houghson RL, Smyth GA. Slower adaptation of VO2 to steady state of submaximal exercise with beta adrenergic blockade. Eur J Appl Physiol 1983;52:107–110.

49. McConnell TR, Clark BA. Prediction of maximal oxygen consumption during handrail-supported treadmill exercise. J Cardiopulm Rehabil 1987;7:324–331.

50. Zeimetz G, McNeill J, Hall J, Moss R. Quantifiable changes in oxygen uptake, heart rate, and time to target heart rate when handrail support is allowed during treadmill exercise. J Cardiopulm Rehabil 1985;5:525–539.

51. Wilkoff B, Corey J, Blackburn G. A mathematical model of the cardiac chronotropic response to exercise. J Electrophysiol 1989;3:176–180.

52. Borg GA. Physiological bases of perceived exertion. Med Sci Sports Exer 1982;14:377–381.

53. Borg G, Linderholm H. Perceived exertion and pulse rate during graded exercise in various age groups. Acta Med Scand 1967;472:194–206.

54. Brubaker PH, Rejeski WJ, Law HC, et al. Cardiac patients' perception of work intensity during graded exercise testing: do they generalize to field settings? J Cardiopulm Rehabil 1994;14:127–133.

55. Robertson RJ, Goss FL, Auble TE, et al. Cross-modal exercise prescription at absolute and relative oxygen uptake using perceived exertion. Med Sci Sports Exer 1990;22:653–659.

56. Oldbridge NB, Pashkow FJ. Adherence and motivation in cardiac rehabilitation. In: Pashkow FJ, Dafoe WA, eds. Clinical Cardiac Rehabilitation: a Cardiologist's Guide. Williams and Wilkins, Baltimore, 1999, pp. 467–503.

9 Obesity and Coronary Artery Disease
Implications and Interventions

Kristine Napier, RD, MPH

CONTENTS

INTRODUCTION
DEFINITION AND PREVALENCE OF OBESITY
METABOLIC COMPLICATIONS OF OBESITY
GENESIS OF OBESITY
WEIGHT PATTERNS VS OVERALL ADIPOSITY IN CAD
EPIDEMIOLOGICAL EVIDENCE FOR OBESITY IN CAD
WEIGHT CONTROL STRATEGIES: A POSITIVE RATHER
   THAN A NEGATIVE SPIN
CONCLUSION
REFERENCES

INTRODUCTION

Obesity increases the risk of disease and death. With now one-third of Americans classified as obese *(1,2)*, and the prevalence increasing, it is evident that obesity and its consequences have become one of the country's most urgent health care concerns. As we move into the 21st century, obesity-induced diseases will claim an increasing percentage of health care resources, as well as medical efforts.

It has been clearly demonstrated that obesity greatly increases the risk of diabetes mellitus, hypertension, dyslipidemia, coronary artery disease (CAD) *(3)*, and some cancers. Women who are more than 40% overweight have higher rates of fatal endometrial, ovarian, cervical, breast, and gallbladder cancers *(4)*. According to the American Cancer Society, increasing weight is directly related to risk of cancer in men who have never smoked.

This chapter discusses the relationship of obesity to CAD, reviewing the epidemiological evidence that obesity increases the potency of risk factors for CAD. Although there has been general agreement that extreme obesity increases the risk of CAD as well as all-cause mortality *(5)*, it is only in more recent years that there is a consensus that even modest degrees of weight gain and obesity significantly increase the risk of CAD. The

From: *Contemporary Cardiology: Preventive Cardiology:*
Insights Into the Prevention and Treatment of Cardiovascular Disease, Second Edition
Edited by: J. M. Foody © Humana Press Inc., Totowa, NJ

chapter also reviews the proposed mechanisms by which obesity inflates these risks, and the association of body fat distribution vs total body fat content with respect to CAD risk. The chapter concludes with practical and candid strategies for weight reduction.

DEFINITION AND PREVALENCE OF OBESITY

Officially, in the United States, a person is said to be obese when body mass index (BMI) exceeds 27.8 kg/m^2 in men and 27.3 kg/m^2 in women *(1)*, which corresponds to 120% of desirable body weight *(6)*. According to these standards, the National Health and Nutritional Examination Survey found 24% of adult men and 28% of adult women to be obese in the survey period from 1978 to 1980 *(7)*. Just a decade later, in the survey period from 1988 to 1991, the percentages rose alarmingly to 31% and 34%, respectively *(1,8)*. Prevalence varies by race, with rates considerably higher among black women and Hispanics of both genders *(1,9)*.

It is important to differentiate between the official definition of obesity and the metabolic point in time at which being overweight contributes to CAD risk. The latter occurs at lower body weights than are defined by the official definitions of obesity, especially with central or truncal adiposity. Taking into account such metabolic consequences, it seems more appropriate to define three stages of obesity and institute more aggressive weight-loss strategies accordingly. According to these more aggressive standards, a person is said to be moderately obese when BMI is in the range of 25 to 26.9 kg/m^2; obese when BMI is 27 to 30.9 kg/m^2; and markedly obese when BMI equals or exceeds 31 kg/m^2 *(10)*.

Refer to Tables 1–3 for ideal body weights, and Table 4 for BMIs; BMI is a far more powerful tool in describing how body weight impacts disease risk.

Weight patterning, or fat distribution, can lower the threshold at which the cardiovascular consequences of adiposity begin. Persons with truncal or central adiposity are at significantly greater risk. In addition, in persons genetically predisposed to cardiovascular disease, gaining weight accentuates their genetically programmed risk factors, rendering weight gain for them of far greater consequence *(11)*. For example, a certain subset of genetically susceptible people will become hypertensive after gaining weight; another subset will become dyslipidemic; and another subset will acquire type 2 diabetes, each a potent risk factor for CAD.

METABOLIC COMPLICATIONS OF OBESITY

Many of the metabolic abnormalities engendered by obesity occur in the cardiovascular system, increasing the risk for developing CAD. The major metabolic changes, and, therefore, risk factors, for CAD resulting from obesity include:

1. Atherogenic dyslipidemia, which includes:
    a. Elevated total cholesterol.
    b. Increased serum triglyceride.
    c. Decreased low-density lipoprotein (LDL) particle size.
    d. Reduced serum high-density lipoprotein (HDL).
2. Hypertension.
3. Insulin resistance and glucose intolerance.
4. Abnormalities in the coagulation system (procoagulant state) *(12)*.

Some investigators think that insulin resistance is the root cause of this group of risk factors; hence, they favor the term *insulin-resistance syndrome (13–15)*. A reduction in

Table 1
Desirable Weights for Men

Height without shoes	Frame size[a]	Desirable weight (pounds)	Overweight (≥20% over desirable weight)	Obese (≥30% over desirable weight)
5'5"	Small	124–133	≥155	≥168
5'5"	Medium	130–143	≥164	≥178
5'5"	Large	138–156	≥176	≥191
5'6"	Small	128–137	≥160	≥173
5'6"	Medium	134–147	≥169	≥183
5'6"	Large	142–161	≥182	≥198
5'7"	Small	132–141	≥164	≥178
5'7"	Medium	138–152	≥174	≥189
5'7"	Large	147–156	≥188	≥204
5'8"	Small	136–145	≥169	≥183
5'8"	Medium	142–156	≥179	≥194
5'8"	Large	151–170	≥193	≥209
5'9"	Small	140–150	≥174	≥189
5'9"	Medium	146–160	≥184	≥200
5'9"	Large	155–174	≥198	≥214
5'10"	Small	144–154	≥179	≥194
5'10"	Medium	150–165	≥190	≥205
5'10"	Large	159–179	≥203	≥220
5'11"	Small	148–158	≥184	≥199
5'11"	Medium	154–170	≥194	≥211
5'11"	Large	164–184	≥209	≥226
6'0"	Small	152–162	≥188	≥204
6'0"	Medium	158–175	≥200	≥217
6'0"	Large	168–189	≥215	≥233
6'1"	Small	156–167	≥194	≥211
6'1"	Medium	162–180	≥205	≥222
6'1"	Large	173–194	≥221	≥239
6'2"	Small	160–171	≥199	≥216
6'2"	Medium	167–185	≥211	≥229
6'2"	Large	178–199	≥227	≥246
6'3"	Small	164–175	≥204	≥221
6'3"	Medium	172–190	≥217	#235
6'3"	Large	182–204	≥232	≥302

[a]Use Table 3 to calculate frame size. (Adapted from ref. *16*.)

insulin sensitivity, however, may be but one of several abnormalities resulting from a generalized metabolic derangement induced by obesity. Thus, a more generic term for the syndrome of multiple metabolic risk factors, *metabolic syndrome (16)*, seems more appropriate and is used in this chapter to denote the constellation of risk factors commonly associated with obesity.

The genesis of metabolic syndrome begins with energy imbalance leading to energy overload, which results in excess fat being stored inertly in adipose tissue *(17–19)*. However, an energy overload state also results in high fasting concentrations of

Table 2
Desirable Weights for Women

Height without shoes	Frame size[a]	Desirable weight (pounds)	Overweight (≥20% over desirable weight)	Obese (≥30% over desirable weight)
5'0"	Small	102–110	≥127	≥138
5'0"	Medium	107–119	≥136	≥147
5'0"	Large	115–131	≥148	≥160
5'1"	Small	105–113	≥131	≥142
5'1"	Medium	110–122	≥139	≥151
5'1"	Large	118–134	≥151	≥164
5'2"	Small	108–116	≥134	≥146
5'2"	Medium	113–126	≥143	≥155
5'2"	Large	121–138	≥155	≥168
5'3"	Small	111–119	≥138	≥150
5'3"	Medium	116–130	≥148	≥160
5'3"	Large	125–142	≥160	≥173
5'4"	Small	114–123	≥142	≥153
5'4"	Medium	120–135	≥152	≥165
5'4"	Large	129–146	≥164	≥178
5'5"	Small	118–127	≥146	≥159
5'5"	Medium	124–139	≥157	≥170
5'5"	Large	133–150	≥169	≥183
5'6"	Small	122–131	≥151	≥164
5'6"	Medium	128–143	≥162	≥176
5'6"	Large	137–154	≥174	≥188
5'7"	Small	126–135	≥156	≥169
5'7"	Medium	132–147	≥167	≥181
5'7"	Large	141–158	≥179	≥194
5'8"	Small	130–140	≥162	≥176
5'8"	Medium	136–151	≥172	≥186
5'8"	Large	145–163	≥185	≥200
5'9"	Small	134–144	≥167	≥181
5'9"	Medium	140–155	≥176	≥191
5'9"	Large	149–168	≥190	≥205
5'10"	Small	138–148	≥172	≥186
5'10"	Medium	144–159	≥181	≥196
5'10"	Large	153–173	≥196	≥212

[a]Use Table 3 to calculate frame size. (Adapted from ref. 16.)

nonesterified fatty acids. Several tissues bear the brunt of the effects of excess nonesterified fatty acids, including skeletal muscle; it is the major site of nonesterified fatty acid use (18). According to Randle and colleagues (20), increased muscle uptake of nonesterified fatty acids in obese persons shifts energy use from carbohydrates to fatty acids. This shift leads to resistance to the action of insulin in muscle (21,22), which creates a tendency for hyperglycemia.

In turn, peripheral insulin resistance secondary to obesity is accompanied by hyperinsulinemia (23,24). High nonesterified fatty acid concentrations may act directly

Table 3
Frame Size According to Wrist Measurement

Height (in.)	Wrist size that indicates small frame (in.)	Wrist size that indicates medium frame (in.)	Wrist size that indicates large frame (in.)
Under 5'3"	<5.5"	5.5–5.75	>5.75"
5'3" to 5'4"	<6"	6–6.75	>6.25"
Over 5'4"	<6.25"	6.25–6.5	>6.5"

Adapted from ref. *16*.

on the pancreatic β-cells to prime them for enhanced insulin secretion in response to any given increasing serum glucose concentration *(25)*. Prolonged overstimulation of insulin secretion by β-cells may eventually impair β-cell function, thereby reducing insulin secretion and leading to type 2 diabetes *(26,27)*.

A third major target of energy overload is the liver *(28–31)*. The increased concentration of very LDL particles entering the bloodstream raise both plasma triglycerol and cholesterol concentrations *(12,29)*. The higher triglycerol concentrations, in turn, cause the creation of smaller LDL particles *(32,33)*, and decrease the concentrations of HDL cholesterol *(34)*. In addition, obesity apparently increases the activity of hepatic triglycerol lipase *(35,36)*. This change may also reduce LDL particle size *(37)* and lower HDL cholesterol concentrations further *(38,39)*.

GENESIS OF OBESITY

The cause of obesity is multifaceted and complex, but shares a common global link: industrialization and the adoption of a Western lifestyle. This industrialization of Asia and even Africa and the Middle East show a trend toward obesity *(40–43)*. Asians, for example, have traditionally lived in rural environments with a lifestyle that supported a lean habitus: they commonly performed heavy physical labor and had a limited food supply. Their lifestyle is changing, however, as their societies grow more urbanized and industrialized. Today, with an increasingly generous food supply and decreasingly physical labor-intensive employment, their incidence of weight gain is increasing steadily *(44)*. In tandem, a steady and proportionate rise in several CAD risk factors is observed, including increasing LDL cholesterol, insulin resistance, and glucose intolerance, as well as a definite increased frequency of CAD *(45)*.

Although industrialization is a significant factor for weight gain around the world, increasing age is another. Certainly, the two causes are interrelated, with industrialization being the root of some of the factors leading to the weight gain of aging. In the United States, the average American gains approx 10 kg (22 lb) between age 20 and age 50 *(46)*. Several factors are thought to contribute to what has been termed the weight gain of aging, including a decline in metabolic rate, decreased physical activity, and genetics. Although, at one time, high-fat diets were thought to contribute to weight gain, this is now a point of considerable controversy.

The major reason for the well-documented age-associated decrease in resting metabolic rate (RMR) *(47–51)* is most likely the decline in muscle mass that also occurs with

Table 4
Body Mass Index and How to Calculate

Height (in.)	19	20	21	22	23	24	25	26	27	28	29	30	31	32	33	34	35
	Normal Weight						*Moderately Obese*		*Obese*				*Markedly Obese*				
	Body weight (lbs)																
58	91	96	100	105	110	115	119	124	129	134	138	143	148	153	158	162	167
59	94	99	104	109	114	119	124	128	133	138	143	148	153	158	163	168	173
60	97	102	107	112	118	123	128	133	138	143	148	153	158	163	168	174	179
61	100	106	111	116	122	127	132	137	143	148	153	158	164	169	174	180	185
62	104	109	115	120	126	131	136	142	147	153	158	164	169	175	180	186	191
63	107	113	118	124	130	135	141	146	152	158	163	169	175	180	186	191	197
64	110	116	122	128	134	140	145	151	157	163	169	174	180	186	192	197	204
65	114	120	126	132	138	144	150	156	162	168	174	180	186	192	198	204	210
66	118	124	130	136	142	148	155	161	167	173	179	186	192	198	204	210	216
67	121	127	134	140	146	153	159	166	172	178	185	191	198	204	211	217	223
68	125	131	138	144	151	158	164	171	177	184	190	197	203	210	216	223	230
69	128	135	142	149	155	162	169	176	182	189	196	203	209	216	223	230	236
70	132	139	146	153	160	167	174	181	188	195	202	209	216	222	229	236	243
71	136	143	150	157	165	172	179	186	193	200	208	215	222	229	236	243	250
72	140	147	154	162	169	177	184	191	199	206	213	221	228	235	242	250	258
73	144	151	159	166	174	182	189	197	204	212	219	227	235	242	250	257	265
74	148	155	163	171	179	186	194	202	210	218	225	233	241	249	256	264	272
75	152	160	168	176	184	192	200	208	216	224	232	240	248	256	264	272	279
76	156	164	172	180	189	197	205	213	220	230	238	246	254	263	271	279	287

Body mass index[a]

[a]Body mass index (BMI) is usually measured with the Quetelet index as follows: weight diveded by height squared *W/H_2 [kg/m^2]). To use the table, find your height in the left-hand column. Move across the row to your weight; the number at the top of the column is the BMI for your height and weight. (Adapted from ref. *16*.)

aging. Muscle mass has a much higher RMR than fat mass, and when muscle mass falls, so, too does RMR. Other factors may also contribute to age-associated declines in RMR, including the possibility that, as we age, we waste less metabolic energy *(52,53)*. Fortunately, increases in physical activity, especially in weight training, can counter the decline in RMR, as is discussed later in the Weight Control Strategies: A Positive Rather Than a Negative Spin section.

According to the National Institutes of Health (NIH) Consensus Development Panel on Physical Activity and Cardiovascular Health, physical activity is at an all-time low in the United States *(54)*. The latest Surgeon General's report, Physical Activity and Health, found that more than 60% of American adults are not regularly active; in fact, 25% of adults report absolutely no physical activity. Of even greater concern is the trend toward decreased physical activity at younger ages. The Surgeon General's report found that nearly half of American youths 12 to 21 yr of age are not vigorously active on a regular basis, and that physical activity declines dramatically during adolescence. Now that high school students have a choice regarding physical education classes, daily enrollment in physical education classes has declined from 42% in 1991 to 25% in 1995. In terms of decreased calorie expenditure, this is disastrous in combination with an increasingly enhanced industrialized society relying more on mechanization rather than physical labor.

Body weight is not influenced solely by behavior and culture. Two lines of research support the theory that body weight is under genetic control: studies in identical twins *(55)* and genetic epidemiology *(56)*. The latter suggests that as much as one-fourth to one-half of the variability on body weight in the general population is explained by genetics. Currently, it is unknown whether genetic factors influence appetite and the amount of food ingested, the rate of energy expenditure, or both *(57)*. It should be emphasized that although simply having the genetic profile that predisposes to obesity does not imply that such people will automatically become obese. In this population, environment and behavior also play significant roles in the determination of body weight.

WEIGHT PATTERNS VS OVERALL ADIPOSITY IN CAD

Body fat distribution seems to play an important and independent role in enhancing cardiovascular disease risk factors. People with more central fat accumulation have a heightened risk of CAD risk factors than those with fat in the peripheral regions, such as the gluteal–femoral area. Central adiposity is strongly related to insulin resistance and the associated metabolic abnormalities, including insulin resistance, hyperinsulinemia, and elevated triglycerides. As a result, the risks of type 2 diabetes, dyslipidemia, and hypertension are increased *(52)*. Cancer mortality also seems to be related to central adiposity *(58)*.

Two measures are used to describe the risk associated with central adiposity: the waist-to-hip ratio (WHR) and the waist circumference. Traditionally, the WHR was the more commonly used method, and, in fact, most studies published to date have used that measure. According to the 1998 Evidence Report on obesity from the NIH, however, the waist circumference has recently been found to be the better marker of abdominal fat content and carries greater prognostic significance. Ideal waist circumference varies by gender. Men should strive for a waist circumference of less than 40 in. (102 cm) and women of less than 35 in. (88 cm). Waist circumference may not applicable in people under 5 ft tall *(52)*.

Whether central adiposity remains a risk factor after taking total adiposity into account has been a subject of controversy. The Nurses' Health study evaluated this issue, studying the relationship in 44,702 women aged 40 to 65 yr of age. Researchers adjusted for BMI and other cardiac risk factors, and confirmed an independent association between the risk of CAD in women and central adiposity as measured by WHR and waist circumference. Women with a WHR of 0.88 or higher had a relative risk (RR) of 3.25 for CAD compared with women with a WHR of less than 0.72. A waist circumference of 96.5 cm (38 in.) or greater was associated with a RR of 3.06. After adjustment for reported hypertension, diabetes, and high cholesterol level, a WHR of 0.76 or higher or waist circumference of 76.2 cm (30 in.) or more was associated with more than a twofold higher risk of coronary heart disease (CHD) (59).

EPIDEMIOLOGICAL EVIDENCE FOR OBESITY IN CAD

A number of studies have confirmed the association of obesity with increased CAD risk in several populations. In the late 1960s and early 1970s, epidemiologists noted that CAD was higher in heavier persons, but there was little evidence that any obesity index made an additional contribution to risk once coexisting risk factors were taken into account (60–62). Until the early 1980s, the consensus was that the increased CAD risk among the obese was caused primarily by the influence of the associated risk factor profile and not to obesity itself.

In 1983, investigators from the Framingham Heart Study and the National Heart, Lung and Blood Institute reexamined data from a subset of patients in the Framingham Heart Study specifically to study the obesity–CAD risk question. The initial analysis had suggested that the degree of obesity is not a potent independent risk factor for CAD, particularly in women (63,64). The researchers were spurred to reanalyze the data for two reasons: there were upward revisions to the Metropolitan Life Insurance Company desirable weight tables, essentially because of new data suggesting that it was healthier to be heavier than once thought. In addition, the researchers realized that the original analysis of the Framingham Heart Study data was based on analyses of the influence of relative weight during shorter periods of follow-up and may not have conveyed the true impact of disease risk (65).

The reanalysis examined data from 5209 men and women from the original Framingham study, a population followed biennially for 26 yr for the development of CAD. The reanalysis showed that obesity was a significant independent predictor of CAD, particularly among women. Percentage of desirable weight predicted the 26-yr incidence of CAD, coronary death, and congestive heart failure, after controlling for age, cholesterol, systolic blood pressure, cigarette smoking, left ventricular hypertrophy, and glucose intolerance. Relative weight in women was also positively and independently associated with coronary disease, stroke, congestive failure, and coronary and CAD death. In addition, the reanalysis showed that weight gain after the early adult years conveyed an increased risk of CAD in both men and women, a risk that could not be attributed to initial weight or the levels of the risk factors that may have resulted from weight gain. So, nearly two decades ago, researchers first confirmed that obesity is an independent risk factor for CAD (65).

Five years later, investigators from the Framingham Heart Study reported on the relationship of obesity and CAD risk in a subset of older, nonsmoking persons. At that time, there were 3630 people from the original Framingham study who survived to age

65 yr by the 16th biennial examination. Current and exsmokers were excluded from the study, resulting in a final study population of 1723 people who had been followed from 1 to 23 yr. The major independent variable was BMI, based on weight measurements taken at the examination at which an individual attained age 65 yr and on height measurements taken closest to that examination. Among men, four classes of BMI were created:

1. BMI less than 23.0 kg/m^2.
2. BMI between 23.0 and 25.2 kg/m^2.
3. BMI between 25.3 and 28.3 kg/m^2.
4. BMI 28.4 kg/m^2 and greater.

For women, the four groups were:

1. BMI less than 24.2 kg/m^2.
2. BMI between 24.2 and 26.1 kg/m^2.
3. BMI between 26.2 and 28.6 kg/m^2.
4. BMI of 28.7 kg/m^2 or greater *(66)*.

The researchers found that men with a BMI of 28.4 kg/m^2 and greater had a RR for all-cause mortality of 1.7, and men with a BMI between 25.3 and 28.3 kg/m^2 had a RR of 1.3. Among women, the RR for all-cause mortality was 2.0 for those with a BMI of 28.7 kg/m^2 or greater and 1.4 for women with a BMI between 26.2 and 28.6 kg/m^2. The authors concluded that, after controlling for cardiovascular risk factors, being overweight is a serious health problem for older people. This relationship was even stronger for those with long-standing weight problems.

As noted earlier, there are significant differences in the prevalence of both CAD and obesity by race. As such, it is important to determine whether there are differences in the impact of risk factors, such as obesity, on CAD. Investigators from the University of Minnesota examined the relationship between obesity and CAD in blacks and whites in two populations, young and middle-aged adults *(67)*.

One sample was the Coronary Artery Risk Development in Young Adults study, which consisted of 5115 adults aged 18 to 30 yr of age living in three cities (Birmingham, AL; Chicago, IL; and Minneapolis, MN); there were approximately equal numbers of whites and blacks in this study. The second sample, the Atherosclerosis Risk in Communities investigation studied 12,681 people aged 45 to 64 yr from Forsyth County, NC; Jackson, MS; suburban Minneapolis, MN; and Washington County, MD. In both populations, obesity was defined as the sum of subscapular and triceps skinfold measurements. Prevalence of CAD in blacks aged 45 to 65 yr was associated with obesity; after adjusting for age and cigarette smoking, the odds ratio was 1.3 for both black men and women. Further analysis showed that central adiposity conferred increased risk.

The authors also examined the relationship between the sum of subscapular and triceps skinfold measurements and levels of atherogenic plasma lipids, systolic blood pressure, serum glucose, serum insulin, and the prevalence of diabetes mellitus, finding a positive association. Interestingly, although they found that the strength of these relationships was similar in blacks and whites, the also found that, with each unit increase in sum of skinfold thicknesses, plasma triglyceride concentrations in blacks seemed to increase only one-third to one-half as much as in whites.

In contrast, the Charleston Heart Study did not find that BMI nor fat patterning predicted mortality in black women, although it did in the cohort of white women in the study *(68)*. BMI and body girths were examined as predictors of all-cause and CHD mortality

during 25 to 28 yr of follow-up in a subset of 312 white and 243 black women. Body girth was measured at the chest, abdomen, and midarm. The black women had a significantly greater mean BMI than the white women (27.7 vs 24.7 kg/m^2), which meant that 25% of the white and 46% of the black women were obese. All of the girths in the black women were greater than in the white women, although white women had more central adiposity than did the black women.

BMI was associated with both all-cause and coronary heart disease mortality in white, but not black women. After controlling for differences in BMI, the risk of all-cause mortality was greater in white women with larger chest and abdominal girths. In black women, the girths were not predictive of either all-cause or CHD mortality.

The relationship of adiposity to CAD and stroke risk was studied in Japanese men in the Honolulu Heart Program, a study that followed 8006 Japanese men for 18 to 20 yr; all men were of Japanese ancestry, born between 1900 and 1919, and living on the island of Oahu in 1965. BMI, subscapular skinfold thickness, and centrality index (subscapular skinfold thickness/triceps skinfold thickness) were measured at baseline and at follow-up. After controlling for other cardiovascular risk factors, the authors found that all three indicators of obesity were predictive of CAD risk, indicating an independent contribution of body fat to CAD risk (69).

Of particular interest is the study by Fraser and colleagues (70), examining the association of traditional risk factors on Seventh Day Adventists, a population at low-risk of CAD because of their characteristically low-risk lifestyle, which also found a clear association of obesity on CAD risk. This was the first study to examine the association between traditional risk factors and CAD events in Seventh Day Adventists. More than 10,000 men and 17,000 women, ranging in age from 25 to 99 yr, with approximately one-quarter older than age 65 yr, were followed for 6 yr for the occurrence of myocardial infarction and CAD-related deaths. Overall, the authors found that even in this low-risk lifestyle population, traditional coronary risk factors (hypertension, diabetes mellitus, body height, body weight, smoking, and exercise habits) exhibit their usual associations with the risk of CAD-associated events. Obesity, examined by weight tertiles, was more clearly associated with myocardial infarction than with fatal events. The RRs were 1.0, 1.18, and 1.83 for increasing tertiles of obesity.

The impact of modest degrees of overweight was examined in a cohort of 115,818 women from the Nurses' Health Study (71). The women were between the ages of 30 and 55 yr at enrollment in 1976, and were followed for 14 yr for changes in weight and the incidence of CAD, which the investigators defined as nonfatal myocardial infarction or fatal CAD. After controlling for age, smoking, menopausal status, postmenopausal hormone use, and parental history of CAD, the authors found that even modest increases in weight increase the risk of CAD. Among women within the BMI range of 18 to 25 kg/m^2, weight gain after 18 yr of age remained a strong predictor of CAD risk. Comparing women with stable weight after age 18 (defined as ±5 kg of weight at age 18 yr), women who gained 5 to 7.9 kg had a RR of CAD of 1.25; those who gained 8 to 10.9 kg had a RR of 1.64; those who had a 11 to 19 kg weight gain had a RR of 1.92; and weight gain greater than 20 kg had a RR of 2.65. The authors emphasize that even modest weight gains during adult life, and levels of body weight not generally considered to be overweight are associated with important increases in the risk of CAD.

This study by researchers from the Harvard School of Public Health and the Brigham and Women's Hospital was one of the first to call to attention the dangerously false

reassurance that small amounts of weight gain are "normal" and expected, a reassurance fueled by the 1990 upward changes in US weight guidelines that allowed for weight gain with age. The revisions were increased to correspond to so-called normal BMIs of 21 to 27 kg/m^2, in contrast to the 1985 guidelines, which corresponded to a BMI between 19 and 24 kg/m^2. The 1990 changes in weight tables implied that weight gains of 4.5 to 6.8 kg were consistent with good health. Also of concern was the other implication of the revised weight tables: that a BMI less than 21 kg/m^2 is unhealthy. Finally, these 1990 changes brought false reassurance regarding overweight in one additional way: they indicated that the seriousness of a person's degree of overweight should be evaluated by the presence of comorbid conditions such as hypertension and diabetes—rather than respond to the degree of overweight to prevent such complications (72,73).

The Harvard researchers also examined the effect of obesity and body fat distribution in a cohort of 29,122 US middle-aged and older men from the Health Professionals Follow-up Study, a prospective study of 51,529 US male health professionals who were 40 to 75 yr old in 1986 (74). They confirmed that weight is an independent risk factor for CAD, but also found that although BMI predicted CAD risk in men younger than age 65 yr, body fat distribution (as measured by WHR) was more predictive of risk in men aged 65 yr and older.

The investigators measured BMI, WHR, and height at entrance into this study in 1987, and also inquired about weight gain since age 21 yr. They then followed the men for 3 yr for the occurrence of CAD events, defined as fatal CAD, nonfatal myocardial infarction, coronary artery bypass grafting, or percutaneous transluminal coronary angioplasty. Men were excluded if they had a history of myocardial infarction, angina, stroke, coronary artery bypass graft, or coronary angioplasty; the authors controlled for alcohol use, vitamin E supplementation, smoking, total energy intake, family history of myocardial infarction, profession, and three dietary factors (intake of total and type of fat, cholesterol, and fiber).

The authors found that BMI, WHR, short stature, and weight gain since age 21 yr were associated with an increased risk of CHD. They reported their results by age of study participants at time of enrollment: men younger than age 65 yr and those age 65 and older, comparing both with lean men with a BMI less than 23.0 kg/m^2. The association of increased weight (as described by increasing BMI) was strongest for the younger men. Among men younger than 65 yr, after adjusting for the other coronary risk factors noted, the RR for CAD events was 1.72 for men with BMI 25 to 28.9 kg/m^2; 2.61 for BMI 29 to 32.9 kg/m^2, and 3.44 for BMI at least 33 kg/m^2. Although the RRs were much lower in the group of men aged 65 yr and older in each BMI category, the WHR was a much stronger predictor of risk. Those with WHRs in the highest quintiles had a RR 2.76 compared with men with WHRs in the lowest quintile.

WEIGHT CONTROL STRATEGIES: A POSITIVE RATHER THAN A NEGATIVE SPIN

Helping patients lose weight is difficult. Assisting them in maintaining lost weight is certainly the more difficult task, with recidivism rates exceptionally high, often greater than 95%, depending on the series one examines. Still, given the cardiovascular and other disease burdens imposed by obesity, it is essential to try new strategies to help patients achieve and maintain weight loss. Health care professionals, especially nutrition pro-

fessionals, are challenged to redefine efforts that historically have not worked to help patients achieve and maintain weights compatible with better health. The following is a candid, practical discussion of strategies that should improve your patients' odds of success.

Imposing a positive spin on dietary changes necessary in controlling weight is the basis of all efforts. Historically, nutrition counseling has been negatively focused, with advice centered on what patients should avoid. For the patient, this translates into deprivation. This author maintains that nutrition counseling must have a positive focus. As such, our program of nutrition intervention in the Preventive Cardiology and Rehabilitation Program is named "The Nutrition Enhancement Project," after the concept that nutritional intervention should enhance rather than deprive patients' lifestyles. Certainly, CAD patients must be instructed on how to limit dietary fats, especially saturated fats, but this too can be accomplished under the guise of enhancing one's lifestyle rather than avoiding the forbidden fruit.

This author divides weight loss strategies into three categories: behavioral, food, and exercise. The first two are certainly intimately related to each other, but for purposes of discussion, they are discussed separately here.

Behavioral Strategies

APPROPRIATE WEIGHT GOAL SETTING

Weight loss goal setting is dual pronged: health care professionals must help patients set both reasonable weight loss goals and an appropriate and flexible calorie level. Although the ultimate goal is to help patients achieve a BMI below that which defines obesity (27.8 kg/m^2 for men and 27.3 kg/m^2 for women), this may not be a reasonable initial goal. This is especially true when it translates into weight loss needs in excess of 20% of a person's current weight. Some clients may consider such weight loss demands daunting and unachievable, feelings that prevent some people from making any changes at all. Instead, set smaller weight loss increments for patients, encouraging them to approach weight loss in smaller goals. According to the NIH Evidence Report on Obesity, a weight loss goal of 10% is realistic and achievable. It is better, says the NIH Evidence Report, to maintain a moderate weight loss during a prolonged period than to regain weight after a marked weight loss. After maintaining a moderate weight loss for 6 mo, patients with more weight to lose should be encouraged to lose an additional 10%; if necessary, they can take another break and continue as needed to achieve the healthiest weight for them.

In addition to changing a seemingly impossible task to an achievable one, the benefits of losing 10% of body weight have been well-documented in their ability to reduce obesity-associated risk factors *(52)*.

APPROPRIATE CALORIE GOAL SETTING

As health care professionals, we have failed to communicate one of the most critical pieces of the weight loss algorithm: only modest reductions in calorie intake are necessary to achieve weight loss. We are guilty of handing out 1200 or 1300 calorie diet sheets, calorie levels too low to maintain during any extended period. Not only are such calories levels exceedingly difficult to maintain, but they are unnecessary to achieve weight loss goals.

Grundy *(75)* has noted that the degree of energy imbalance leading to obesity is relatively small. He calculates, from standard estimates of energy requirements per kilogram of body weight, that an excess of only 300 calories per day (1255 kJ/d) of excess energy maintains approx 10 kg (22 lb) of excess weight. In other words, the middle-aged person who has gained 10 kg of excess weight since age 25 yr has only 300 calories of energy imbalance. Grundy similarly calculates that 600 calories per day (2510 kJ) sustains approx 20 kg (44 lb) of excess weight.

Calorie levels in the range of 1400 to 1700 are far more reasonable to sustain, and will result in the desired weight loss during the long haul. This may be difficult to convey to patients once they become motivated and want to realize immediate results. It may be useful to have them work with a registered dietitian, who can calculate with them the caloric content of the diet they had been following, and the relatively insignificant daily changes necessary to achieve a 300-calorie deficit. Empowering patients with this type of knowledge is quintessential in helping them achieve both their short-term goal of losing weight steadily and their long-term goal of maintaining lost weight.

THREE IMPORTANT MOTIVATION STRATEGIES

Persevering with weight loss requires an inordinate amount of self-motivation. This author finds three strategies particularly important to convey and continuously review with patients in need of losing weight.

1. Help patients realize that tomorrow is today, or, simply put, helping them not wait for the proverbial tomorrow to begin the lifestyle modifications necessary to lose weight. Be aware that some clients may not want to begin weight loss efforts for fear of failing.
2. Give patients permission to forgive their transgressions. Help clients realize ahead of time that their weight loss program will not be perfect and strategize with them on how they will deal with such transgressions. Research confirms that people who recover quickly from their transgressions realize more weight loss success. This author suggests a simple scheme to use with patients in teaching them how to handle transgressions: help patients learn that they can fall forward (i.e., learn from their mistake and move forward), or fall backward (i.e., fall down and never recover) after eating something they had not planned to.
3. The final behavioral strategy bridges to the food strategies: encourage patients to eat only food they enjoy, and to enjoy every bite they eat. The last strategy is so important that it warrants additional discussion.

Nutrition professionals know from experience that one of the most expedient ways for clients to surrender dieting motivation is to eat food they do not like. A recent survey, the 1999 Health Focus Trend Report *(76)*, found that fewer shoppers than ever before are willing to compromise taste for health benefits. Also, the survey reported that fewer shoppers are willing to avoid favorite foods to eat healthier.

Practically speaking, health care professionals wishing to help clients achieve success must find ways to make this a reality, including becoming students themselves of gourmet healthy cooking and eating. This facilitates assisting patients in seeking gourmet healthy food and cooking classes.

Food Strategies

This author encourages the use of food strategies for losing weight that shift the focus from the negative to the positive. The Health Focus Trend Report confirms the consumer

demand for this paradigm shift to positive-based nutrition information, with consumers reporting they want "Positive nutrition, with little or no downside." The Trend Report also noted that consumers want to understand the science behind the advice, and in a format they can assimilate: understandable bites. In fact, the survey found that the market for health and nutrition information is less satisfied and more demanding than ever before. This provides support for empowering patients with another critical piece of the weight loss algorithm: how food affects their disease. It follows, then, that consumers, with their focus on longevity with good health and good quality of life, believe that prevention benefits are about health management through disease and symptom prevention.

Given this important background information, we take a brief look at the main food strategies that should be addressed with CAD patients embarking on weight loss programs:

1. Include protein at each meal and snack. Research confirms that of the three macronutrients, protein is the most satiating *(77)*, which may help avoid excessive eating. Clients should be instructed in how to choose protein foods, which tend to be sources of fat, especially saturated fat. Vegetable and marine sources of protein should be encouraged. Clients should be advised to include at least two fish meals and two vegetable protein meals weekly; all lunch protein should be vegetable based.
2. Increase fiber intake. Including high-fiber foods is advantageous to clients with CAD for several reasons. From a weight loss point of view, there is now evidence that increasing fiber intake may decrease the metabolizable energy content of the diet, especially of fat *(78)*. In addition, high-fiber foods lead to earlier satiety and also to decreased unplanned snacking *(79)*. High-fiber foods tend to be replete with the nutrients and phytochemicals that may help decrease CAD risk factors, including folate, B6, vitamin C, vitamin E, carotenoids, flavonoids, potassium, and other minerals.
3. Front-load calories. Dieters tend to start the day with their greatest willpower, which often works against them. Practically speaking, this means they often eat a very low-calorie breakfast and lunch. Often, this brings them to midday or early evening with excessive hunger; in turn, this leads to overeating at day's end. By front-loading calories, or eating the calorically heavier meals at the beginning of the day, patients are more satisfied at the end of the day. Taking in enough calories at the beginning of the day may reduce the feeling of fatigue that often troubles dieters.
4. Divide calories into six meals rather than three. Preliminary evidence indicates that consuming calories in six smaller meals rather than three larger ones may assist with weight loss. Researchers from Tufts University studied the fat-burning ability of two groups of women: one in their twenties and another that was postmenopausal. Each age group of women was fed three test-size meals of varying calories—250, 500, and 1000 calories, respectively. After each test meal, the researchers measured the amount of energy each age group burned. The metabolic response to the 250- and 500-calorie meals was similar between the two groups, but quite disparate after the 1000-calorie meal. The postmenopausal women burned about 30% less fat than the younger women. In addition to giving clients the metabolic edge in losing weight, eating six smaller meals may also help reduce total and LDL cholesterol levels.

EXERCISE STRATEGIES

Clients need to engage regularly in two forms of exercise to improve the chances of weight loss success and maintain lost weight: aerobic and weight training. According to the latest Surgeon General's report on Physical Activity and Health, all Americans should

exercise 30 min most, and preferably all, days of the week to improve cardiovascular fitness *(80)*. In addition, concludes the report, there may become additional benefit gained through engaging in even greater amounts of exercise. This is also the minimum amount of exercise needed to maintain muscle mass. Cross-training, or performing more than one type of aerobic exercise, helps build muscles throughout the body, and therefore keeps total muscle mass greater and metabolism higher.

Although the Surgeon General's report concluded that consumers can derive much the same benefit from dividing 30 min of exercise into two or three shorter sessions, it also states that people who can maintain a regular regiment of activity that is of longer duration or of more vigorous intensity are likely to derive greater benefits.

It is worthwhile to review with clients the multiple benefits of exercise. In addition to boosting metabolism and assisting with weight loss, physical activity greatly reduces the risk of premature mortality, in general, and of CAD, hypertension, colon cancer, and diabetes mellitus, in particular. Physical activity also improves mental health and is important for the health of muscles, bones, and joints.

The second form of physical activity—weight training or resistance training—is also key to maintaining muscle mass, especially with increasing age. According to the American College of Sports Medicine, resistance training should be progressive in nature, and provide a stimulus to all major muscle groups; it should also be individualized. The American College of Sports Medicine recommends performing one set of 8 to 10 exercises 2 to 3 d per week; if time allows, clients are advised to perform a second set of the same exercise, which may provide greater benefits. Older and more frail persons (those older than age 50–60 yr) may benefit from 10 to 15 repetitions using less weight *(81)*.

CONCLUSION

In most people, weight gain is insidious. Health care professionals should take this as a positive factor and also a call to action. Rather than waiting for patients to reach obesity, health care professionals should follow their weight over time and encourage patients to act early when weight loss is not so daunting. Because the health consequences of being overweight begin before being defined as obesity, it is critically important for the health care professional to follow patients' weight over time and assist them in preventing the excessive weight gain that defines obesity.

REFERENCES

1. Kuczmarski RG, Flegal KM, Campbell SM, Johnson CL. Increasing prevalence of overweight among US adults. The National Health and Nutrition Examination Surveys, 1960–1991. JAMA 1994;273:205–211.
2. Federation of American Societies for Experimental Biology Life Sciences Research Office. Third report on nutrition monitoring in the United States. US Government Printing Office, Washington, DC, 1995.
3. Solomon CF, Manson JE. Obesity and mortality: a review of the epidemiologic data. Am J Clin Nutr 1997;66(Suppl):1044S–1050S.
4. Lew EA, Garfinkel L. Variations in mortality by weight among 750,000 men and women. J Chronic Dis 1979;32:564–576.
5. Manson JE, Stampfer MH, Hennekens CH, et al. Body weight and longevity, a reassessment. JAMA 1987:257:353–358.
6. Metropolitan Life Insurance Company. 1983 height and weight tables. Stat Bull Metropol Insur Co 1984:64:2–9.
7. Najjar MF, Rowland M. Anthropometric reference data and prevalence of overweight, United States, 1976–1980. Vital Health Stat 1987;11:238.

8. Federation of American Societies for Experimental Biology Life Sciences Research Office, 1995.
9. Federation of American Societies for Experimental Biology Life Sciences Research Office, 2004.
10. Metropolitan Life Insurance Company. Metropolitan height and weight tables. Stat Bull Metropol Life Insur Co 1983:64:1–9.
11. Garrison RJ, Kannel WB. A new approach for estimating healthy body weights. Int J Obes 1993:17:417–423.
12. Grundy SM. Atherogenic dyslipidemia and the metabolic syndrome: pathogenesis and the challenge of therapy. In: Gotto AM Jr, ed. Drugs Affecting Lipid Metabolism. Kluwer Academic Publishers, Dordrecht, Netherlands, 1996, pp. 237–247.
13. Reaven GM. Insulin resistance and its consequences: non-insulin-dependent diabetes mellitus and coronary heart disease. In: LeRoith D, Taylor SI, Olefsky JM, eds. Diabetes Mellitus. Lippincott-Raven, Philadelphia, 1966, pp. 509–519.
14. DeFronzo RA. The triumvirate: β-cell, muscle, liver. A collusion responsible for NIDDM. Diabetes 1998;37:667–687.
15. Howard G, O'Leary DH, Zaccaro D, et al. Insulin sensitivity and atherosclerosis. Circulation 1996:93:1809–1817.
16. The National Institutes of Health. Clinical Guidelines on the identification, evaluation, and treatment of overweight and obesity in adults: the evidence report. June 1998. US Department of Health and Human Services.
17. Bjorntorp P. Bergman H, Varnauskas E. Plasma free fatty acid turnover rate in obesity. Acta Med Scand 1969;185:351–356.
18. Jenson MD, Haymond MW, Rizza RA, et al. Influence of body fat distribution on free fatty acid metabolism in obesity. J Clin Invest 1989:83:1168–1173.
19. Campbell PJ, Carlson MG, Nurjhan N. Fat metabolism in human obesity. Am J Physiol 1994:266:E600–E605.
20. Randle PI, Priestman DA, Mistry S, Halsall A. Mechanisms modifying glucose oxidation in diabetes mellitus. Diabetologia 1994:37:S155–161.
21. Abate N, Garg A, Peshock RM, et al. Relationship of generalized and regional adiposy to insulin sensitivity in men. J Clin Invest 1995:96:88–98.
22. Abate N, Garg A, Peshock RM, et al. Relationship of generalized and regional adiposy to insulin sensitivity in men with NIDDM. Diabetes 1996:45:1684–1693.
23. Elahi D, Nagulesparan N, Herscopf, RJ. Feedback inhibition of insulin secretion by insulin: the hyperinsulinemia of obesity. N Engl J Med 1989;306:1196–1202.
24. Saad MF, Knowler WC, Pettitt DJ, et al. The natural history of impaired glucose tolerance in the Pima Indians. NJEM 1998;319:1500–1506.
25. Stein DT, Esser V, Stevenson BE, et al. Essentiality (sic) of circulating fatty acids for glucose-stimulated insulin secretion in the fasted rat. J Clin Invest 1996;97:2728–2735.
26. Zimmet P, Dowse G, Bennett PH. Hyperinsulinemia is a predictor of non-insulin-dependent diabetes mellitus. Diabetes Metab Rev 1991:17:101–118.
27. Garg A, Chandalia M, Vuituh F. Severe islet amyloidosis in congenital generalized lipodystrophy. Diabetes Care 1996;19:28–31.
28. Grundy SM, Mok HY, Zech L, et al. Transport of very low density lipoprotein triglycerides in varying degrees of obesity and hypertriglyceridemia. J Clin Invest 1979:63:1274–1283.
29. Kesaniemi YA, Bells WF, Grundy SM. Comparison of metabolism of apolipoprotein B in normal subjects, obese patients, and patients with coronary heart disease. J Clin Invest 1985;76:586–595.
30. Egusa G, Beltz WP, Grundy SM, Howard BV. Influence of obesity on the metabolism of apolipoprotein B in man. J Clin Invest 1985;76:596–603.
31. Miettinen TA. Cholesterol production in obesity. Circulation 1971;44:842–250.
32. Austin MA, Kokanson JE, Brunzell JD. Characterization of low-density lipoprotein subclasses: methodologic approaches and clinical relevance. Curr Opin Lipidol 1994;5:395–403.
33. Richards EG, Grundy SM, Cooper K. Influence of plasma triglycerides on lipoprotein patterns in normal subjects and in patients with coronary artery disease. Am J Cardiol 1989:63:1214–1220.
34. Schaefer EJ, Levy RI, Anderson DW, et al. Plasma triglycerides in regulation of HDL-cholesterol. Lancet 1978:2:391–393.
35. Katzel LI, Coon PJ, Busby MJ, et al. Reduced HDL2 cholesterol subspecies and elevated postherapin hepatic lipase activity in older men with abdominal obesity and asymptomatic myocardial ischemia. Arterioscler Thromb 1992:12:814–823.

36. Depres JP, Ferland M, Joorjani S, et al. Role of hepatic-triglyceride lipase activity in the association between intra-abdominal fat and plasma HDL cholesterol in obese women. Arteriosclerosis 1989:9:485–492.
37. Zambon A, Austin MA, Brown BG, et al. Effect of hepatic lipase on LDL in normal men and those with coronary artery disease. Arterioscler Thromb 1993;13:147–153.
38. Kuusi T. Saarinen P, Nikkila EA. Evidence for the roll of hepatic endothelial lipase in the metabolism of plasma high density lipoprotein 2 in man. Atherosclerosis 1980;36:589–593.
39. Blades B, Vega GL, Grundy SM. Activities of lipoprotein lipase and hepatic triglyceride lipase in postheparin plasma of patients with low concentrations of HDL cholesterol. Arterioscler Thromb 1993;13:1227–1235.
40. Gopinath N, Chadu SL, Jain P, et al. An epidemiological study of obesity in adults in the urban population of Delhi. J Assoc Physicians India 1994:42:212–215.
41. Popkin BM, Paeratakul S, Zhai F, Ge K. A review of dietary and environmental correlates of obesity with emphasis on developing countries. Obes Res 1995:3(Suppl 2):89S–93S.
42. el Mugamer IT, Alizayat AS, Hossain MM, Pugh RN. Diabetes, obesity, and hypertension in urban and rural people of Bedouin origin in the United Arab Emirates. J Trop Med Hyg 1995:98:407–415.
43. Amine EK, Samy M. Obesity among female university students in the United Arab Emirates. J Royal Soc Health 1996;116:91–96.
44. Singh RB, Niza MA, Agarwal P, et al. Epidemiologic study of central obesity, insulin resistance and associated disturbances in the urbal (sic) population of North India. Acta Cardiol 1995:50:215–225.
45. Bhatnager D, Anand IS, Durrington PN, et al. Coronary risk factors in people from the Indian subcontinent living in West London and their siblings in India. Lancet 1997;331:397–398.
46. The National Institutes of Health. The Lipid Research Clinics population studies data book: the prevalence study. NIH, Bethesda, MD, 1979 (Publication no 79-1527).
47. Visser M, Deurenberg P, van Staveren WA, Hautvast JGAJ. Resting metabolic rate and diet-induced thermogenesis in young and elderly subjects: relationship with body composition, fat distribution, and physical activity level. Am J Clin Nutr 1995:61:772–778.
48. Tzankoff SP, Norris AH. Longitudinal changes in basal metabolism in man. J Appl Physiol 1978;45:536–539.
49. Poehlman ET, Toth MJ. Mathematical ratios lead to spurious conclusions regarding age and sex-related differences in resting metabolic rate. Am J Clin Nutr 1995:61:482–485.
50. Poehlman ET, Berke EM, Joseph JR, et al. Influence of aerobic capacity, body composition, and thyroid hormones on the age-related decline of resting metabolic rate. Metabolism 1992:41:915–921.
51. Poehlman ET. Regulation of energy expenditure in aging humans. J Am Geriatric Soc 1993:41:552–559.
52. NIH Clinical Guidelines on the identification, evaluation, and treatment of overweight and obesity in adults: the evidence report. June 1998. US Department of Health and Human Services.
53. Garrow JS. Modern methods of measuring body composition. In: Whitehead RG, Prentice A. New Techniques in Nutritional Research. Academic, San Diego, 1991, pp. 233–239.
54. NIH Consensus Development Panel on Physical Activity and Cardiovascular Health. Physical activity and cardiovascular health. JAMA 1996;276:241–246.
55. Bouchard C, Tremblay Y, Despres J. The response to long-term overfeeding on identical twins. N Engl J Med 1990:322:1477–1482.
56. Bluchard (sic) C, Perusse L. Genetics of obesity. Annu Rev Nutr 1993:13:337–354.
57. Grundy SM. Multifactorial causation of obesity: implications for prevention. Am J Clin Nutr 1998; 67(Suppl):563S–572S.
58. Folsom AR, Kay SA, Sellers TA, et al. Body fat distribution and 5-year risk of death in older women. JAMA 1993;269:483–487.
59. Rexrode KM, Carey VJ, Hennekens CH, et al. Abdominal adiposity and coronary heart disease in women. JAMA 1998;280:1843–1848.
60. Rabkin SW, Mathewson FA, Hsu PH. Relation of body weight to development of ischemic heart disease in a cohort of young North American men after a 26 year observation period: the Manitoba Study. Am J Cardiol 1977:39:452–458.
61. Robertson TL, Kato H, Gordon TM, et al. Epidemiologic studies of coronary heart disease and stroke on Japanese men living in Japan, Hawaii, and California: prevalence of coronary and hypertensive heart disease and associated risk factors. Am J Epidemiol 1975;102:514–525.
62. Chapman JM, Coulson AH, Clark VA. Borun ER. The differential effect of serum cholesterol, blood pressure and weight on the incidence of miocardial infarction and angina pectoris. J Chronic Dis 1971;23:631–645.

63. Truett J, Cornfield J, Kannel W. A multivariate analysis of the risk of coronary heart disease in Framingham. J Chronic Dis 1967;20:511–524.
64. Kannel WB, Gordon T. Obesity and cardiovascular disease. The Framingham Study. In; Burland WL, Samuel PD, Yudkin J, eds. Obsesity Symposium. Proceedings of a Survier Research Institute Symposium, Churchill-Livingstone, Edinburgh, 1974, p. 24.
65. Hubert HB, Feinleib M, McNamara PM, Castelli WP. Obesity as an independent risk factor for cardiovascular disease: a 26-year follow-up of participants in the Framingham Heart Study. Circulation 1983;67:968–977.
66. Harris T, Cook F, Garrison R, et al. Body mass index and mortality among nonsmoking older persons. The Framingham Heart Study. JAMA 1988;259:1520–1524.
67. Folsom AR, Burke GL, Byers CL, et al. Implications of obesity for cardiovascular disease in blacks: the CARDIA and ARIC studies. Am J Clin Nutr 1991;53:1604S–1611S.
68. Steven J, Keil JE, Rust PF, et al. Body mass index and body girths as predictors of mortality in black and white women. Arch Intern Med 1992;152:1257–1262.
69. Curb JD, Marcus EB. Body fat, coronary heart disease, and stroke in Japanese men. Am J Clin Nutr 1991;53:1612S–1615S.
70. Fraser GE, Strahan M, Sabate J, et al. Effects of traditional coronary risk factors on rates of incident coronary events in a low-risk population. Circulation 1992;86:406–413.
71. Willett WC, Manson JE, Stampfer MJ, et al. Weight, weight change and coronary heart disease in women. JAMA 1995;273:461–465.
72. US Department of Agriculture, US Department of Health and Human Services. Nutrition and Your Health: Dietary Guidelines for Americans, 3rd ed. Washington DC: US Government Printing Office, 1990.
73. US Department of Agriculture, US Department of Health and Human Services. Nutrition and Your Health: Dietary Guidelines for Americans, 2nd ed. Washington DC: US Government Printing Office, 1985.
74. Rimm EB, Stampfer MJ, Giovannucci E, et al. Body size and fat distribution as predictors of coronary heart disease among middle-aged and older US men. Am J Epidemiol 1995;141:1117–1127.
75. Grundy SM. Multifactorial causation of obesity: implication for prevention. Am J Clin Nutr 1998;67(Suppl):563S–572S.
76. HealthFocus, Inc. 1999 HealthFocus Trend Report. Published by HealthFocus, Inc. P.O. Box 7174, Des Moines, IA 50309-7174.
77. Poppitt SD, McCormack D, Buffenstein R. Short-term effects of macronutrient preloads on appetite and energy intake in lean women. Physiol Behav 1998;64:279–284.
78. Baer DJ, Rumpler WV, Miles CW, Fahey GC. Dietary fiber decreases the metabolizable energy content and nutrient digestibility of mixed diets fed to humans. J Nutr 1997;127:579–586.
79. Delargy HJ, O'Sullivan KR, Fletcher RJ, Blundell JE. Effects of amount and type of dietary fibre (soluble and insoluble) on short-term control of appetite. Int J Food Sci Nutr 1997;48:67–77.
80. US Department of Health and Human Services, Centers for Disease Control and Prevention. Physical Activity and Health: A Report of the Surgeon General Executive Summary.
81. Pollock ML, Gaesser GA, Butcher JD, et al. The recommended quantity and quality of exercise for developing and maintaining cardiorespiratory and muscular fitness and flexibility in health adults. Med Sci Sports Exer 1998, pp. 975–991.

10   Tobacco as a Cardiovascular Risk Factor

*Robyn Bergman Buchsbaum, MHS, CHES
and Jeffrey Craig Buchsbaum, MD, PhD*

CONTENTS

INTRODUCTION

Tobacco use in the form of cigarettes has long been established as a major risk factor for coronary heart disease (CHD). It is the most preventable cause of mortality. Each year, cigarette smoking causes more than 400,000 deaths in the United States alone, more than the number of American lives lost during World War I, Korea, and Vietnam combined *(1,2)*. Not only does this modifiable behavior cause pain and suffering, but it poses a significant economic burden. Total US Medicaid expenses caused by tobacco use are more than $6 billion a year *(3)*. Total direct health care costs are in excess of $75 billion a year. Indirect losses, usually because of lost productivity, increase that figure by another $80 billion a year *(3,4)*. For every cigarette pack sold in the United States, the country spends approx $7.18 in health care-related and lost productivity costs *(5)*. In the mid-1990s, state attorneys general participated in legal action with tobacco companies in hopes of winning back money spent on Medicaid expenses. In 1998, an out-of-court settlement was reached giving states billions of dollars upfront and billions more in annual payments *(6)*. Since then, most states have failed to allocate the Centers for Disease Control and Prevention-recommended funding for tobacco prevention, despite the fact that states are taking in record amounts of tobacco-generated revenue from the settlement and from increased cigarette taxes *(7)*.

Despite the legal battles taking place on state and federal levels, personal battles with tobacco are still being waged. Although smoking prevalence is the lowest it has been in

From: *Contemporary Cardiology: Preventive Cardiology:*
Insights Into the Prevention and Treatment of Cardiovascular Disease, Second Edition
Edited by: J. M. Foody © Humana Press Inc., Totowa, NJ

decades, approx 22.5% *(8)* of Americans still smoke. This percentage is still higher than the 12% national goal outlined in Healthy People 2010 *(9,10)*. Additionally, the decrease in smoking prevalence is not being seen across all groups. Specifically, cigarette smoking continues to be a problem with young African-American men and women, whose rates are increasing or maintaining, respectively, at their current levels. An inverse relationship between education level and smoking status has also been observed. Prevalence of smoking among college graduates is far less than among those with less than a high school education *(11)*. Although more than 40 million Americans have quit smoking, each day approx 4000 teenagers try smoking for the first time and another 2000 children who previously had experimented with smoking become regular smokers *(11,12)*. Worldwide, cigarette smoking is linked to the deaths of some 3 million people each year. Because of tobacco's allure, it is fast becoming one of the leading killers in developing countries *(13)*.

HISTORY

Cigarette smoking reached its fashionable peak in the 1950s when smoking was advertised as a health benefit. In fact, physicians were the primary endorsers. Ads portrayed cigarettes as "physician tested" or the "brand of physicians" *(14)*. These ads had some truth to them. Physicians and other allied health workers continued to smoke tobacco despite early evidence that cigarettes were linked to increased incidence of carcinoma *(15)*. Even in the early 1950s, cigarette ads were still prominent in leading medical journals, such as the *Journal of the American Medical Association*, *The Lancet*, and the *British Medical Journal (15)*.

Cigarettes were fashionable and trendy. Soon smoking became what some call "the most overpracticed addiction in the world" *(16)*. It was around that time in 1964 that the Surgeon General and his advisory committee released their report, entitled "Smoking and Health," a strong condemnation of tobacco use. The committee had reviewed 7000 scientific articles in the process of developing the report. Since then, there have been more than 30,000 articles published connecting tobacco use with a vast array of medical problems *(17)*.

In 1998, the major tobacco companies, although not admitting any wrongdoing, did agree to the Master Settlement Agreement between themselves and 46 states, the District of Columbia, and several territories. The agreement essentially ended any current or future litigation between the states and the tobacco companies for health care expenses related to tobacco use. The participating states received money to allocate as they chose and the tobacco companies agreed to follow certain restrictions regarding youth access and public health *(6)*. However, the tobacco companies continue to be under careful scrutiny. Despite the agreement to prohibit marketing to children, the tobacco companies have recently introduced candy-flavored cigarettes, such as R. J. Reynolds "Kauai Kolada," "Twista Lime," and "Warm Winter Toffee" *(18)*.

BIOCHEMISTRY AND PATHOPHYSIOLOGY

Since the Surgeon General's first report in 1964, subsequent reports have found tobacco use to be associated with a long list of medical issues, not the least of which is CHD. The various mechanisms related to smoking and cardiac disease cross broad categories, including decreased oxygen-carrying capacity secondary to carbon monoxide's direct

effects on hemoglobin *(19)*, vasoconstriction, platelet adhesion and hypercoagulability, catecholamine release, and endothelial dysfunction secondary to complex molecular mechanisms *(20)*. Of the thousands of ingredients *(21)* contained within a cigarette, nicotine and carbon monoxide seem to be the most lethal culprits. By smoking a single cigarette, the body reacts by increasing myocardial oxygen demand secondary to increased heart rate, blood pressure, peripheral resistance, and cardiac output *(22,23)*. Yet, the very same cigarette decreases the amount of coronary blood flow and myocardial oxygen supply. The elevated carboxyhemoglobin levels caused by smoking decrease the oxygen-carrying capacity of the blood resulting in myocardial ischemia *(22,24)*. Studies have shown that smoking increases the blood's ability to coagulate, and also enhances platelet aggregation and adhesiveness *(25–27)*, even in the presence of aspirin *(28)*. In addition, smoking causes endothelial cell dysfunction, thus, potentiating possible injury to the blood vessel wall *(22,29)*. The smoking of one cigarette seems to cause acute endothelial dysfunction for at least 60 min, without the development of tolerance *(22)*. Recent data shows that smoking causes decreased wall thickness and impaired endothelium-dependent dilation of arterial walls long before atherosclerosis is present *(30)*.

Additionally, chronic exposure to cigarette smoke has been shown to cause localized hypoxia, allowing for subendothelial edema and lipid accumulation in the vessel walls. Chronic smoking also lowers fibrinolytic function, allowing further plaque formation *(31)*. Because chronic smoking is also associated with increased serum cholesterol and reduced high-density lipoproteins, the damage to the blood vessel walls provides ample opportunity for exposure to lipids and thrombosis. Smoking has been shown to lower the amount of endothelial derived nitric oxide produced *(32–34)*. Many current areas of pathophysiological investigation relating heart disease and smoking go beyond the scope of this chapter, including both traditional approaches in areas such as the role of homocysteine *(35,36)* and an increasing role for molecular biology, pharmacokinetics, and genetics *(37,38)*. Passive smoking studies, although limited, are pointing to the same mechanisms for causing disease in adults, children, and even newborns *(39–42)*.

EPIDEMIOLOGY

Cigarette smoking has been proven to be a powerful predictor of cardiovascular mortality. The Framingham Study showed a 10-fold increase in relative risk (RR) of sudden cardiac death in men who smoked than in nonsmoking men. This also held true for women, with a RR 4.5 times higher in women smokers *(43,44)*. Risk from cigarette smoking is dose-dependent. Quantity and duration of a smoking habit are the factors most contributory to the development of disease. An individual's risk for cardiac events depends on the age at which the person started smoking, the number of cigarettes smoked per day, and the depth of inhalation *(24)*. Studies have shown that low-yield cigarettes make little difference in regard to risk *(29)*. Although even younger smokers have more raised plaque lesions than do nonsmokers *(30)*, middle age is when both men and women's risk for CHD doubles that of their nonsmoking counterparts *(24)*.

Patients who have established heart disease and yet continue to smoke suffer severe consequences. The Coronary Artery Surgery Study provided evidence showing that 5-yr mortality is significantly higher for smokers than quitters, 22 vs 15% *(45)*. Patients who had quit smoking had a survival rate of approx 80% compared with a 69% survival rate for those who continued to smoke *(46)*. In addition, after a 10-yr follow-up, smokers had

a lower quality of life compared with former or nonsmokers. Smokers were more likely to have angina, be limited in their activity level, be unemployed, and, overall, have more hospital admissions *(46)*.

In a study by Daly and associates *(46)*, smokers were observed for longer than 7 yr after their hospital admission, either for myocardial infarction (MI) or unstable angina. Mortality in individuals who continued smoking was 82%, whereas those who stopped smoking had mortality rates of approx 37%. The continuation of smoking was most pronounced in patients with unstable angina, in whom higher rates of sudden death were seen *(47)*.

Although the evidence for increased morbidity and mortality resulting from cigarette smoking is overwhelming, there are some areas in which smoking use is not associated with increased risk, emphasizing the need for more understanding of the pathophysiology of smoking. There is mixed evidence regarding smoking and postangioplasty restenosis. Several studies have shown no relationship between smoking status and restenosis, whereas two other studies have shown that smoking was an independent predictor of restenosis *(48–52)*. Additionally, smoking has a questionable relationship with the incidence of angina *(53)*. In both the Framingham Study and the Goteborg Primary Prevention Study, the risk of angina was not significantly higher for smokers than nonsmokers *(53,54)*. Additionally, although it is strongly thought that there is a synergistic interaction between smoking and other major risk factors, the exact relationship is not clearly understood *(1,53)*.

PASSIVE SMOKING

Recently, the issue of environmental exposure to cigarette smoke has gotten a great deal of attention. For years, observational data suggested that environmental tobacco smoke was related to a host of medical problems, including CHD. Until recently, however, no definitive studies were published linking environmental tobacco smoke to morbidity and mortality. The problem was the difficulty in proving causality in exposed people. In 1986, after the US Surgeon General and the National Academy of Sciences determined that this was clearly an issue that needed to be resolved, epidemiological studies began showing a definite negative relationship between environmental tobacco smoke and CHD *(55)*. In almost all of these studies, the RRs and/or odds ratios for nonsmoker spouses of smokers were greater than 1 *(55)*.

One of the strongest studies to date, published by Kawachi and colleagues *(55)*, followed more than 32,000 nonsmoking women between the ages of 36 and 71 yr for 10 yr. The results were clear. For nonsmoking women exposed to cigarette smoke in either the work-place or at home, RR of developing CHD increased. Specifically, for women who reported only occasional exposure to cigarette smoke, the RR rose to 1.58. For those with regular exposure to cigarette smoke, the RR increased to 1.91 *(56)*. This study was vitally important for two reasons. First, as opposed to previous studies, this study was prospective. Second, this was one of the first rigorous studies in which a causal relationship between passive smoke and CHD was seen *(56)*.

Although the major epidemiological studies have differed regarding endpoints and/or methodology, the results have been consistent. Passive smoke increases a person's risk of CHD, most likely in a dose-dependent manner. All of the major studies controlled for one or more confounding factors, such as age, high blood pressure, high cholesterol, body mass, socioeconomic status, and education. Despite this attempt to disprove the relation-

ship, the consistent outcome is that environmental tobacco smoke increases RR for CHD with nonsmokers.

Translated into numbers, approx 37,000 deaths a year from CHD are attributable to passive smoking in the United States (55). Beyond our borders, it is estimated that 18% of people living in developed nations will die from the effects of environmental smoke exposure (13).

The mechanisms by which environmental tobacco smoke cause morbidity and mortality are similar to those of current smokers. Nonsmokers exposed to tobacco smoke on a regular basis are found to have an increased myocardial oxygen demand, oftentimes resulting in ischemia and increased platelet aggregation. Although this increase in oxygen demand is considerably smaller than that of primary smokers, the effects can clearly be seen during exercise, a time in which the body uses large amounts of its oxygen from the blood (55). In a study by Leone and colleagues, healthy young adults were more easily exhausted during exercise after being experimentally exposed to tobacco smoke (53,57,58). For adults with established heart disease, exposure to passive smoke results in decreased ability to exercise and a greater likelihood of developing arrhythmias during exercise (55). During the same time that there is an increase in oxygen demand, the carbon monoxide in tobacco smoke reduces the oxygen-carrying ability of the blood by forming carboxyhemoglobin. In addition, the oxygen that is received is not as efficiently used by the myocardium after repeated exposure to passive smoke (55). Other deleterious effects from environmental tobacco smoke include increased resting heart rate and blood pressure (both systolic and diastolic) (55).

Blood platelets are negatively impacted by environmental tobacco smoke, increasing the risk of thrombus, damaging the lining of the coronary arteries, and contributing to plaque lesion formation (59). In a study done by Burghuber and associates (59), smokers and nonsmokers were exposed to cigarette smoke for 20 min in a waiting room. The results found that nonsmokers had significant changes in their platelet activity, almost equal to that of a smoker. The smoker, on the other hand, had very few changes in their platelet activity after additional exposure to smoke (60). This study, in addition to other similar studies (60–62), have found that nonsmokers' platelet activity is much more sensitive to even low levels of passive smoke than platelet activity of smokers (59).

There has also been evidence that passive smoking causes damage to the endothelial cells, leaving them open to increased platelet adherence and eventually increased atherosclerosis. Additionally, it has been shown that passive smoking negatively affects high-density lipoprotein cholesterol, leaving exposed nonsmokers at higher risk of developing CHD than nonexposed nonsmokers (59).

In a study by Howard and coworkers (63), 10,814 carotid ultrasounds were compared by smoking classification and passive smoking classification. In addition to finding higher rates of atherosclerosis progression among current smokers, as expected, the results also showed a 20% increase in atherosclerosis progression in individuals exposed to passive smoke. The effects of passive smoke in this study seemed to be cumulative and irreversible, prompting more debate regarding banning smoking in all public places (64).

In the ATTICA study, Panagiotakos and colleagues looked at the effect of passive smoke on inflammatory markers. In study subjects exposed to passive smoke three or more days per week, white blood cell counts, C-reactive protein, homocysteine, fibrinogen, and oxidized low-density lipoprotein cholesterol levels were all elevated. These findings remained even after adjusting for confounders (65).

SMOKING CESSATION

It has long been understood that nicotine is one of the all-time most addictive substances. No doubt that is the reason so many people continue to smoke. Since 1964, when the landmark Surgeon General's report on smoking and health was released, the number of ex-smokers has increased tremendously, allowing for thorough study of smoking cessation. In 1990, the Surgeon General released another report entitled, "The Health Benefits of Smoking Cessation." There were four major conclusions regarding heart disease in the report:

1. Smoking cessation results in immediate, substantial health benefits with people of all age groups and differing disease states.
2. Those who quit smoking live longer.
3. Smoking cessation decreases the risk of lung cancer, other cancers, heart attack, stroke, and chronic lung disease.
4. The health benefits resulting from smoking cessation far outweigh the risks of gaining a small-to-moderate amount of weight after quitting (66).

The benefits from quitting smoking are staggering. In a study looking at women, smoking and incidence of MI, those who had not smoked for 3 to 4 yr had an RR virtually identical to nonsmokers' RR. This remained true, regardless of the amount smoked, the duration of smoking, the age of the woman, or the presence of other cardiac risk factors (66,67). Many studies have come to the same conclusions (68,69). Other studies have suggested upward of 10 yr smoke free to see a significant decrease in risk (56).

Clearly, smoking cessation is essential in maintaining health. Despite all of the information regarding benefits to quitting, millions continue to smoke. According to a recent study by Ayanian and Cleary (69), smokers do not see themselves at increased risk of heart disease or cancer, despite the general knowledge that smoking "is not good"(70). Yet, it is estimated that approx 70% of current smokers desire to quit, but only 8% a year have some success. Of those 8%, only 10% will maintain their new nonsmoking status (71). Physician involvement in the cessation process is a key factor. Several studies have shown that encouragement from the physician regarding smoking cessation is effective (72,73). However, according to a study in the early 1980s, less than half of all smokers had received advice from their physician to quit, a figure that still holds true today (74–78). More disturbing is the fact that there are clear demographic differences between smokers who are counseled and those who are not. Specifically, men with heart disease were counseled more often than women with heart disease. Non-Hispanic whites also had higher rates of smoking cessation counseling than their Hispanic counterparts. Adolescents were very rarely counseled, although they had more potential opportunities compared with adult smokers. Income level was a significant predictor of counseling, with white collar workers receiving advice more often than blue collar workers. On a positive note, two-thirds of people who smoked more heavily were counseled despite the fact that they had fewer physician visits per year than people who smoked more lightly (74). In a meta-analysis study looking at 39 controlled smoking cessation trials, the results showed that there is nothing novel about successful intervention programs. Personalized advice and assistance from the physician and other members of the staff during a long period of time was the key to increasing cessation rates (79). It also seems that withdrawing this assistance after cessation results in higher rates of relapse than if the message continues to be given at each physician visit (79).

Stages of Change and the Physician

The stages-of-change model, well-accepted within the field of public health, has long been the basis for smoking-cessation intervention. Understanding and working within the model's framework allows both the patient and the physician a guide through the "jungle" of cessation. Many physicians think that success on their parts is cessation on the patient's. This kind of thinking only leads to frustration for both the patient and the physician. Within the stages-of-change framework, there is a middle ground. The stages-of-change model includes five stages; precontemplation, contemplation, preparation, action, and maintenance *(61)*. As opposed to other models that are linear in thinking, the stages-of-change model is circular. All smokers fit into one of the following categories:

1. Precontemplation. The patient has no intention of trying to quit in the next 6 mo. He or she avoids communication regarding the topic and is usually uninformed or underinformed regarding personal risk.
2. Contemplation. The patient is fairly aware of the risks and is seriously thinking of quitting within the next 6 mo. However, the patient is still not convinced of the long-term benefits and thinks more about the short-term costs. Many patients get stuck in the "thinking" phase without impetus to move forward.
3. Preparation. The patient is getting ready to quit within the next month. He or she is already making small changes in preparation for his or her quit date.
4. Action. The patient has made major and substantial change to his or her risky behavior and is most at risk of relapse during this time period, lasting about 6 mo.
5. Maintenance. The patient is actively working on maintaining a smoke-free environment *(80)*.

It is important to assess a patient's stage at each visit so that the physician can tailor the smoking cessation message. Instead of defining success as cessation, success becomes moving the patient forward on the road to cessation *(80)*. Patients who are precontemplative are not interested in setting quit dates or hearing about nicotine replacement. A more effective use of the physician's time is to discuss the patient's personal risk from smoking. Oftentimes patients get stuck in the contemplative stage. They know the risks of smoking in abstract, but the discomfort and irritation that comes with cessation is too high a price to pay *(80)*. These patients need firm warnings from the physician as well as information on programs and nicotine replacement.

The reality of smoking cessation is that for every 100 patients counseled to cessation, 75 will relapse *(80)*. The circular nature of the stages-of-change model is important because patients who relapse will return usually to the precontemplative or contemplative stage. On average, it takes a smoker three to four cycles through the stages before true cessation occurs *(80)*. With this understanding, physicians can reduce the frustration associated with cessation advice and continue to help the patient move along toward the ultimate goal of cessation. Prochaska and Goldstein *(79)* suggest the following simple three-question assessment of a patient's stage regarding smoking cessation.

Assessment of Patient's Stage Regarding Smoking Cessation

1. Are you intending to quit smoking in the next 6 mo? If the answer is no, the patient is precontemplative.
2. Are you intending to quit smoking in the next month? If the answer is no but the patient answered yes to question one, the patient is contemplative.
3. Did you try to quit smoking in the past year? If yes, and the patient is planning to quit within the next month, the patient is in the preparation stage *(79)*.

For persons who have already quit, it is important not to stop asking about their smoking status. Patients need to be asked how long ago they quit and if this is less than 6 mo, they are in the action stage and are at high risk for relapse. If they are more than 6 mo smoke-free, they are in maintenance and support needs to continue *(80)*.

The Public Health Service Guidelines

In addition to using the stages-of-change model described previously, The Public Health Service has expanded on the model with the "5 As." The recommendation is that at every visit, the physician use the 5As to help smokers. The 5As are Ask, Advise, Assess, Assist, and Arrange. This allows for the physician to determine the patient's stage of change, to deliver concise messages regarding the health risks of smoking, and to assist the smoker in following through on any attempts agreed on *(81)*.

INTERVENTIONS

The American Heart Association, the American Cancer Society, and the American Lung Association, along with thousands of local programs, offer behavior modification programs trying to help the millions of people wanting to quit smoking every year. These techniques are useful and can be initiated in the physician's office. In fact, physician advice to smokers increases quit rates and abstinence rates in a dose–response fashion *(81)*. Although highly intensive counseling is more effective than less-intensive counseling, even a small amount of advice can help motivate smokers to quit *(82)*. Techniques such as logging each cigarette smoked in a diary and noting the "triggering" event or the feelings associated with the cigarette (e.g., stress, coffee consumption, and so on) are useful in helping patients understand when they smoke most. Helping the patient set a quit date is often effective in moving them into a state of action. Preparing patients for what they and their families can expect during nicotine withdrawal is also important. Insufficient social support is one of the leading predictors of relapse *(83)*. In addition to behavior modification, physicians now have at their disposal a variety of pharmacological smoking cessation aids. Research shows that using any of the approved nicotine replacement therapies increases quit rates by 50 to 100%. Unfortunately, only one in five smokers trying to quit actually uses these aids *(84)*.

Nicotine Gum

Nicotine gum (nicotine polacrilex) was the first pharmacological aid for those attempting to quit smoking, and was approved by the Food and Drug Administration in 1985. The gum comes in two different doses, 2 mg, the more common dose, and 4 mg, and is now sold over the counter. The goal of nicotine gum is to deliver a short burst of nicotine to overcome nicotine cravings and helping the patient to discontinue the habit of smoking. In early studies looking at 2- vs 4-mg dose gum, the results showed the two doses to be comparable in efficacy *(85,86)*. In later studies, however, when smokers who were more nicotine-dependent were analyzed separately, it was found that the 4-mg dose of the gum was much more effective *(86)*. It is thought that the 2-mg dose of gum actually translates into 0.8 to 1.0 mg of nicotine being bioavailable to the smoker. For smokers with increased levels of nicotine dependence, this is inadequate to control nicotine cravings *(87)*. In a study by Herrera and associates *(87)*, the 6-wk, 1-, and 2-yr chemically verified quit rates for high nicotine level-dependent smokers on the 4-mg gum were 60, 39, and 34%, respectively *(88)*. Side effects noted with all doses of nicotine gum use include

gastric upset, hiccups, and/or jaw ache *(89)*. In addition, it has also been noted that coffee and carbonated beverages can block absorption of nicotine from the gum, a concern for some patients *(90)*.

Nicotine Patch

The transdermal nicotine patch was first available for prescription in late 1991, approved for over-the-counter use in 1996, and has since become one of the most widely used pharmacological aids in smoking cessation. The patch delivers a steady dose of nicotine to the bloodstream, eliminating the nicotine cravings that accompany smoking cessation. In 1994, Fiore and colleagues *(90)* conducted a meta-analysis of 23 clinical trials involving the nicotine patch. Overall, the study observed a 22% abstinence rate 6-mo after the study vs a 9% abstinence rate of subjects using placebo. Additionally, the researchers found that the nicotine patch was fairly effective without intense adjuvant therapy, although subjects involved in behavioral counseling were more likely to be abstinent at 6 mo after the study *(91)*. The study also found that both the 16- and 24-h patches were effective. Various versions of the patch are now sold over the counter, after multiple studies proved its efficacy, safety, and cost effectiveness *(92)*.

The biggest benefit of patch use as opposed to gum use is the steady stream of nicotine delivered into the blood system. Contrary to preliminary data, smoking cigarettes while wearing the patch is not cardiotoxic. Instead, the risk associated with simultaneous use of patch and cigarettes is no more than risk from cigarette smoking alone. Although cigarette smoking increases blood coagulability, transdermal nicotine does not seem to have the same effect *(20)*. However, it is advised that caution be taken with patients having acute cardiovascular incidents, such as post-MI patients or those with serious arrhythmias *(82)*.

The nicotine gum and patch are commonly used together and have shown greater success in achieving smoking cessation than either alone. However, very few studies have looked at the combination use *(93)*. The patch comes over the counter as Nicotrol® and Nicoderm CQ® and now is also available in generic forms. Nicotrol is a one-dose patch, whereas Nicoderm CQ is a stepped approach with three varied-dose patches. There has not been any evidence that one brand is more effective than the other, because there are pros and cons to each *(93)*.

Nicotine Nasal Spray

The nicotine nasal spray was first approved by the Food and Drug Administration for prescription use in 1996. The goal of its introduction was to deliver nicotine more rapidly so as to better handle smokers' cravings. Studies have consistently found that the nasal spray doubles the quit rates of smokers when compared with the use of placebo *(93)*. The spray is successful at increasing peak levels of nicotine faster than either the nicotine gum or the patch, yet not as rapidly as a cigarette *(94)*. The dose is one spray into each nostril or 1 mg of nicotine. It is recommended that patients start with 1 to 2 doses per hour with a minimum of 8 doses per day and a maximum of 40 doses per day. This should be reduced after 6 to 8 wk of continuous treatment *(95)*. The side effects from the nasal spray are significant. The most common are runny nose, nasal irritation, throat irritation, watery eyes, sneezing, and coughing *(96)*. However, most side effects disappear within 1 wk. There has been some concern regarding treatment dependence with the nicotine nasal spray because of its rapid nature. Recent studies have not shown abuse liability *(97,98)*.

Nicotine Inhaler

In 1997, the inhaler became the fourth addition to the nicotine replacement family. As with other nicotine replacement products, the inhaler doubles quit rates when compared with placebo *(96,99)*. It is currently available only by prescription. The inhaler is a small plastic rod containing a nicotine plug that delivers a nicotine vapor each time a patient takes a "puff." Although resembling a cigarette, the inhaler contains considerably less nicotine than a true cigarette. It takes approx 80 puffs from the inhaler to equal the amount of nicotine in one cigarette. Patients are instructed to take frequent continuous "puffs" each time they have a nicotine craving, using the inhaler for approx 20 min per craving *(96)*. The vapors are then absorbed through the lining of the mouth. The major benefit associated with the inhaler is the similar hand–mouth ritual to which smokers are accustomed *(93)*. For a pack-a-day smoker, this hand–mouth action is repeated almost 200 times a day *(100)*, sometimes making the habit more difficult to break than the nicotine addiction. Although the inhaler has shown efficacy in cessation, mixed long-term studies suggest that the inhaler's best use may be as an immediate nicotine replacement aid and that, after the initial withdrawal, other pharmacotherapies should be used *(82)*. The side effects of the nicotine inhaler are relatively mild, with mouth and throat irritation being the most common *(93)* (*see* Table 1 for additional information and usage guidelines).

Bupropion and Other Nonnicotine Pharmacotherapy

Bupropion, or Zyban®, is a slow-release formulation of the antidepressant more commonly known as Welbutrin® *(101)*. For many years, researchers thought that there was a relationship between dopamine, norepinephrine, other neurotransmitters, and nicotine *(102)*. Early studies with doxepin, clonidine, and nortriptyline showed promise as adjuncts to smoking cessation therapy *(103–105)*. In the early 1990s, two small double-blind studies using the immediate-release version of 300 mg bupropion found efficacy *(102)*. Bupropion, an inhibitor of neuronal uptake of norepinephrine and dopamine, is thought to help smokers quit in two ways *(102)*. The first is by affecting dopaminergic activity in the brain, where reinforcement of addictive drugs occurs. The second is by working on noradrenergic activity affecting nicotine withdrawal *(102)*.

As with other nicotine replacement treatments, clinical studies found that bupropion consistently doubled quit rates when compared with placebo *(102,106)*. Interestingly enough, extended-release bupropion worked equally well for smokers with and without a history of depression, bolstering the notion that bupropion works differently for each condition *(93)*. In a study by Jorenby and associates *(106)*, higher quit rates were seen with a combination of bupropion and the nicotine patch *(107)*. The recommended dosage of bupropion for smoking cessation is 300 mg per day for 7 to 12 wk, beginning 1 wk before smoking cessation. The most common side effects include dry mouth, insomnia, and headache. Hurt and colleagues *(101)* also found reduced weight gain for patients on a higher dose of bupropion (300 mg). This seemed only to last for the duration of the drug treatment *(102)*. Earlier trials with bupropion found evidence of increased seizures *(105,108)*. However, studies that are more recent have found that risk to be no more than with other antidepressants. It is recommended, however, to screen patients for seizure possibility before bupropion treatment. It is advised that patients with seizure disorders, anorexia, heavy alcohol use, or head trauma use other pharmacological agents for smoking cessation *(93)*.

Table 1
Pharmacotherapy Summary

Product	Dosage	Guidelines	Duration of use	Advantages	Disadvantages
Nicotine gum	2 or 4 mg Persons who smoke less than 25 cigarettes a day should use the 2-mg gum, otherwise use the 4-mg gum. No more than 24 pieces per day	Bite the gum slowly until it tingles, then park it in between the cheek and gum for a minute. No chewing and parking for 30 min.	Weeks 1–6, one piece every 1–2 h weeks 7–9, one piece every 2–4 h, weeks 10–12	The gum is convenient, sold over the counter, and flexible to the patient.	Nicotine is slow to absorb in the system. Must be chewed correctly to avoid gastric distress and to achieve nicotine levels. those with jaw or dental problems.
Nicotine patch	Stepped-dose approach = 21, 14, and 7 mg. One-dose approach = 15 mg.	The patch must be rotated to different locations on the body that have minimal hair	6–10 wk depending on the brand. No study has found one brand to be more effective than another	There are few side effects to the patch. It is easy to use and only needs to be applied once a day.	Nicotine is delivered slowly to the brain with no flexibility in dose. In addition, skin rashes can occur.
Nicotine nasal spray	1 or 2 sprays per hour.	The nasal spray works best with a minimum of 8 doses per day and a maximum of 40 doses per day. risks from continued cigarette use for hightly dependent smokers.	6–8 wk is appropriate use. Abuse liability does not seem t o be a problem. Risks of long-term use are less than during use	The nasal spray delivers nicotine quickly for rapid relief of cravings. It is easy to use and it may decrease weight gain disappear within about 1 wk.	The side effects (nose and throat irritation, sneezing coughing, watery eyes) can be hard t o tolerate, although they typically
Nicotine inhaler	One cartridge equals 80 deep draws or 300 shallow puffs per craving. No more than 16 cartridges should be used per day.	Twenty minutes of continuous, active puffing was found to be most effective in achieving appropriate nicotine levels.	Up to 3 mo with gradual reduction over 6–12 wk if neede.	The inhaler substitutes the hand–mouth behavior to which smokers have been habituated.	It must be used frequently throughout the day. Mild side effects (mouth and throat irritation) may occur.

(continued)

189

Table 1 (Continued)

Product	Dosage	Guidelines	Duration of use	Advantages	Disadvantages
Bupropion	150 mg, 300 mg	Patients should start with 150 mg daily 3 d prior to quitting. Patients should then increase the dose to 150 mg twice a day.	7–12 wk is the recommended treatment period.	Bupropion is nonnicotinic and can be used with the patch. It is a pill and is taken may be less with bupropion.	There is a slight risk of seizure and should not be taken if there is a history of seizure, anorexia, heavy trauma. Dry mouth and insomnia are the most common side effects
Nicotine lozenge	2 or 4 mg	The lozenge is placed in the mouth and moved from side to side while it dissolves (approx 20–30 min). Avoid eating or drinking 15 min prior to use. Limit use to 20 lozenges per day.	12-wk schedule: 1 lozenge every 1–2 h for first 6 wk, 1 lozenge every 2–4 h for next 3 wk, 1 lozenge every 4–8 h last 3 wk.	Lozenges are easy, convenient, and sold over the counter. There are few side effects.	Lozenges must be used correctly to be effective and to avoid heartburn and indigestion. Because eating and drinking prior to use limits the effectiveness of the lozenge, patient must plan lozenge accordingly.

With such favorable results using bupropion, researchers began looking at other nonnicotine pharmacotherapies. Clonidine was one such drug indicated in an early study as having promise for smoking cessation use. It is a centrally acting α_2-adrenergic agonist that lowers sympathetic nervous system activity. It is typically used to treat hypertension but has been shown to be somewhat effective used as a smoking cessation aid. Several studies have been conducted to examine the effectiveness of clonidine, and most have shown promise. However, the dosing ranges varied significantly, the side effects were severe enough to impact the clinical trials, and there were concerns regarding the ability to taper patients off clonidine gradually. Because of this mixed bag of results and no clear dosing information, clonidine currently is only recommended as a second-line agent for smoking cessation *(81)*.

Nortriptyline is another example of an antidepressant that looks promising as a smoking cessation aid. Nortriptyline is a tricyclic antidepressant that blocks reuptake of norepinephrine and serotonin *(82)*. In the two studies completed to date, nortriptyline doubled or tripled the abstinence rates of smokers regardless of smokers' histories of depression. It also did not reduce withdrawal symptoms, suggesting, as with other nonnicotine pharmacotherapies, that the mechanism of action is not fully understood *(81)*. Nortriptyline, as of now, is only indicated to treat depressive symptoms and is still considered a second-line treatment for smoking cessation *(82)*.

Nicotine Lozenges

A newcomer to the cessation field is the nicotine lozenge, also known as the Commit® Lozenge. Nicotine lozenges work much the same way as other nicotine products, yet offer the smoker an alternative to gum, patches, or sprays. The lozenge is placed in the mouth and allowed to dissolve while the patient moves the lozenge from side to side. The whole process takes approx 20 to 30 min. If the lozenge is chewed or swallowed, the dose of nicotine will be ineffective and can lead to heartburn or indigestion *(109)*. Eating or drinking should be avoided 15 min before using a lozenge, and no more than 20 lozenges should be used per day. The lozenge comes in two different strengths, 2 mg and 4 mg. People who smoke heavily, those who smoke within 30 min of waking, are encouraged to use the stronger dose. No matter which strength, the makers of Commit encourage patients to follow a 12-wk schedule. Patients are advised to use one lozenge every 1 to 2 h for the first 6 wk, one lozenge every 2 to 4 h for the next 3 wk, and one lozenge every 4 to 8 h the last 3 wk. Studies have shown that the lozenge is effective in helping patients maintain abstinence from smoking and in reducing cravings. The adverse events associated with lozenge use were comparable to those observed with nicotine gum *(110,111)*. They include nausea, hiccups, coughing, insomnia, heartburn, headache, and flatulence *(109)*.

REFERENCES

1. Fielding JE. Smoking: health effects and control. N Engl J Med 1985;313:491–498.
2. Fielding J. Practical solutions to smoking control. Corp Comment 1985;1:46–49.
3. Centers for Disease Control and Prevention. Medical care expenditures attributable to cigarette smoking—United States, 1993. MMWR 1994;43:469–472.
4. Centers for Disease Control and Prevention. Targeting Tobacco Use: The Nation's Leading Cause of Death 2004, US Department of Health and Human Services, ed. 2004, US Government.
5. Centers for Disease Control and Prevention. Annual smoking-attributable mortality, years of potential life lost and economic costs—United States, 1995–1999. MMWR, 2002;51:300–303.
6. National Conference of State Legislatures. Summary of the Attorneys General Master Tobacco Settlement Agreement. 1999, US Government.

 7. Campaign for Tobacco-Free Kids. A Broken Promise to Our Children: The 1998 Tobacco Settlement 6 Years Later. 2004.
 8. US Department of Health and Human Services. Progress Review, Tobacco Use, ed. 2003.
 9. US Department of Health and Human Services. Healthy People 2010 Goal 27-1 Reduce Tobacco Use by Adults, ed. 2005.
10. Office of Disease Prevention and Health Promotion. Healthy people 2000: midcourse review and 1995 revisions. 1995, US Department of Health and Human Services: Washington, DC.
11. Pierce JP, et al. Trends in cigarette smoking in the United States. Projections to the year 2000. JAMA 1989;261:61–65.
12. Substance Abuse and Mental Health Service Administration. Results from the 2001 National Household Survey on Drug Abuse, US Department of Health and Human Services, ed. 2002.
13. Peto R, Lopez A, Boreham, J, et al. Mortality from smoking worldwide. Br Med Bull 1996;52:12–21.
14. Mahaney FX Jr. Oldtime ads tout health benefits of smoking: tobacco industry had doctors' help. J Natl Cancer Inst 1994;86:1048–1049.
15. Bartrip P. Pushing the weed: the editorializing and advertising of tobacco in the Lancet and the British Medical Journal, 1880–1958. Clio Med 1998;46:100–126; discussion 127–129.
16. DeNelsky G. Smoking: what it's all about, what to do about it. in Preventive Cardiology and Rehabilitation Group Conference. Cleveland Clinic, 1998.
17. Terry LL. The Surgeon General's first report on smoking and health. A challenge to the medical profession. NY State J Med 1983;83:1254–1255.
18. Campaign for Tobacco-Free Kids. Big Tobacco Still Targeting Kids, Special Report. 2005, Washington, DC.
19. Adams KF, et al. Acute elevation of blood carboxyhemoglobin to 6% impairs exercise performance and aggravates symptoms in patients with ischemic heart disease. J Am Coll Cardiol 1988;12:900–909.
20. Benowitz NL, Gourlay SG. Cardiovascular toxicity of nicotine: implications for nicotine replacement therapy. J Am Coll Cardiol 1997;29:1422–1431.
21. Johnstone RA, Plimmer JR. The chemical constituents of tobacco and tobacco smoke. Chem Rev 1959;59:885–936.
22. Lekakis J, et al. Effects of acute cigarette smoking on endothelium-dependent arterial dilatation in normal subjects. Am J Cardiol 1998;81:1225–1228.
23. Thomas CB, Murphy EA. Circulatory responses to smoking in healthy young men. Ann NY Acad Sci 1960;90:266–276.
24. Tresch DD, Aronow WS. Smoking and coronary artery disease. Clin Geriatr Med 1996;12:23–32.
25. Nowak J, et al. Effect of nicotine infusion in humans on platelet aggregation and urinary excretion of a major thromboxane metabolite. Acta Physiol Scand 1996;157:101–107.
26. Gleerup G, Winther K. Smoking further increases platelet activity in patients with mild hypertension. Eur J Clin Invest 1996;26:49–52.
27. de Padua Mansur A, et al. Smoking and lipoprotein abnormalities on platelet aggregation in coronary heart disease. Int J Cardiol 1997;62:151–154.
28. Hung J, et al. Cigarette smoking acutely increases platelet thrombus formation in patients with coronary artery disease taking aspirin. Circulation 1995;92:2432–2436.
29. Reinders JH, et al. Cigarette smoke impairs endothelial cell prostacyclin production. Arteriosclerosis 1986;6:15–23.
30. Esen AM, et al. Effect of smoking on endothelial function and wall thickness of brachial artery. Circ J 2004;68:1123–1126.
31. Allen RA, Kluft C, Brommer EJ. Effect of chronic smoking on fibrinolysis. Arteriosclerosis 1985;5:443–450.
32. Rangemark C, Wennmalm A. Smoke-derived nitric oxide and vascular prostacyclin are unable to counteract the platelet effect of increased thromboxane formation in healthy female smokers. Clin Physiol 1996;16:301–315.
33. Ichiki K, et al. Long-term smoking impairs platelet-derived nitric oxide release. Circulation 1996;94:3109–3114.
34. Randi ML, et al. Cerebral vascular accidents in young patients with essential thrombocythemia: relation with other known cardiovascular risk factors. Angiology 1998;49:477–481.
35. Jensen OK, Ingerslev J. Increased p-homocysteine—a risk factor for thrombosi. Ugeskr Laeger 1998;160:4405–410.
36. Miller GJ, et al. Activation of the coagulant pathway in cigarette smokers. Thromb Haemost 1998;79:549–553.
37. Nagai R. Cardiovascular research in the era of genome medicine and EBM. Rinsho Byori 2003;51:208–213.

38. Winkelmann BR, et al. Rationale and design of the LURIC study—a resource for functional genomics, pharmacogenomics and long-term prognosis of cardiovascular disease. Pharmacogenomics 2001;2(1 Suppl 1):S1–73.
39. Taylor BV, et al. Clinical and pathophysiological effects of active and passive smoking on the cardiovascular system. Can J Cardiol 1998;14:1129–1139.
40. Nelson E. The miseries of passive smoking. Hum Exp Toxicol 2001;20:61–83.
41. Sherman J, et al. Prenatal smoking and alterations in newborn heart rate during transition. J Obstet Gynecol Neonatal Nurs 2002;31:680–687.
42. Kahn A, et al. Sudden infant deaths: from epidemiology to physiology. Forensic Sci Int 2002;130(Suppl):S8–20.
43. Kannel WB, D'Agostino RB, Belanger AJ. Fibrinogen, cigarette smoking, and risk of cardiovascular disease: insights from the Framingham Study. Am Heart J 1987;113:1006–1010.
44. Kannel WB. Update on the role of cigarette smoking in coronary artery disease. Am Heart J 1981;101:319–328.
45. Cavender JB, et al. Effects of smoking on survival and morbidity in patients randomized to medical or surgical therapy in the Coronary Artery Surgery Study (CASS): 10-year follow-up. CASS Investigators. J Am Coll Cardiol 1992;20:287–294.
46. Daly LE, et al. Long term effect on mortality of stopping smoking after unstable angina and myocardial infarction. Br Med J (Clin Res Ed) 1983;287:324–326.
47. Macdonald RG, et al. Patient-related variables and restenosis after percutaneous transluminal coronary angioplasty—a report from the M-HEART Group. Am J Cardiol 1990;66:926–931.
48. Arora RR, et al. Restenosis after transluminal coronary angioplasty: a risk factor analysis. Cathet Cardiovasc Diagn 1990;19:17–22.
49. Benchimol D, et al. Risk factors for progression of atherosclerosis six months after balloon angioplasty of coronary stenosis. Am J Cardiol 1990;65:980–985.
50. Galan KM, et al. Increased frequency of restenosis in patients continuing to smoke cigarettes after percutaneous transluminal coronary angioplasty. Am J Cardiol 1988;61:260–263.
51. Myler RK, et al. Multiple vessel coronary angioplasty: classification, results, and patterns of restenosis in 494 consecutive patients. Cathet Cardiovasc Diagn 1987;13:1–15.
52. Wilhelmsen L. Coronary heart disease: epidemiology of smoking and intervention studies of smoking. Am Heart J 1988;115(1 Pt 2):242–249.
53. Glantz SA, Parmley WW. Passive smoking and heart disease. Mechanisms and risk. JAMA 1995;273:1047–1053.
54. Kannel WB, D'Agostino RB, Belanger AJ. Update on fibrinogen as a cardiovascular risk factor. Ann Epidemiol 1992;2:457–466.
55. Kawachi I, et al. A prospective study of passive smoking and coronary heart disease. Circulation 1997;95:2374–2379.
56. Dwyer T, et al. Evaluation of the Sydney "Quit. For Life" anti-smoking campaign. Part 2. Changes in smoking prevalence. Med J Aust 1986;144:344–347.
57. Glantz SA, Parmley WW. Passive smoking and heart disease. Epidemiology, physiology, and biochemistry. Circulation 1991;83:1–12.
58. Glantz SA, Parmley WW. Passive smoking causes heart disease and lung cancer. J Clin Epidemiol 1992;45:815–819.
59. Burghuber OC, et al. Platelet sensitivity to prostacyclin in smokers and non-smokers. Chest 1986;90:34–38.
60. Davis JW, et al. Cigarette smoking—induced enhancement of platelet function: lack of prevention by aspirin in men with coronary artery disease. J Lab Clin Med 1985;105:479–483.
61. Davis JW, et al. Effects of tobacco and non-tobacco cigarette smoking on endothelium and platelets. Clin Pharmacol Ther 1985;37:529–533.
62. Davis JW, et al. Lack of effect of aspirin on cigarette smoke-induced increase in circulating endothelial cells. Haemostasis 1987;17:66–69.
63. Howard G, et al. Cigarette smoking and progression of atherosclerosis: The Atherosclerosis Risk in Communities (ARIC) Study. JAMA 1998;279:119–124.
64. US Public Health Service, Office of the Surgeon General. The health benefits of smoking cessation: Report of the Surgeon General. Washington, DC, 1990.
65. Panagiotakos DB, et al. Effect of exposure to secondhand smoke on markers of inflammation: the ATTICA study. Am J Med 2004;116:145–150.
66. Rosenberg L, Palmer JR, Shapiro S. Decline in the risk of myocardial infarction among women who stop smoking. N Engl J Med 1990;322:213–217.

67. Rosenberg L, et al. The risk of myocardial infarction after quitting smoking in men under 55 years of age. N Engl J Med 1985;313:1511–1514.
68. Dobson AJ, et al. How soon after quitting smoking does risk of heart attack decline? J Clin Epidemiol 1991;44:1247–1253.
69. Ayanian JZ, Cleary PD. Perceived risks of heart disease and cancer among cigarette smokers. JAMA 1999;281:1019–1021.
70. US Department of Health and Human Services. Smoking cessation: clinical practice guideline. Department of Health and Human Services: Washington, DC, 1996.
71. Ockene JK, et al. Increasing the efficacy of physician-delivered smoking interventions: a randomized clinical trial. J Gen Intern Med 1991;6:1–8.
72. Glynn TJ, Manley MW, Pechacek TF. Physician-initiated smoking cessation program: the National Cancer Institute trials. Prog Clin Biol Res 1990;339:11–25.
73. Frank E, et al. Predictors of physician's smoking cessation advice. JAMA 1991;266:3139–3144.
74. Kottke TE, et al. Attributes of successful smoking cessation interventions in medical practice. A meta-analysis of 39 controlled trials. JAMA 1988;259:2883–2889.
75. Kottke TE, et al. A comparison of two methods to recruit physicians to deliver smoking cessation interventions. Arch Intern Med 1990;150:1477–1481.
76. Kottke TE, et al. A controlled trial to integrate smoking cessation advice into primary care practice: Doctors Helping Smokers, Round III. J Fam Pract 1992;34:701–708.
77. Kottke TE. Smoking cessation therapy for the patient with heart disease. J Am Coll Cardiol 1993;22:1168–1169.
78. Kottke TE. Observing the delivery of smoking-cessation interventions. Am J Prev Med 1998;14:71–72.
79. Prochaska JO, Goldstein MG. Process of smoking cessation. Implications for clinicians. Clin Chest Med 1991;12:727–735.
80. Hughes JR, Hatsukami D. Signs and symptoms of tobacco withdrawal. Arch Gen Psychiatry 1986;43:289–294.
81. Fiore MC. Treating tobacco use and dependence: an introduction to the US Public Health Service Clinical Practice Guideline. Respir Care 2000;45:1196–1199.
82. Centers for Disease Control and Prevention. Reducing tobacco use: a report of the Surgeon General. Department of Health and Human Services, ed. US Government, 2000.
83. Kornitzer M, et al. A double blind study of 2 mg versus 4 mg nicotine-gum in an industrial setting. J Psychosom Res 1987;31:171–176.
84. Cummings KM, Hyland A. Impact of nicotine replacement therapy on smoking behavior. Annu Rev Public Health 2005;26:583–599.
85. Tonnesen P, et al. Two and four mg nicotine chewing gum and group counseling in smoking cessation: an open, randomized, controlled trial with a 22 month follow-up. Addict Behav 1988;13:17–27.
86. Benowitz NL, Jacob P 3rd, Savanapridi C. Determinants of nicotine intake while chewing nicotine polacrilex gum. Clin Pharmacol Ther 1987;41:467–473.
87. Herrera N, et al. Nicotine gum, 2 and 4 mg, for nicotine dependence. A double-blind placebo-controlled trial within a behavior modification support program. Chest 1995;108:447–451.
88. Lee EW, D'Alonzo GE. Cigarette smoking, nicotine addiction, and its pharmacologic treatment. Arch Intern Med 1993;153:34–48.
89. Henningfield JE, et al. Drinking coffee and carbonated beverages blocks absorption of nicotine from nicotine polacrilex gum. JAMA 1990;264:1560–1564.
90. Fiore MC, et al. The effectiveness of the nicotine patch for smoking cessation. A meta-analysis. JAMA 1994;271:1940–1947.
91. Wasley MA, et al. The cost-effectiveness of the nicotine transdermal patch for smoking cessation. Prev Med 1997;26:264–270.
92. Hughes JR, et al. Recent advances in the pharmacotherapy of smoking. JAMA 1999;281:72–76.
93. Schneider NG, et al. Clinical pharmacokinetics of nasal nicotine delivery. A review and comparison to other nicotine systems. Clin Pharmacokinet 1996;31:65–80.
94. Pfizer Inc. Nicotrol nasal spray prescribing information. Pfizer Consumer Healthcare, Morris Plains, NJ, 2005.
95. Sutherland G, et al. Randomised controlled trial of nasal nicotine spray in smoking cessation. Lancet 1992;340:324–329.

96. Hughes J. Dependence on and abuse of nicotine replacement: an update. In: N. Benowitz, ed. Nicotine Safety and Toxicity. New York, Oxford University Press, 1999, pp. 147–160.

97. Schuh KJ, et al. Nicotine nasal spray and vapor inhaler: abuse liability assessment. Psychopharmacology (Berl) 1997;130:352–361.

98. Leischow SJ, Nilsson F, Franzon MA. Efficacy of the nicotine inhaler as an adjunct to smoking cessation. Am J Health Behav 1996;20:364–371.

99. Tonnesen P, et al. A double-blind trial of a nicotine inhaler for smoking cessation. JAMA 1993;269:1268–1271.

100. Glaxo Wellcome. Zyban prescribing information. Glaxo Wellcome: Research Triangle Park, NC, 1998.

101. Hurt RD, et al. A comparison of sustained-release bupropion and placebo for smoking cessation. N Engl J Med 1997;337:1195–1202.

102. Prochazka AV, et al. Transdermal clonidine reduced some withdrawal symptoms but did not increase smoking cessation. Arch Intern Med 1992;152:2065–2069.

103. Prochazka AV, et al. A randomized trial of nortriptyline for smoking cessation. Arch Intern Med 1998;158:2035–2039.

104. Edwards NB, et al. Doxepin as an adjunct to smoking cessation: a double-blind pilot study. Am J Psychiatry 1989;146:373–376.

105. Ferry L, Johnston JA. Efficacy and safety of bupropion SR for smoking cessation: data from clinical trials and five years of postmarketing experience. Int J Clin Pract 2003;57:224–230.

106. Jorenby DE, et al. A controlled trial of sustained-release bupropion, a nicotine patch, or both for smoking cessation. N Engl J Med 1999;340:685–691.

107. Ascher JA, et al. Bupropion: a review of its mechanism of antidepressant activity. J Clin Psychiatry 1995;56:395–401.

108. Haller CA, Benowitz NL. Adverse cardiovascular and central nervous system events associated with dietary supplements containing ephedra alkaloids. N Engl J Med 2000;343:1833–1838.

109. GlaxoSmithKline Inc. Nicotine lozenge patient information. King of Prussia, PA, 2002.

110. Shiffman S, et al. Efficacy of a nicotine lozenge for smoking cessation. Arch Intern Med 2002;162:1267–1276.

111. Shiffman S, Dresler CM, Rohay JM. Successful treatment with a nicotine lozenge of smokers with prior failure in pharmacological therapy. Addiction 2004;99:83–92.

11 The Implications of Mental Stress for Cardiovascular Disease

Brendon L. Graeber, MD, Aaron Soufer,
Matthew M. Burg, PhD, and Robert S. Soufer, MD

INTRODUCTION

Evidence points to a significant role for psychological factors in the pathogenesis of cardiovascular disease (CVD). Mental stress, including psychological, psychosocial, or emotional stress, is recognized as a risk factor for the development of CVD. It also seems to contribute to the onset of—and can directly precipitate—acute coronary syndromes (ACS), fatal arrhythmias, and acute heart failure.

The association of emotions with the heart goes back as far as classical times and the teachings of Aristotle, who asserted that the heart was the seat of emotions. His belief that the heart was both the physical progenitor and the effector of emotional states was incorrect, and we now know that, in all matters of thought and consciousness, the brain is supreme. But Aristotle and his followers may be forgiven for thinking otherwise, because, in fact, the heart is an essential component of any response to emotions. Unfortunately, it may suffer negative, potentially catastrophic, consequences as a part of this response. The volatile and irascible cardiovascular surgeon, Sir John Hunter, neatly summarized this relationship more than two centuries ago when he famously said, "My life is in the hands of any rascal who chooses to put me in a passion." His subsequent death by heart attack during a heated argument with a colleague fulfilled his own prophecy. Indeed, popular memory is full of anecdotes describing those who have died suddenly from fury or fear.

From: *Contemporary Cardiology: Preventive Cardiology:*
Insights Into the Prevention and Treatment of Cardiovascular Disease, Second Edition
Edited by: J. M. Foody © Humana Press Inc., Totowa, NJ

The association of chronic stressors with disease of the cardiovascular system has been a comparatively recent discovery. As a result, investigations of the relationship between the two are diminishing the relative importance of the classic, anecdotal paradigm of sudden anger or distress leading to an acute heart attack. These dramatic events, even when they occur today, are imbued with something of a sensational nature because of their relative rarity. By contrast, the experience of chronic mental stress is unavoidable and universal. At its worst, chronic stress seems to whittle away insidiously at the integrity of the cardiovascular system, exploiting a relationship with traditional risk factors to initiate disease and particularly to worsen existing disease. This combination of universality and potentially amenable causes means that chronic stress may be suited to preventive interventions. The forms that these interventions may take are only beginning to be determined.

Mental stress is known to have a wide variety of effects on the cardiovascular system. Epidemiological and laboratory studies have documented that both acute and chronic stressors can cause cardiovascular perturbation, damage, and acute events. Moreover, an understanding of stress and its effects on the cardiovascular system is beginning to take shape within a conceptual model of the brain–heart, or neurocardiac, interaction. This model is being described and clarified through recent studies in functional neuroimaging, myocardial perfusion imaging, and vasomotor dynamics. These studies have defined some of the effects of mental stress on the heart and are beginning to describe the pathways in the brain that mediate the experience of stress and to elucidate the pathophysiology of its effects. Finally, a deepening understanding of the importance of mental stress in CVD and of the mechanisms behind its effects is leading to the testing of novel treatment strategies designed to ameliorate or prevent the damage mental stress may cause.

As this understanding grows, it will be increasingly important for clinicians to consider stress and the societal and individual factors that contribute to its occurrence as targets for treatment and prevention in patients. There exists the possibility of preventing mental stress-induced heart disease. Conceptually, this could be accomplished by helping patients to manage stressors in their lives and by intervening with psychological or pharmacological therapies to modify patients' personal experience of stress.

EPIDEMIOLOGY

Cohort studies of mortality and cardiac outcomes have revealed that both acute and chronic stressors have negative effects on the heart. Although a single acute stressor may precipitate myocardial ischemia ranging in severity from subclinical to catastrophic, the repetitive occurrence of individually subtle stressors or a pattern of persistent stress can also damage the cardiovascular system. This damage creates a predisposition to acute cardiovascular events, as indicated by the relationship between cardiac mortality and chronic stress.

Acute Stress

Perhaps our earliest and most intuitive understanding of the role of stress in CVD has come from the association of myocardial infarction (MI) with the experience of sudden emotional stress (Fig. 1). This anecdotal association has been shown to have a scientific basis. For example, a recent study demonstrated a 2.5-fold increased risk of MI for up to 2 h after the experience of moderate-to-extreme anger (1). Earthquakes have also served

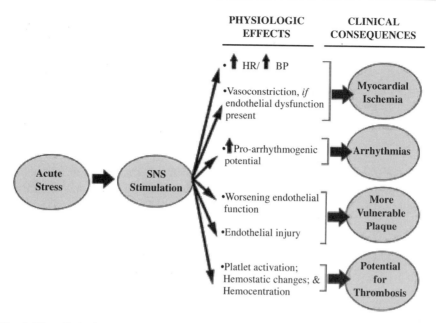

Fig. 1. The clinical consequences of acute stress. SNS, sympathetic nervous system.

as a useful example of an acute mental stressor experienced by many people in a similar manner. The potential of such a stressor to provoke MI had been reported as early as 1983, in a study of fatal heart attacks after the Athens earthquake of 1981 *(2)*. Subsequent studies have confirmed the association between these two phenomena *(3,4)*. Additionally, acute stressors of this magnitude have been found to cause perturbations of heart rate variability (HRV), which may contribute to arrhythmogenesis and sudden cardiac death *(5)*.

Mental stress may directly cause cardiac arrhythmias as well. Patients experiencing psychological stress can experience life-threatening ventricular arrhythmias in the absence of underlying structural heart disease, an effect which may be related to increased sympathetic activation *(6)*. Two studies examined the triggering of shocks to correct ventricular tachyarrhythmias in patients with implanted cardioverter–defibrillators after the terrorist attacks of September 11, 2001. These studies found that, in the weeks immediately after the attacks, ventricular arrhythmias increased significantly in patients both near to and far removed from the area of the attacks *(7,8)*. These findings indicate that the deleterious effects of acute mental stress are not limited to stressors that pose an immediate, tangible risk, as in the example of an earthquake. Mental stress unrelated to a survival risk, when acutely experienced, is sufficient to trigger cardiac arrhythmia.

The effects of an acute episode of emotional stress are not limited to the hours or days immediately after the exposure. One long-term prospective study of individuals who had lost a child found that their relative risk of a fatal MI from 7 to 17 yr after the event was 1.58 compared with matched controls, suggesting that, in addition to triggering acute cardiac events, a severe stressor may cause long-term damage as well, possibly through chronic sequelae arising out of an acute, emotionally traumatic experience *(9)*.

A syndrome of acute heart failure in response to a severe, acute mental stressor has been described in several case reports and case series *(10,11)*. It is marked by severe ventricular dysfunction and wall motion abnormalities. In contrast to precipitation of MI or arrhythmia, in which the acute stressor exploits the already diseased heart and coronary

arteries, this syndrome may occur in otherwise healthy hearts that lack evidence of significant coronary or electrophysiological disease. It therefore seems to occur directly as a result of the stressor. This syndrome of myocardial stunning after acute mental stress is not yet well understood. There is some evidence that it may be caused by extreme activation of the sympathetic nervous system and marked by supraphysiological levels of catecholamine release. At such high levels, the catecholamines become cardiotoxic and appear to induce the syndrome *(11)*.

Chronic Stress

The chronic frustrations and annoyances of everyday life are far more common, insidious, and potentially damaging for many people than the abrupt experiences just described. Chronic psychosocial stress in all its forms has been extensively investigated as a risk factor in CVD *(12)*. Broadly considered, the experience of chronic stress is a combination of individual stressors; the social support mechanisms that help us to deal with them; and the host factors of the individual that ameliorate or worsen the experience of stress *(13)*. In this equation it is important to consider that absent or insufficient social support is in itself a source of chronic stress, even as this condition worsens the impact of other external stressors. Host factors, as a function of the internal life of the individual, will be considered subsequently; stress and support, which are essentially universal and external, will be considered next.

Chronic mental stressors may arise from many sources, including any situations that seem to tax the ability of the individual to achieve desired aims or goals. These range from minor annoyances, such as traffic and unhelpful customer service personnel, to more serious problems, such as excessively long hours at work. Stressors may also arise from, or be exacerbated by, a lack of social and emotional support from spouses, friends, family, and coworkers. Finally, stress can arise from real or perceived difficulties related to the ability to obtain and use resources ranging from essentials, such as food and shelter, to luxuries, such as disposable income and free time.

The interactions among these factors are necessarily complex, but their effect on CVD and related mortality is well-illustrated by the example of low socioeconomic status, which is considered to be a composite psychosocial stressor incorporating many of the elements of chronic stress *(14)*. There is an inverse relationship between socioeconomic status and coronary artery disease (CAD) mortality, and this gradient is only partially accounted for by the fact that traditional cardiac risk factors, such as smoking and poor diet, tend disproportionately to afflict the lower end of the socioeconomic scale *(15)*. The balance of that relationship is, presumably, attributable in part to the increased psychosocial stress that accrues as wealth and privilege decline.

This relationship holds when the components of psychosocial stress are considered separately in studies of their effects on CAD progression and mortality *(16)*. Interestingly, insufficient social support, which relates particularly to the composition, extent, and quality of social and familial networks, seems to play a particularly prominent role in the progression and mortality of CAD *(16–18)*. This likely indicates that social support is essential in the prevention of the cardiovascular effects of chronic mental stress. It also points to an important preventive intervention, that of assessing patients' support networks and encouraging their development.

The risk that chronic psychosocial stress poses for an initial MI is comparable to that of traditional risk factors, underscoring its importance for cardiovascular risk. The

INTERHEART study, a large, international case–control study, showed that a standardized index of psychosocial risk factors carried a relative risk for first MI of 3.49 for women and 2.58 for men *(19)*. The psychosocial index included elements of work stress, home stress, financial stress, and recent stressful life events. The relative risks associated with it were comparable to those observed for diabetes, hypertension, obesity, and current smoking.

Chronic mental stress is a universal experience, and so its effects are also of widespread concern. Those effects are perhaps not of the dramatic nature associated with acute stress, but, although they are subtle, they are of much greater significance among populations than the relatively rare occurrences of cardiac sudden death associated with acute stress. They are also amenable to preventive measures, as previously mentioned, and therefore assume great importance for the field of preventive cardiology.

Host Factors

An essential element in the experience of stress is the person who does the experiencing. Regarding stress, there are wide variations in the subjective experiences of people that could be considered to have normal psychology, and these experiences are profoundly affected by an individual's psychological traits. These variations comprise a continuum; at the far end of that continuum are those who have psychopathologies, such as anxiety or depression, that may worsen the experience of stress or may themselves be stressors. The presence of particular traits or psychopathologies has ramifications for CVD.

Research on depression has increased ever since studies began to show that it is a risk factor for increased cardiac mortality. There is a strong relationship between depression and both the occurrence and the progression of CVD *(20)*. Depression has been shown to be a risk factor for a first MI, and its presence is also associated with increased mortality and recurrence after MI, these associations having been established in multiple studies *(12)*. Depression likely worsens the progression of CVD indirectly by contributing to lifestyle habits that have a deleterious effect on cardiovascular health. Examples of this are overeating and a lack of exercise, both of which may be associated with depression. However, depression is also associated with chronically heightened sympathetic activation, as demonstrated by circulating levels of catecholamines and cortisol, alterations in autonomic tone as demonstrated by fluctuations in HRV, and chronically elevated levels of inflammatory markers that have been implicated in the pathogenesis of CVD.

Anxiety, both in the form of frank disorders and as a trait, also seems to play a role. In one study, symptoms of anxiety were associated with an increased incidence of cardiac events during a period of 3 yr after MI *(21)*. Anxiety also may contribute to cardiac sudden death, both as a general symptom and as part of a specific phobia *(22,23)*.

Anger and hostility have been implicated in the progression of CVD. The traditional association of CVD and MI with "type A" behavior pattern has evolved into a more meaningful assessment of anger and hostility as psychological traits and of their contributions to CVD *(24)*. This assessment differentiates between the universal experience of anger and those who have a particular predilection to anger and are perhaps more likely to evince anger or hostility in response to everyday life situations. The presence of anger and hostility as traits is associated with an increased risk for MI and a worse prognosis after MI. Anger and hostility are also associated with an increased likelihood of experiencing both ventricular dysfunction *(25)* and potentially fatal ventricular arrhythmias during periods of mental stress *(26,27)*.

STUDIES OF THE HEART AND VESSELS DURING MENTAL STRESS

The conditions of acute and chronic mental stress have been replicated in the laboratory. Acute mental stress has been modeled in both animals and humans in a number of different ways, but these different modalities have all succeeded in provoking derangements of normal function in the cardiovascular system. Chronic stress, although difficult to model in humans, has been successfully modeled in animals by exploiting challenging social or behavioral circumstances.

Acute Stress

Acute mental stress is known to cause elevations in several measures of cardiovascular function, including heart rate, blood pressure, rate–pressure product, and cardiac index *(28)*. What is unusual about acute mental stress, in contrast to exercise stress, is that it is accompanied by an increase in systemic vascular resistance (SVR) that contributes to a concomitant drop in left ventricular (LV) ejection fraction in healthy individuals without evidence of CVD *(28)*. This phenomenon also occurs in patients with CAD *(29,30)*.

In 1984, Deanfield et al. reported that a mental stress task performed in the laboratory could provoke asymptomatic myocardial ischemia *(31)*. By subjecting patients with stable angina to a mathematical arithmetic stress task, the investigators were able to elicit abnormalities of myocardial perfusion using Rb-82 positron tomography. In 50% of those demonstrating ischemia, there were no accompanying symptoms or obvious electrocardiographic changes. This phenomenon has been extensively observed in patients with CAD, and it has been found to occur in anywhere from 30 to 60% of patients with CAD *(32)*. The decline in LV ejection fraction that occurs during mental stress is, in part, attributable to an increase in SVR. However, mental stress also has the ability to cause local abnormalities in cardiac wall motion during the ventricular beat *(30,33)*. These may result from increased afterloading, from segmental myocardial ischemia, or from a combination of the two. Although these wall-motion abnormalities provide a functional measurement of myocardial ischemia, their concordance with absolute myocardial ischemia as observed with perfusion imaging is not well described.

These deficits of function and perfusion are accompanied by deficits of vasomotor function in the coronary arteries during mental stress. In 1991, Yeung et al. reported that, in diseased coronary arteries, a mental arithmetic stress task caused vasoconstriction that decreased coronary blood flow. The degree of constriction correlated with paradoxical constriction of diseased arteries in response to an infusion of acetylcholine *(34)*. Such abnormal responses to normally vasodilatory stimuli have come to be understood as endothelial dysfunction, so-called because they represent a deficiency of endothelium-dependent relaxation of vascular smooth muscle. This phenomenon has also been observed in peripheral arteries *(35,36)*, using brachial artery reperfusion dilation (commonly called flow-mediated dilation) as a surrogate measurement that correlates with coronary endothelial dysfunction *(37)*.

Mental stress may induce frank myocardial ischemia, but its effects on the coronary arteries may also be more subtle. In some subjects with CAD, the response to mental stress may be marked not by ischemia but by a relative diminution of coronary function. Although these subjects do not become frankly ischemic, they do not exhibit the same increase in myocardial blood flow that accompanies mental stress in healthy subjects *(38,39)*. This failure of the coronary arteries to normally augment myocardial blood flow

during mental stress does not correlate with the presence of significant stenoses in the epicardial coronary arteries, and it has been postulated that this effect may result from dysfunction of the coronary microvasculature.

Mental stress also affects the electrophysiology of the heart and may contribute to cardiac arrhythmias. It has been shown to destabilize ventricular arrhythmias and worsen ventricular tachycardia in the laboratory *(40)*. This destabilization apparently occurs through effects on two electrophysiological parameters. First, HRV is decreased by mental stress, likely through a pathway mediated by the central nervous system (CNS) that affects vagal tone and, therefore, beat-to-beat period variation *(41)*. Second, abnormal myocardial repolarization seems to increase during mental stress, as measured by indices of T-wave parameters on ECG that correspond to heterogeneity of repolarization *(42)*.

Finally, the presence of ischemia or LV dysfunction in response to mental arithmetic stress or recall of a previous anger-provoking incident has prognostic implications. In a longitudinal study, 30 patients with stable angina pectoris and ischemia on stress perfusion imaging underwent continuous LV functional monitoring during stress induced by serial subtraction. They were then followed for 2 yr for occurrences of MI or unstable angina. Of the 15 patients with LV dysfunction during stress, 10 went on to experience one of these events during the follow-up period, whereas only 4 of the 15 patients without LV dysfunction experienced an event *(43)*. This finding has been replicated by three other studies, with the most recent demonstrating a statistically significant 3.0 rate ratio for death during a 5-yr follow-up among CAD patients with ischemia during laboratory mental stress *(44)*.

Chronic Stress

A strong association exists between chronic mental stress and CVD in human populations, as documented in epidemiological studies. However, the conditions of chronic mental stress are extremely difficult to replicate in the laboratory for human study groups, both from an ethical and a practical perspective. Chronic stress models have therefore been developed in animals through stimuli that cause discomfort or disrupt normal social and behavioral patterns. These stressful disruptions have been known for many years to contribute to cardiovascular dysfunction and atherogenesis in several different animal models *(45)*. The methodologies of these studies have become more advanced, allowing researchers to derive from them useful insights into the effects of chronic stress. In particular, models of chronic psychosocial stress that take advantage of the complex social structures of primates are providing valuable information regarding how stress effector pathways may operate in humans.

One method of attempting to model chronic stress in humans has been through repeated applications of a single acute stress task, separated by days or weeks. In the laboratory setting, there seems to be some degree of habituation of stress responses to a task. One such study used a social stress task repeated three times at 4-wk intervals, and found that responsiveness of heart rate and cortisol to the same task declined with time. However, the neurohormonal responses of the sympathetic nervous system were preserved despite familiarity with the task *(46)*. This suggests a role for sympathetic effectors in mediating the long-term effects of mental stress, although cortisol is known to be elevated in the setting of chronic stress as well.

This is reinforced by studies in cynomolgus monkeys, which provide a useful primate model for studies of psychosocial stress *(47)*. This is because they have complex social

dominance hierarchies that in some ways mimic human social organization, and that their cardiovascular and endothelial physiology is similar to our own. Cynomolgus monkeys can be chronically stressed by frequent manipulation of colony membership, thereby providing a context for the continued establishment of dominance hierarchies. Those monkeys who are psychosocially stressed by this method demonstrate greater development of atherosclerosis and greater endothelial damage than those who are not exposed to this chronic stress *(48)*. They also suffer disruptions of normal vasomotor function, and particularly of endothelially mediated dilation, which correlate with psychosocial stress *(49)*. Of note, the monkeys most affected by this manipulation are those that continuously rise to the top of the dominance hierarchy after each manipulation. When monkeys undergoing this stress exposure are treated chronically with β-adrenergic antagonists, the severity of their resulting endothelial damage and atherosclerotic disease is reduced *(50)*. These results provide direct evidence that chronic mental stress causes atherogenesis and endothelial damage in an animal model with many similarities to humans. They further point to a direct role for sympathetic activation in the pathophysiology of CVD induced by chronic stress.

PHYSIOLOGY AND PATHOPHYSIOLOGY

Research is moving beyond the descriptive effects of mental stress on the cardiovascular system and into a nascent understanding of the pathophysiology of mental stress. This work encompasses all areas of the experience of mental stress, from its initial processing and manifestations in the brain to its ultimate effects on the heart and blood vessels.

The various systems in the brain responsible for interpreting and manifesting the experience of stress are being described through the use of functional neuroimaging modalities in humans. Differences in mood and emotional coping mechanisms across human subjects make it implausible to detect highly consistent patterns of cortical activation across different neuroimaging studies of mental stress. Furthermore, different induction methods of mental stress through cognitive and emotional tasks elicit activity across incongruent areas of the brain *(51)*. Nevertheless, the totality of neuroimaging studies in healthy normal subjects imply that the stress response is mediated by limbic structures—such as the amygdala, hippocampus, hypothalamus, and cingulate cortex— in addition to prefrontal regions, the insular cortex, and other brainstem nuclei *(51–53)* (Fig. 2). These results point to a complex, integrated response involving centers dealing with emotion, reason, affect, and executive function. Furthermore, some of these areas are implicated in autonomic control of the cardiovascular system *(54)*, and therefore these findings are significant because our understanding of the subsequent effects of mental stress—after it has been processed and interpreted as stress—focuses on the autonomic nervous system and its physiological effects.

One study assigned a mixed-gender group of 41 healthy right-handed subjects to recall either two emotional events or a series of neutral events associated with a normal day while undergoing positron emission tomography (PET) scanning. Subjects involved in the emotional recall condition demonstrated activity in the subcortical structures of the pons, midbrain, and hypothalamus relative to those in the neutral condition. They also demonstrated bilateral activation along the anterior and posterior cingulate and insular cortices. There was also deactivation detected along the orbitofrontal and dorsal lateral prefrontal cortices *(53)*.

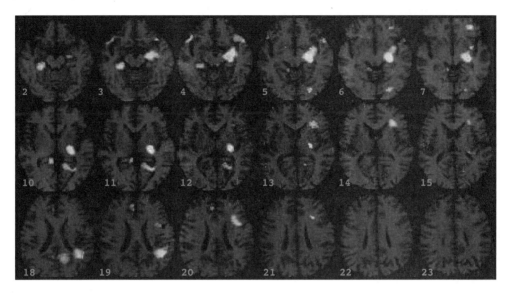

Fig. 2. Cortical hyperactivation in CAD with mental stress ischemia. (Reprinted with permission from ref. *52*.)

Another smaller study of normal male subjects assessed cortical activation during stress induced by aversive images. The subjects viewed aversive and nonaversive images during functional magnetic resonance imaging and then were asked to subjectively score their responses to the images. The results showed that activation in the medial prefrontal cortex and the amygdala correlated with the subjects' ratings of their own unpleasant emotional states provoked by the aversive pictures *(51)*.

Significantly, the CNS activations observed in normal subjects are also observed and are even more pronounced in subjects who have various psychopathologies that represent extreme susceptibilities to mental stress. Patients with anxiety disorders, such as post-traumatic stress disorder, obsessive–compulsive disorder, and social phobia, exhibit significantly heightened activation in limbic and cortical regions associated with the emotional stress response, and sometimes exhibit incongruent cortical function with respect to normal subjects *(55–58)*.

Stress-induced activation of the limbic cortex has also been associated with myocardial ischemia in patients with CAD. Soufer et al. induced acute mental stress through an arithmetic serial subtraction task in healthy human subjects and patients with CAD. Cortical activation and LV function were monitored during mental stress in both experimental groups via PET imaging and transthoracic echocardiography. Patients with CAD exhibited elevated activity in corticofrontal and limbic regions associated with emotion and cognition, and decreased activation in the right cerebral hemisphere during mental stress with respect to healthy subjects *(59)*. Those CAD subjects who experienced asymptomatic myocardial ischemia exhibited increased activation in the left hippocampus and bilateral deactivation of the anterior cingulate cortex, which is associated with pain and the experience of emotion *(52)*.

The limbic and frontal cortices project to centers of autonomic control, whereas the hypothalamus is an integral part of limbic circuits. These areas of the brain are relays of the experience of mental stress, and the neural pathways into which they project are

essential mediators of the peripheral responses to stress, through the widespread effects of their signal molecules on the body. Thus, measurements of neural and neurohormonal output provide the next link in the chain connecting the experience of stress to its peripheral effects. The hypothalamic–pituitary–adrenal (HPA) axis and the autonomic nervous system are two essential pathways that mediate stress responses.

The HPA axis is mediated through three cortical regions that are involved in the emotional stress response: the amygdala, which integrates information from other brain structures and provides a mechanism for classical conditioning; the hypothalamus, which controls various biological functions; and the hippocampus, which places stressful situations in context through the storage of memories. Activation of the HPA axis proceeds when an acute stressor stimulates the central nucleus of the amygdala, which signals the hypothalamus to release corticotrophin-releasing hormone (CRH). This, in turn, stimulates release of adrenocorticotropin from the pituitary gland and then cortisol, a glucocorticoid, from the adrenal gland *(60)*. Cortisol stimulates glucocorticoid receptors on the hippocampus, enhancing long-term memory consolidation *(61)*. Cortisol also increases calcium conductance through voltage-gated ion channels *(62)*, which may contribute to consolidation of long-term memory. Paradoxically, this may also explain the mechanism by which glucocorticoids wither hippocampal neurons—through calcium-induced excitotoxicity. Corticotropic activation of the hippocampus serves as a feedback mechanism to halt hypothalamic release of CRH. Thus, hippocampal cell death caused by chronic stress makes the HPA axis less sensitive to negative feedback inhibition, which perpetuates cortisol release. The self-deteriorating and perpetuating nature of the HPA axis is relevant because cortisol enhances the vasoconstrictive effects of catecholamines and the retention of serum electrolytes, effectively increasing blood pressure in the setting of chronic stress.

The output of the HPA axis and the autonomic nervous system can be measured either by surrogate measures of efferent tone, or by direct measurement of their component molecules. Important methods using these two strategies include muscle sympathetic nerve activity (MSNA), an invasive method of measuring sympathetic tone; HRV, the high-frequency component of which can be used as a noninvasive measure of vagal, or parasympathetic, tone; direct measurement of plasma and saliva cortisol, the latter providing a convenient and noninvasive method for measuring HPA output; and direct measurement of serum catecholamines.

Studies of both MSNA and serum catecholamines have shown that sympathetic output is increased during stress, regardless of stimulus. A large prospective study of outcomes in patients with stable CAD and exercise-induced myocardial ischemia measured sympathetic responses to various mental stressors by measuring serum catecholamines in both a study group of 196 subjects with CAD and in a healthy reference group of 29 subjects *(28,29)*. Both groups experienced increases in serum catecholamines during mental stress, and epinephrine in particular was correlated with increases in blood pressure, heart rate, cardiac output, and SVR in the CAD group *(29)*. Serum cortisol was measured in the reference group, and no significant differences were found in cortisol levels between baseline and any of the acute stress conditions. However, salivary cortisol has been shown to be increased in the setting of chronic job stress and ongoing daily stressful events *(63)*.

Using MSNA as well as measurements of heart rate and blood pressure, one group of researchers assessed responses to mental stress mediated by sympathetic tone by block-

ing sympathetic output centrally with the drug, monoxidine. They found that increases in heart rate, blood pressure, and MSNA during a mental arithmetic stress task were all attenuated by a central sympathetic blockade *(64)*.

Increased sympathetic tone may also contribute to stress-induced arrhythmia. T-wave alternans, a particular measure of heterogeneous myocardial repolarization, is increased during mental stress, and this correlates with increases in epinephrine seen during mental stress *(42)*. Interestingly, the study that demonstrated this relationship found that changes in myocardial repolarization did not correlate with changes in parasympathetic tone as measured by high-frequency HRV. This suggests that mental stress contributes to arrhythmogenesis through an effect of sympathetic mediators on the myocardium itself, as well as through an effect of parasympathetic tone on rate control and pacing. The physiological contribution of decreased parasympathetic tone to the pathology of mental stress remains unclear, although there is some early evidence that parasympathetic tone may play a protective, anti-inflammatory role in CVD *(65)*.

The increases in SVR and coronary vascular tone and the changes in the electrophysiological properties of the myocardium observed during mental stress seem to be related to changes in neurohormonal output from the CNS. The molecules that affect the myocardium, endothelium, and vascular smooth muscle to cause these changes are the final link in the physiological chain that connects mental stress to adverse cardiovascular events. Catecholamines and cortisol clearly have a role in this, although it is not well defined. However, mental stress also causes endothelial dysfunction in both healthy subjects *(35)* and in patients with CAD *(34)*. Consequently, endothelially derived molecules are receiving increasing attention as mediators of mental stress-induced cardiovascular pathology. These autonomic and endothelial mediators are the subject of continuing investigation, because the ability to block the effects of mental stress peripherally has implications for pharmacotherapy of CVD.

The consequences of mental stress-induced activation of these neurohormonal pathways are therefore in have at least four parts. First, chronic mental stress leads to a reduction in parasympathetic tone, which perhaps causes a proinflammatory condition in the vessels that contributes to atherogenesis. Second, mental stress increases both blood pressure and SVR, leading to increased afterloading of the ventricle, which may have both acute and chronic effects on its function as a pump. Third, changes in autonomic tone affect vascular tone, leading to vasoconstriction or even vasospasm in diseased large arteries and in the microcirculation. Ischemia and myocardial damage then ensue as a direct result of vasoconstriction, plaque disruption, or both. Finally, changes in the balance of autonomic tone affect the electrophysiology of the heart. This predisposes the heart to fatal arrhythmias that can cause sudden cardiac death (Fig. 3).

A CONCEPTUAL MODEL OF THE BRAIN–HEART INTERACTION

The links between the CNS and the heart are largely understood in terms of autonomic interactions. The heart is innervated by sympathetic and parasympathetic efferents that regulate both the rate and contractility of the cardiac pump itself and the vascular dynamics of the coronary vessels that nourish it. However, there are higher levels of functioning within the CNS that serve to control both tonic autonomic output and the particular bursts of activity that accompany physical or psychological stimuli. We are personally familiar with the autonomic effects of pain on cardiac function, and even those of physical fear,

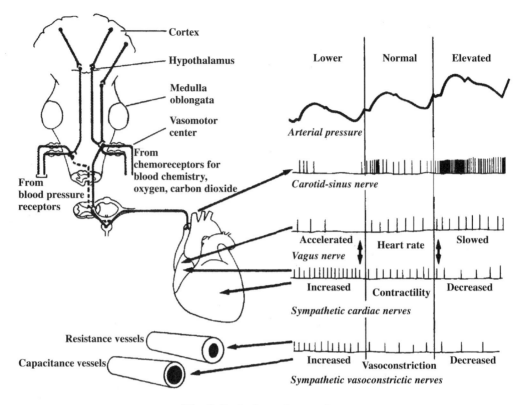

Fig. 3. Brain–heart interaction.

perhaps after a confrontation or a car accident. But far more obscure to our anciently evolved sense of self-preservation are some of the other psychosocial stressors that are nevertheless able to produce robust autonomic responses throughout our bodies, and particularly in our cardiovascular system. Consider the tachycardia, inotropy, tachypnea, and even nausea that can accompany a forgotten meeting suddenly remembered, but with no chance of arriving at the appointed time. This capacity to process a stimulus, generate a fearful response to it, and then signal the appropriate autonomic outputs to initiate the effects of that response requires complicated interactions among higher cortical areas that then feed into and modulate the downstream responses in more primitive CNS regions.

A hypothetical model of the brain's response to stress and of the neurocardiac interaction that mediates that response is beginning to take shape. According to this model, stress is experienced as the perception of a situation or event that makes demands of the survival resources of the individual. These perceptions are mediated by frontal and prefrontal cortical regions in combination with the limbic system. The former are thought to mediate an evaluative component of stress, namely the ability to appropriately assess a threat and shape a response; the latter mediates the experience of stress and the emotional responses associated both with the urgency of a particular threat and with the ability—or inability—to address it. The experience of a stressor as determined by these rational and emotional components then initiates a physiological response that is transduced through subcortical neuronal pathways. Noradrenergic projections from the locus coeruleus to the hypothalamus and the cortex serve to integrate the stress response and,

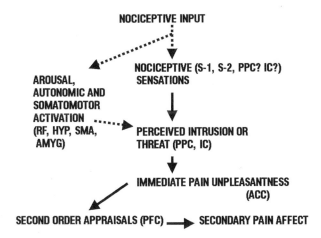

Fig. 4. Typical response patterns to stress. (Reprinted with permission from ref. *66*). ACC, anterior cingulate cortex; AMYG, amygdala; HYP, hypothalamus; IC, insular cortex; PFC, prefrontal cortex; PPC, posterior parietal complex; S-1, S-2, first and second somatosensory cortical areas; SMA, supplementary motor area.

in turn, to modulate the outflow of neurohormonal responses via the HPA axis and the autonomic nervous system. These responses are mediated through peripheral release of stress hormones, as well as through described changes in sympathetic and parasympathetic tone (Fig. 4).

Any response to stress must necessarily be a complex interaction between the stimulus and the individual. There is a wide variety in physiological responses among individuals to even highly standardized psychological stimuli. Conceptually, these represent variations in emotional, psychological, and even biochemical factors that control the experience, interpretation, and responses associated with stress. Elements of experience and interpretation that control the response may be understood as a balance between executive frontal function and emotional limbic function. A tip in the balance favoring emotional, or limbic, forces is in turn associated with a more robust and possibly harmful physiological response. Posttraumatic stress disorder provides an illustrative example of the extreme case, in which, in response to specific stimuli, the balance has been shifted decisively in favor of a marked emotional, physiological response. The ability to hear a loud noise, recognize and process it appropriately as harmless and not as a survival threat, and modulate the attendant startle response, has been lost, and a potentially debilitating response to the stimulus ensues. However, an upsetting of this balance may occur in many far less dramatic cases. Repeated exposure to heavy traffic, long lines, or financial insecurity may cause a chronic processing of these stimuli or anything associated with them as survival threats and may lead to a physiological stress response not commensurate with the actual threat.

The ability to interpret stressors and place them in context thus becomes essential to coping with stress. This ability may be altered in various ways: decreased by exposure to stress, or by associations of otherwise benign circumstances with perceived survival threats; or increased by innate coping skills and the presence of external social support networks that allow us to share and diffuse our stressful experiences, or to have them diminished through the material assistance of others. Furthermore, acute stressors that

represent very real and immediate threats, or are perceived as such, may overwhelm the ability to contextualize and limit the stress response, leading to immediate pathology. This is of particular concern in the setting of existing CVD; acute mental stress seems to induce ACS in most cases by exploiting underlying disease.

Whether the inability to cope with stress or the accumulation of stress-related pathology occurs during a lifetime or instantaneously, the end result is a series of changes in the output of efferent neurohormonal pathways, marked generally by the following sequelae: increased stress hormones, particularly glucocorticoids; increased sympathetic tone, with surges in catecholamines that range from modest to dramatic; and decreased parasympathetic tone. These may lead to a slow degradation of endothelial integrity via increased inflammation. They may cause changes in vascular tone, affecting the ability of the coronary arteries to perfuse the heart or the ability of the heart to pump adequately into the circulation. Alternatively, they may acutely disrupt the normal electrical function of the myocardium, causing arrhythmia.

ISSUES IN TREATMENT AND MANAGEMENT

Although mental stress has an important role in the occurrence and progression of CVD, it presents some unique treatment challenges. The nature of a stressful experience provides two areas of potential focus for clinical intervention: the stressor itself, which may be prevented or lessened; and the host factors of the patient, which may worsen the experience of stress. The former is challenging because it may not be within the power of the treater to significantly alter the stressful circumstances of the patient, and especially to prevent acute stressors that may trigger cardiac events. The latter is challenging because the psychological factors that contribute to the experience of stress have traditionally been outside of the established field of practice for physicians, leading to causing unfamiliarity with those factors and how to treat them. Nevertheless, the importance of the psychology and experience of mental stress to the care of patients with CVD continues to increase. Attempts have been made to address both elements through different therapeutic modalities. The results of therapeutic studies have been promising, offering evidence that psychological interventions can be of benefit in preventing stress-induced myocardial damage.

A number of studies have tested whether treating stress-related factors in patients with CVD improves emotional well-being, quality of life, and event-free survival. A meta-analysis of these studies found that the addition of psychosocial interventions to standard cardiac rehabilitation significantly reduced medical morbidity and mortality and psychological distress, and positively influenced risk factors such as blood pressure, cholesterol level, and heart rate during the 2-yr follow-up (67).

The Recurrent Coronary Prevention Project was a controlled intervention trial in which 1021 post-MI patients were randomly assigned to either cardiac counseling or cardiac counseling with stress reduction counseling for up to 4 yr. Treatment was focused on the development of a greater awareness of personal stress responses, on the learning of strategies for physical and psychological relaxation, and on the modification of attitudes, thoughts, and beliefs that reinforced stressful responses. By the third year of treatment, coronary recurrence rate, defined as both fatal and nonfatal events, was 7.2% for the stress counseling vs 13% for the cardiac counseling-only condition, with the difference being significant only for nonfatal events. Marked reductions in stressful

behavior also resulted from the stress counseling (31.7%) compared with the cardiac counseling (7.2%). Patients received follow-up evaluations 4 to 5 yr after the intervention, and significant differences in coronary recurrences remained.

Another comprehensive intervention designed for patients with CAD was the Lifestyle Heart Trial *(68)*. The intervention condition consisted of a diet and exercise program, stress management, and social support. The stress management component included stretching exercises, diaphragmatic breathing techniques, meditation, progressive muscle relaxation, and imagery. Patients engaged in individual relaxation exercises and structured biweekly group discussions that provided social support and were designed to facilitate patient adherence to lifestyle changes. At the end of the year-long intervention, the average percentage of arterial stenosis in the intervention group decreased from 40 to 37.8%, whereas it increased from 42.7 to 46.1% in the control group. These differences were further magnified when examining only coronary lesions that were of greater than 50% stenosis. Improvements were most pronounced in patients demonstrating the highest levels of treatment adherence. The experimental group also experienced significant decreases in total and low-density lipoprotein cholesterol and reduced complaints of angina.

In the Ischemic Heart Disease Life Stress Monitoring Study, 461 male post-MI patients were randomized to a standard care or intervention and followed for up to 5 yr *(69)*. All received monthly phone monitoring of stress, and when stress levels were high, patients in the treatment group received nurse-delivered, home-based interventions, consisting of support, education, and individually tailored referrals. High-stress patients in the intervention group had significantly fewer recurrent MIs than patients who received standard medical care.

Two studies assessed the value of stress management in patients known to experience myocardial ischemia during mental stress. In the first study, 107 patients with CAD received either usual care, exercise training, or stress management. The stress management group had a 0.26 relative risk for a major cardiac event over 3+ yr of follow-up compared with the usual care group *(70)*. In the second study, 134 patients with ischemic heart disease were also randomized to receive usual care, exercise training, or stress management over 16 wk. The stress management group showed greater improvement in both LV function and HRV at the end of treatment relative to the usual care group *(71)*.

Pharmacological strategies for treatment of CAD related to mental stress show promise as well. Recently, the Sertraline Antidepressant Heart Attack Randomized Trial (SADHEART; *72*) assessed the safety and efficacy of the antidepressant sertraline for treatment of major depression in patients with unstable angina or recent MI *(72)*. The study found that sertraline was safe and effective for treatment of depression in the setting of CAD. However, the study also showed that the incidence of death and severe cardiovascular events was lower among those patients in the treatment group than in the control group during the 24-wk follow-up period. This effect was not significant and the study was not powered to show significance. Nevertheless, it suggests that treatment of depression after MI may improve secondary prevention of cardiac outcomes.

As understanding of the pathophysiology of stress-induced CVD grows, the physiological end-effectors of the experience of stress that act on the heart and blood vessels will present themselves as targets for intervention. The ramifications of research in this area are unclear, but studies that show a role for the endothelium in contributing to the deleterious effects of stress may point to a role for drugs that can interdict this process and protect the blood vessels against the ravages of chronic stress. However, this line of

investigation has not yet succeeded in identifying any specific molecular targets for the interdiction of stress-induced pathology.

The results of these studies demonstrate that it is important for cardiologists to aid their patients in managing risk factors for psychosocial stress, because interventions are effective when provided by appropriately trained professionals. The picture of mental stress in CVD is one of an interaction between the host and the environment, as it is with so many traditional risk factors. Mental stress in all its forms is analogous to traditional risk factors in another important way: both tend to cluster together *(73)*. Even as social–environmental stress may cluster with depression and anxiety, so too any one of these may contribute to behaviors that worsen traditional risk factors, such as inactivity, smoking, or overeating. These forces represent a gathering storm for those whose socioeconomic circumstances and genetic makeup predispose them to the development of CVD, to say nothing of those in the realm of secondary prevention, for whom the storm already rages.

This situation points to the need for comprehensive and multidisciplinary preventive strategies for CVD. A treatment program that addresses traditional risk factors without also addressing psychosocial ones invites problems with adherence and efficacy, and therefore with overall success. In addition, although assessing and treating the mental health and social well-being of patients is beyond the traditional territorial boundaries of the cardiologist, the confluence of these risk factors argues for multidisciplinary approaches to care.

Steps are already being taken in this direction. Various groups have recommended strategies to screen for psychosocial risk factors and to improve patient adherence to treatment regimens. One recommendation is that cardiologists use a set of screening questions to assess a patient's overall level of stress and the social support networks in place to help deal with that stress *(73)*. Another proposal suggests that cardiologists stratify their patients based on psychosocial risk. Patients at higher levels of risk would receive counseling for stress from professional therapists as part of an integrated care team *(13)*. These strategies seek to improve patient wellness and adherence to more traditional therapies, but they require both vigilance and active participation by the cardiologist to recognize and address stress-related risk.

CONCLUSION

There is increasing recognition in the medical and scientific communities of the importance of behavioral and psychosocial factors in the prevention, development, and treatment of cardiovascular disorders. Both chronic and acute psychosocial stress can be detrimental to the patient with CVD, and preliminary evidence indicates that mental stress testing for ischemia is a predictor of prognosis in these individuals. Moreover, the identification of depression and other psychosocial risk factors for coronary disease progression has led to promising behavioral and psychosocial interventions to aid in the treatment and prevention of coronary disease in high-risk individuals. These data provide a basis for the inclusion of psychosocial treatment components in preventive and cardiac rehabilitation efforts, and suggest that the time may be approaching when evaluation and treatment of psychological stress and depression will be an expected standard of treatment for the patient with CVD. However, additional research is needed to identify the role of mental stress testing in risk assessment in CVD, the most effective types of interventions for particular patients, and the cost-effectiveness of these interventions.

REFERENCES

1. Mittleman MA, Maclure M, Sherwood JB, et al. Triggering of acute myocardial infarction onset by episodes of anger. Determinants of Myocardial Infarction Onset Study Investigators. Circulation 1995;92(7):1720–1725.
2. Trichopoulos D, Katsouyanni K, Zavitsanos X, Tzonou A, Dalla-Vorgia P. Psychological stress and fatal heart attack: the Athens (1981) earthquake natural experiment. Lancet 1983;1(8322):441–444.
3. Kloner RA, Leor J, Poole WK, Perritt R. Population-based analysis of the effect of the Northridge Earthquake on cardiac death in Los Angeles County, California. J Am Coll Cardiol 1997;30(5):1174–1180.
4. Leor J, Poole WK, Kloner RA. Sudden cardiac death triggered by an earthquake. N Engl J Med 1996;334(7):413–419.
5. Huang JL, Chiou CW, Ting CT, Chen YT, Chen SA. Sudden changes in heart rate variability during the 1999 Taiwan earthquake. Am J Cardiol Jan 15 2001;87(2):245-248, A249.
6. Brodsky MA, Sato DA, Iseri LT, Wolff LJ, Allen BJ. Ventricular tachyarrhythmia associated with psychological stress. The role of the sympathetic nervous system. JAMA 1987;257(15):2064–2067.
7. Shedd OL, Sears SF Jr, Harvill JL, et al. The World Trade Center attack: increased frequency of defibrillator shocks for ventricular arrhythmias in patients living remotely from New York City. J Am Coll Cardiol 2004;44(6):1265–1267.
8. Steinberg JS, Arshad A, Kowalski M, et al. Increased incidence of life-threatening ventricular arrhythmias in implantable defibrillator patients after the World Trade Center attack. J Am Coll Cardiol 2004;44(6):1261–1264.
9. Li J, Hansen D, Mortensen PB, Olsen J. Myocardial infarction in parents who lost a child: a nationwide prospective cohort study in Denmark. Circulation 2002;106(13):1634–1639.
10. Sharkey SW, Lesser JR, Zenovich AG, et al. Acute and reversible cardiomyopathy provoked by stress in women from the United States. Circulation 2005;111(4):472–479.
11. Wittstein IS, Thiemann DR, Lima JA, et al. Neurohumoral features of myocardial stunning due to sudden emotional stress. N Engl J Med 2005;352(6):539–548.
12. Rozanski A, Blumenthal JA, Kaplan J. Impact of psychological factors on the pathogenesis of cardio-vascular disease and implications for therapy. Circulation 1999;99(16):2192–2217.
13. Rozanski A, Blumenthal JA, Davidson KW, Saab PG, Kubzansky L. The epidemiology, pathophysiol-ogy, and management of psychosocial risk factors in cardiac practice: the emerging field of behavioral cardiology. J Am Coll Cardiol 2005;45(5):637–651.
14. Baum A, Garofalo JP, Yali AM. Socioeconomic status and chronic stress. Does stress account for SES effects on health? Ann NY Acad Sci 1999;896:131–144.
15. Marmot MG, Bosma H, Hemingway H, Brunner E, Stansfeld S. Contribution of job control and other risk factors to social variations in coronary heart disease incidence. Lancet 1997;350(9073):235–239.
16. Greenwood DC, Muir KR, Packham CJ, Madeley RJ. Coronary heart disease: a review of the role of psychosocial stress and social support. J Public Health Med 1996;18(2):221–231.
17. Brezinka V, Kittel F. Psychosocial factors of coronary heart disease in women: a review. Soc Sci Med 1996;42(10):1351–1365.
18. Frasure-Smith N, Lesperance F, Gravel G, et al. Social support, depression, and mortality during the first year after myocardial infarction. Circulation 2000;101(16):1919–1924.
19. Rosengren A, Hawken S, Ounpuu S, et al. Association of psychosocial risk factors with risk of acute myocardial infarction in 11119 cases and 13648 controls from 52 countries (the INTERHEART study): case-control study. Lancet 2004;364(9438):953–962.
20. Glassman AH, Shapiro PA. Depression and the course of coronary artery disease. Am J Psychiatry 1998;155(1):4–11.
21. Strik JJ, Denollet J, Lousberg R, Honig A. Comparing symptoms of depression and anxiety as predictors of cardiac events and increased health care consumption after myocardial infarction. J Am Coll Cardiol 2003;42(10):1801–1807.
22. Kawachi I, Sparrow D, Vokonas PS, Weiss ST. Symptoms of anxiety and risk of coronary heart disease. The Normative Aging Study. Circulation 1994;90(5):2225–2229.
23. Kawachi I, Colditz GA, Ascherio A, et al. Prospective study of phobic anxiety and risk of coronary heart disease in men. Circulation 1994;89(5):1992–1997.
24. Trigo M, Silva D, Rocha E. Psychosocial risk factors in coronary heart disease: beyond type A behavior. Rev Port Cardiol 2005;24(2):261–281.

25. Burg MM, Jain D, Soufer R, Kerns RD, Zaret BL. Role of behavioral and psychological factors in mental stress-induced silent left ventricular dysfunction in coronary artery disease. J Am Coll Cardiol 1993;22(2):440–448.

26. Lampert R, Joska T, Burg MM, Batsford WP, McPherson CA, Jain D. Emotional and physical precipitants of ventricular arrhythmia. Circulation 2002;106(14):1800–1805.

27. Burg MM, Lampert R, Joska T, Batsford W, Jain D. Psychological traits and emotion-triggering of ICD shock-terminated arrhythmias. Psychosom Med 2004;66(6):898–902.

28. Becker LC, Pepine CJ, Bonsall R, et al. Left ventricular, peripheral vascular, and neurohumoral responses to mental stress in normal middle-aged men and women. Reference Group for the Psychophysiological Investigations of Myocardial Ischemia (PIMI) Study. Circulation 1996;94(11):2768–2777.

29. Goldberg AD, Becker LC, Bonsall R, et al. Ischemic, hemodynamic, and neurohormonal responses to mental and exercise stress. Experience from the Psychophysiological Investigations of Myocardial Ischemia Study (PIMI). Circulation 1996;94(10):2402–2409.

30. Jain D, Shaker SM, Burg M, Wackers FJ, Soufer R, Zaret BL. Effects of mental stress on left ventricular and peripheral vascular performance in patients with coronary artery disease. J Am Coll Cardiol 1998;31(6):1314–1322.

31. Deanfield JE, Shea M, Kensett M, et al. Silent myocardial ischaemia due to mental stress. Lancet 1984;2(8410):1001–1005.

32. Soufer R, Arrighi JA, Burg MM. Brain, behavior, mental stress, and the neurocardiac interaction. J Nucl Cardiol 2002;9(6):650–662.

33. Bairey CN, Krantz DS, Rozanski A. Mental stress as an acute trigger of ischemic left ventricular dysfunction and blood pressure elevation in coronary artery disease. Am J Cardiol 1990;66(16):28G–31G.

34. Yeung AC, Vekshtein VI, Krantz DS, et al. The effect of atherosclerosis on the vasomotor response of coronary arteries to mental stress. N Engl J Med 1991;325(22):1551–1556.

35. Ghiadoni L, Donald AE, Cropley M, et al. Mental stress induces transient endothelial dysfunction in humans. Circulation 2000;102(20):2473–2478.

36. Sherwood A, Johnson K, Blumenthal JA, Hinderliter AL. Endothelial function and hemodynamic responses during mental stress. Psychosom Med 1999;61(3):365–370.

37. Takase B, Uehata A, Akima T, et al. Endothelium-dependent flow-mediated vasodilation in coronary and brachial arteries in suspected coronary artery disease. Am J Cardiol 1998;82(12):1535–1539, A1537–1538.

38. Arrighi JA, Burg M, Cohen IS, et al. Myocardial blood-flow response during mental stress in patients with coronary artery disease. Lancet 2000;356(9226):310–311.

39. Benight CC, Segall GM, Ford ME, Goetsch VL, Hays MT, Taylor CB. Psychological stress and myocardial perfusion in coronary disease patients and healthy controls. J Psychosom Res 1997;42(2):137–144.

40. Lampert R, Jain D, Burg MM, Batsford WP, McPherson CA. Destabilizing effects of mental stress on ventricular arrhythmias in patients with implantable cardioverter-defibrillators. Circulation 2000;101(2):158–164.

41. Madden K, Savard GK. Effects of mental state on heart rate and blood pressure variability in men and women. Clin Physiol 1995;15(6):557–569.

42. Lampert R, Shusterman V, Burg MM, et al. Effects of psychologic stress on repolarization and relationship to autonomic and hemodynamic factors. J Cardiovasc Electrophysiol 2005;16(4):372–377.

43. Jain D, Burg M, Soufer R, Zaret BL. Prognostic implications of mental stress-induced silent left ventricular dysfunction in patients with stable angina pectoris. Am J Cardiol 1995;76(1):31–35.

44. Sheps DS, McMahon RP, Becker L, et al. Mental stress-induced ischemia and all-cause mortality in patients with coronary artery disease: results from the Psychophysiological Investigations of Myocardial Ischemia study. Circulation 2002;105(15):1780–1784.

45. Henry JP. The induction of acute and chronic cardiovascular disease in animals by psychosocial stimulation. Int J Psychiatry Med 1975;6(1–2):147–158.

46. Schommer NC, Hellhammer DH, Kirschbaum C. Dissociation between reactivity of the hypothalamus–pituitary–adrenal axis and the sympathetic-adrenal-medullary system to repeated psychosocial stress. Psychosom Med 2003;65(3):450–460.

47. Clarkson TB, Kaplan JR, Adams MR, Manuck SB. Psychosocial influences on the pathogenesis of atherosclerosis among nonhuman primates. Circulation 1987;76(1 Pt 2):I29–40.

48. Kaplan JR, Manuck SB, Clarkson TB, Lusso FM, Taub DM, Miller EW. Social stress and atherosclerosis in normocholesterolemic monkeys. Science 1983;220(4598):733–735.

49. Williams JK, Kaplan JR, Manuck SB. Effects of psychosocial stress on endothelium-mediated dilation of atherosclerotic arteries in cynomolgus monkeys. J Clin Invest 1993;92(4):1819–1823.

50. Skantze HB, Kaplan J, Pettersson K, et al. Psychosocial stress causes endothelial injury in cynomolgus monkeys via beta1-adrenoceptor activation. Atherosclerosis 1998;136(1):153–161.

51. Phan KL, Taylor SF, Welsh RC, et al. Activation of the medial prefrontal cortex and extended amygdala by individual ratings of emotional arousal: a fMRI study. Biol Psychiatry 2003;53(3):211–215.

52. Soufer RS, Bremner D, Arrighi JA, et al. Cerebral cortical hyperactivation in response to mental stress in patients with heart disease. Proc Natl Acad Sci USA 1998;95:6454–6459.

53. Damasio AR, Grabowski TJ, Bechara A, et al. Subcortical and cortical brain activity during the feeling of self-generated emotions. Nat Neurosci 2000;3(10):1049–1056.

54. Critchley HD, Corfield DR, Chandler MP, Mathias CJ, Dolan RJ. Cerebral correlates of autonomic cardiovascular arousal: a functional neuroimaging investigation in humans. J Physiol 2000;523 Pt 1:259–270.

55. Shin LM, Wright CI, Cannistraro PA, et al. A functional magnetic resonance imaging study of amygdala and medial prefrontal cortex responses to overtly presented fearful faces in posttraumatic stress disorder. Arch Gen Psychiatry 2005;62(3):273–281.

56. Liberzon I, Taylor SF, Amdur R, et al. Brain activation in PTSD in response to trauma-related stimuli. Biol Psychiatry 1999;45(7):817–826.

57. Rauch SL, Savage CR, Alpert NM, Fischman AJ, Jenike MA. The functional neuroanatomy of anxiety: a study of three disorders using positron emission tomography and symptom provocation. Biol Psychiatry 1997;42(6):446–452.

58. Tillfors M, Furmark T, Marteinsdottir I, et al. Cerebral blood flow in subjects with social phobia during stressful speaking tasks: a PET study. Am J Psychiatry 2001;158(8):1220–1226.

59. Bremner JD, Soufer R, McCarthy G, et al. Gender differences in cognitive and neural correlates of remembrance of emotionally valenced words. Psychopharmacology Bulletin 2001;35:55–78.

60. Charney DS. Neuroanatomical circuits modulating fear and anxiety behaviors. Acta Psychiatr Scand Suppl 2003(417):38–50.

61. Nathan SV, Griffith QK, McReynolds JR, Hahn EL, Roozendaal B. Basolateral amygdala interacts with other brain regions in regulating glucocorticoid effects on different memory functions. Ann NY Acad Sci 2004;1032:179–182.

62. Kerr DS, Campbell LW, Thibault O, Landfield PW. Hippocampal glucocorticoid receptor activation enhances voltage-dependent Ca2+ conductances: relevance to brain aging. Proc Natl Acad Sci USA 1992;89(18):8527–8531.

63. Steptoe A, Cropley M, Griffith J, Kirschbaum C. Job strain and anger expression predict early morning elevations in salivary cortisol. Psychosom Med 2000;62(2):286–292.

64. Wenzel RR, Spieker L, Qui S, Shaw S, Luscher TF, Noll G. I1-imidazoline agonist moxonidine decreases sympathetic nerve activity and blood pressure in hypertensives. Hypertension 1998;32(6):1022–1027.

65. Tracey KJ. The inflammatory reflex. Nature 2002;420(6917):853–859.

66. Price DD. Psychological and neural mechanisms of the affective dimension of pain. Science 2000; 288(55472):1769–1772.

67. Linden W, Stossel C, Maurice J. Psychosocial interventions for patients with coronary artery disease: a meta-analysis. Arch Intern Med 1996;156(7):745–752.

68. Ornish D, Brown SE, Scherwitz LW, et al. Can lifestyle changes reverse coronary heart disease? The Lifestyle Heart Trial. Lancet 1990;336(8708):129–133.

69. Frasure-Smith N, Lesperance F, Juneau M. Differential long-term impact of in-hospital symptoms of psychological stress after non-Q-wave and Q-wave acute myocardial infarction. Am J Cardiol 1992;69(14):1128–1134.

70. Blumenthal JA, Jiang W, Babyale MA, et al. Stress management and exercise training in cardiac patients with myocardial ischemia. Effects on prognosis and evaluation of mechanisms. Arch Intern Med 1997; 157(19):2213–2223.

71. Blumenthal JA, Sherwood A, Babyale MA, et al. Effects of exercise and stress management trainingggg on markers of cardiovascular risk in patients with ischemic heart disease: a randomized controlled trial. JAMA 2005;293(13):1629–1634.

72. Glassman AH, O'Connor CM, Califf RM, et al. Sertraline treatment of major depression in patients with acute MI or unstable angina. JAMA 2002;288(6):701–709.

73. Albus C, Jordan J, Herrmann-Lingen C. Screening for psychosocial risk factors in patients with coronary heart disease-recommendations for clinical practice. Eur J Cardiovasc Prev Rehabil 2004;11(1):75–79.

12   Women and Coronary Artery Disease

JoAnne Micale Foody, MD

CONTENTS

INTRODUCTION

Heart disease is the leading cause of mortality among women in the United States—500,000 women each year die of heart disease; more than twice the number of deaths caused by all cancers combined *(1)*. Approximately one out of every two women in the United States will die from some cardiovascular event—most likely, myocardial infarction (MI), hypertensive heart disease, or stroke *(1)*. The clinical presentation of heart disease *(2,3)*, the impact of individual coronary risk factors *(1,4–7)* and the results of their interventions differ dramatically by gender *(8–17)*. This chapter reviews the uniquely female attributes that are associated with differences in disease presentation, that attenuate coronary risk, and that modulate clinical outcomes.

CORONARY ARTERY DISEASE IN WOMEN

Epidemiology

Coronary artery disease (CAD), the progression of atherosclerosis in the coronary vasculature, is the leading cause of mortality among women in the United States—more than all cancers combined (Fig. 1). Half of all women develop CAD, and one in three die from it *(1)*, accounting for more than 300,000 deaths per year *(18)*. Despite major improvements in the mortality rates for men with CAD, mortality rates in women continue to increase (Fig. 2).

From: *Contemporary Cardiology: Preventive Cardiology:*
Insights Into the Prevention and Treatment of Cardiovascular Disease, Second Edition
Edited by: J. M. Foody © Humana Press Inc., Totowa, NJ

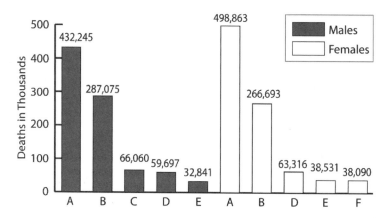

Fig. 1. Leading causes of death for all men and women in the United States, 2001. (From Heart Disease and Stroke Statistics 2005 Update, American Heart Association, with permission.)

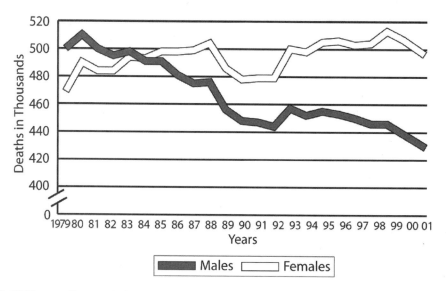

Fig. 2. CVD mortality trends for men and women in the United States, 1979 to 2001. (From Heart Disease and Stroke Statistics 2005 Update, American Heart Association, with permission.)

CAD is not limited to only older women, a significant number of younger women develop CAD *(19,20)*. Among women, rates vary by race/ethnicity. African-American women have higher mortality rates from CAD than white women. The age-adjusted CAD death rate is 25 to 50% higher for black than white women in the United States, with the death rate from MI for African-American women double that for white women. Despite the high prevalence of CAD in women, it has been viewed as a disease of middle-aged men *(3)*.

The increasing rates of CAD are not surprising in view of the fact that coronary risk factors are highly prevalent and increasing in women in the United States. In women aged 20 to 74 yr, 33% have hypertension, more than 25% have hypercholesterolemia, more than 25% are cigarette smokers, more than 25% are overweight, and more than 25%

report sedentary lifestyles *(1)*. Although these risk factors are more prevalent in men than in women, as women age their risk factor profile approaches and, in some instances, surpasses that of their male counterparts.

Although multiple clinical trials have identified important risk factors and effective therapies for CAD, few of these studies have included sufficient numbers of women to draw meaningful conclusions *(21)*.Thus, much of the evidence that supports contemporary recommendations for testing, prevention, and treatment of coronary disease in women is extrapolated from studies conducted predominantly in middle-aged men. Applying the findings of studies in men to management of CAD in women may not be appropriate, because the symptoms of CAD, natural history, and response to therapy may differ in men and women.

CAD Risk Factors in Women

DYSLIPIDEMIA

It is well-established that the higher the level of serum cholesterol, the higher the risk of CAD in both men and women *(22,23)*. In contrast to men, lipid and lipoprotein concentrations vary according to a woman's ovarian function and, therefore, women are at different risks as ovarian function changes. Although the plasma cholesterol (TC) level is similar in both sexes up to 20 yr of age, the TC level increases progressively but at a slower rate for women until the sixth decade, and women have lower total cholesterol than men. After the sixth decade, women's TC levels generally increase faster, exceeding those of men of similar age. Although TC is significantly associated with CAD in women, for a given level of TC, however, women have lower absolute rates of disease than men. For example, the Framingham investigators found that women with total cholesterol levels greater than 295 mg/dL had only 60% the rate of MI compared with men with this same level of TC *(5)*.

Similarly, high-density lipoprotein (HDL)-C is affected by ovarian function. The HDL-C levels of boys are slightly higher than those of girls until puberty, but as girls pass through puberty, HDL-C levels do not fall as they do in boys of the same age. After puberty, HDL-C levels in women increase slowly until before menopause, whereas they remain constant in men. Thus, the average HDL-C values in adult women are approx 20% higher than those of men *(24)*. Although HDL-C levels decline by approx 3.5 mg/dL after menopause, they generally remain higher in women than men throughout life *(25)*.

Elevated HDL-C levels play a key role in protecting both men and women against the development of CAD *(26)*. Data from the Framingham study demonstrate that HDL-C level is also a more powerful predictor in women: for every 10 mg/dL change in HDL-C, a 40 to 50% reduction in coronary risk was noted, and the Framingham investigators suggest that the protective effect of HDL-C in women is approximately twice the atherogenic effect of low-density lipoprotein (LDL)-C *(27–29)*. Both the Framingham study and the Donolo–Tel Aviv Study *(30,31)* have documented increased CAD incidence and mortality in women whose HDL-C levels are greater than 35 mg/dL but less than 50 mg/dL.

LDL-C levels are lower in women than in men throughout the first two-thirds of the life span. After the mid-50s, as a result of menopause, LDL-C levels in women rise abruptly, whereas LDL-C levels in men remain stable. In the last third of life, women generally have higher LDL-C levels *(5)*. Although the National Cholesterol Education Program (NCEP) Adult Treatment Panel III Report indicates an LDL-C level of 130 mg/ dL or higher as a risk factor for CAD in both men and women independent of HDL-C,

the role of LDL-C as a risk factor in women is somewhat controversial. Few prospective studies have examined LDL-C and CAD risk in women. Although very high LDL-C concentrations carry the same poor prognosis in both sexes, mild elevations of LDL-C are not associated with the same risk burden in women compared with men. This may be because of generally higher levels of HDL-C.

Little difference in triglyceride (TG) concentrations is noted between sexes until puberty. Then, TG increases in both sexes with increasing age, although at a much slower rate in women. TG levels in men actually decrease in middle age, whereas they continue to increase gradually in women. Thus, mean levels in women equal those of men by the age of 70 yr. Recent studies have identified TGs as statistically independent predictors of CAD risk even after adjustment for multiple risk factors, including TC levels. Elevated TG levels are likely to be prevalent in older postmenopausal women, in whom they may be markers for the presence of metabolic syndrome, insulin resistance, and associated atherogenic lipoproteins.

DIABETES MELLITUS

Diabetes mellitus is one of the most important risk factors for CAD in women. The presence of diabetes alone or in combination with other risk factors places women at increase risk for subsequent cardiovascular events. This increase risk pertains to women of all ages. Women with diabetes have been found to have twice the risk of MI as nondiabetic women of the same age. In women with diabetes, the incidence of CAD is almost three times that of nondiabetic women, as compared with a twofold increase in incidence in men. The presence of diabetes tends to attenuate any gender-related differences in cardiovascular morbidity and mortality. In fact, the risk of cardiovascular events in women with diabetes is higher than that of both men with diabetes and nondiabetic women, even after adjustment has been made for age and other cardiovascular risk factors.

The higher risk among women with diabetes may be partially explained by the "clustering" of multiple risk factors in individuals with diabetes, such as hypertension, smoking, and obesity. Women with diabetes have significantly higher levels of four cardiovascular risk factors (other than diabetes or high blood glucose levels):

1. Low HDL-C.
2. High TGs.
3. High systolic blood pressure.
4. High body mass index (BMI).

Differences in lipoprotein levels between subjects with diabetes and controls are much more dramatic in women than in men (32). Whether the increased risk associated with diabetes is caused by clustering of other risk factors or is caused by diabetes itself remains to be fully explored in women.

HYPERTENSION

The two other leading causes of cardiovascular mortality and morbidity in women are stroke and hypertension. Stroke is the second leading cause of cardiovascular mortality in women, accounting for nearly 100,000 deaths among women in the United States in 2001 (7). This number is substantially higher than the number of men who died from stroke in that year. The incidence of both fatal and nonfatal stroke rises steadily with age in both genders. Among women aged 30 to 44 yr, the estimated incidence of stroke is only

8000 annually. This figure rises sharply to 50,000 in women between the ages of 45 and 65 yr, and more than triples to 179,000 in women older than 65 yr. Thus, postmenopausal women are at significantly higher risk of stroke than are premenopausal women. Although the incidence of stroke is higher for men of all ages compared with women of all ages, the mortality rate is higher in women. This is caused, in large part, by almost an 80% higher death rate from stoke in black women than in white women.

The epidemiology, natural history, and therapy of hypertension are impacted by gender. Although premenopausal women are less likely than men to have hypertension, one in four white women aged 20 yr or greater have hypertension. The tendency of women to have lower blood pressure than men early in life is counterbalanced by the fact that a women's blood pressure increases more steeply with aging than it does in men. Before menopause, women are at risk for hypertension predominantly because of two gender specific exposures: contraceptive use and pregnancy. With menopause, women (in particular, African-American women) develop hypertension. By age 65 yr, more than half of all women are hypertensive and nearly three-quarters of women older than the age of 75 yr are hypertensive.

OBESITY

The Nurses' Health Study *(33)* showed that, compared with the leanest women, women with a BMI of 25 to 29 kg/m^2 had an age-adjusted relative risk for coronary heart disease (CHD) of 1.8, whereas morbidly obese women (BMI > 29 kg/m^2) had a relative risk for CHD of 3.3. In 115,886 American women, 30 to 55 yr of age, who were followed in the Nurses' Health Study, 40% of coronary events were attributable to excess body weight. Twenty-five percent of American women 35 to 64 yr of age have BMIs of 29 or higher—the category of women having relative risks of nonfatal MI and fatal CHD of 3.2 and 3.5, respectively.

Obesity has been shown to be an independent risk factor for the development of CAD in women. In a 26-yr follow-up of participants in the Framingham Heart Study, relative weight in women was positively and independently associated with coronary disease, and coronary and cardiovascular disease (CVD) death. The study further showed that weight gain after the young adult years conveyed an increased risk of CVD in both genders that could not be attributed either to the initial weight or the levels of the risk factors that may have resulted from weight gain. Based on other epidemiological studies, 30% of the CAD occurring in obese women can be attributed to the excess weight alone, and even mild-to-moderate overweight increases the risk of coronary disease in middle-aged women.

Truncal, android, or male-pattern obesity, manifested as a rise in the waist-to-hip ratio, correlates with higher LDL-C and lower HDL-C levels. Truncal obesity is associated with both higher blood pressure and hyperinsulinemia, which leads to increases in atherogenic lipoproteins and decreases in HDL-C. The mechanism for this is unclear, although it has been hypothesized that it may somehow be related to an increase in peripheral insulin resistance: the portal venous drainage of abdominal fat may induce hepatic insulin resistance, elevated circulating insulin, higher TG levels, and lower HDL-C levels.

Obesity has been strongly associated in women with three major risk factors for CAD: noninsulin-dependent diabetes mellitus, hypercholesterolemia, and hypertension. In multiple studies, obesity was found to be associated with significant modifications of the lipid profile, especially higher TG and LDL-C levels. In fact, more than generalized obesity, an increase in truncal fat (also called "android" or male-pattern obesity) is

manifested as a rise in the waist-to-hip ratio, and correlates with higher LDL-C and lower HDL-C levels. Central or truncal obesity is associated with both higher blood pressure and hyperinsulinemia, which is thought to result in increases in atherogenic lipoproteins and decreases in HDL-C. The mechanism for this is unclear, although it has been hypothesized that it may somehow be related to an increase in peripheral insulin resistance: the portal venous drainage of abdominal fat may induce hepatic insulin resistance, elevated circulating insulin, higher TG levels, and lower HDL-C levels *(34)*.

SMOKING

Although diabetes is the most biologically gender-differentiated risk factor for coronary disease in women, cigarette smoking may be the most psychologically and sociologically distinguishing risk-behavior for men and women. Smoking is deadly, claiming more than 200,000 lives in the United States, or nearly one-fifth of all heart disease deaths. Although smoking prevalence has declined more rapidly among men than women, rates in women have plateaued because young women are now smoking at greater rates than young men. The gender gap in smoking prevalence has narrowed considerably. This is likely to contribute to a substantially greater female burden of CVD.

New evidence points to the significant role of passive smoking in the development of CAD. Women are seriously threatened by this new, emerging risk factor for CAD. Passive smoke reduces the ability of the blood to deliver oxygen to the myocardium and impairs the heart's ability to use oxygen. After inhaling only two cigarettes, nonsmokers' platelet activity matches that of a habitual smoker. Second-hand smoke causes increased intimal wall damage, accelerates atherosclerotic lesions, and increases intimal wall damage after ischemia or MI.

For several decades, it has been clear that smoking is associated with an elevated risk of CHD among men. For some time, it was believed that cigarette smoking was not associated with CHD among women. However, positive correlations have been observed in both case–control and prospective–cohort studies of nonfatal MI, and of fatal coronary disease.

PHYSICAL ACTIVITY

Sedentary lifestyle is now recognized as a major risk for CAD *(34–42)*. Even moderately fit women demonstrate significantly lower blood glucose, blood pressures, and weight, in addition to improved lipid profiles, when compared with women in the lowest fitness category. Thus, the American College of Cardiology/American Heart Association (AHA) guidelines recommend exercise as a key component to any prevention program *(43–45)*. Increasing evidence shows that inactivity and a sedentary lifestyle may be independent risk factors for the development of CAD in both men and women. Few studies have addressed the relationship between physical fitness or habitual activity level to CVD in women.

Cross-sectional studies comparing active and sedentary women report a positive association between exercise and HDL-C in both premenopausal and postmenopausal women. Significant differences between groups remained for HDL-C values when results were adapted for differences in percent of body fat. Two studies compared plasma lipids with menopausal status in female runners. They showed no differences in HDL-C between premenopausal and postmenopausal women who exercised, but when inactive and exercising women were compared, it seemed that younger premenopausal women responded with lipoprotein changes less strongly than older postmenopausal women.

Hence, exercise seemed to attenuate the age-related increase in LDL-C and decrease in HDL-C. Otherwise, in these cross-sectional studies, women taking hormone replacement therapy (HRT) who reported exercising had higher HDL-C levels than sedentary women not taking HRT.

Psychosocial Aspects of Heart Disease in Women

During the past decade, a large body of evidence has accumulated regarding the relationship of socioeconomic status, employment, type A behavior, hostility, depression, and social support to CVD.

Socioeconomic factors, including educational attainment, are an important contributing factor to coronary disease risk. Women with a low educational level had a significantly increased age-specific incidence of angina pectoris. There was no significant correlation between marital status or number of children and incidence of ischemic heart disease or overall mortality. Multivariate analyses showed that the association between low educational level and incidence of angina pectoris was independent of socioeconomic group itself, cigarette smoking, systolic blood pressure, indices of obesity, serum TGs, and serum cholesterol.

As women have assumed different roles in the workplace, the impact of these roles on cardiovascular and women's health in general has come into question. Working women seem to be healthier than nonworking/nonemployed women, according to several health indicators. Several additional studies have confirmed these results. Employed women, in general, have fewer risk factors: they smoke fewer cigarettes, have lower fasting glucose levels, drink less alcohol, and exercise more than their unemployed counterparts. Mean HDL-C level was significantly higher in employed women compared with homemakers.

Menopause as a Risk Factor

No risk factor is as specific for women as hormonal status. Menopause, or the permanent cessation of menses resulting from the loss of ovarian function, coincides with an increase in several comorbidities, including CVD. As defined by the World Health Organization, menopause is clinically defined as the absence of menses for at least 1 yr. The perimenopause is the period immediately before menopause that is characterized by progressive alterations in endocrine and reproductive functions.

Menopause evokes several endocrine changes that have a dramatic impact on postmenopausal health. Ovarian secretion of estrogen, progesterone, and inhibin progressively decline as ovarian function ceases. As a result, the secretion of both follicle-stimulating hormone and luteinizing hormone is altered. In contrast to estrogen, androgen production from the ovary is less affected by menopause. The adrenal gland continues to secrete large amounts of the precursor steroids, such as dehydroepiandosterone-sulfate and androstenedione, which can be converted into androgens and/or estrogens in the peripheral tissues. The conversion of these precursor steroids to estrone by adipose tissue is the major source of estrogen in postmenopausal women. As a result of these modifications, the ratios of estrone and estradiol and of androgens to estrogens is increased in the postmenopausal woman.

The increase in the prevalence of CVD in the postmenopausal years has been partially attributed to the adverse effects of estrogen deficiency on plasma lipid and lipoprotein levels, to direct effects of estrogen deficiency on the cardiovascular system, and finally, to an increase in central obesity. Multiple studies show that a direct relationship does exist between menopause and risk of CAD in women.

More recently, investigators have focused on the role of menopause in the development of the constellation of metabolic abnormalities, including central obesity and insulin resistance. Review of cross-sectional and longitudinal studies suggest that the menopause transition is associated with an increase in abdominal and visceral adipose tissue accumulation. These results seem to be independent of the aging process and total body fat distribution. The majority of interventional studies involving the use of HRT show that HRT attenuates the accumulation of central fat in postmenopausal women compared with controls. Retrospective comparisons of users and nonusers of HRT also demonstrate a protective effect of HRT on fat distribution. In general, little data exist regarding the role of menopause in the development of insulin resistance. However, there seems to be a moderate effect of menopause on its development. Moderate effects of estrogen therapy on were found on insulin resistance in postmenopausal women, although long-term clinical trials are lacking. Treatment with progestins seems to have a deleterious effect on insulin sensitivity. It has been hypothesized that a portion of the adverse cardiovascular risk associated with menopause may be associated with metabolic derangements, resulting in an increase in central obesity and insulin resistance.

Prevention of CAD in Women

The recently released AHA guidelines for the prevention of CVD in women (46) provide an evidence-based approach to risk factor modification in women. In an effort to provide interventions tailored to individual patient risk, the guidelines provide a scoring sheet for physicians to calculate a woman's 10-yr risk of having a coronary event based on the Framingham Risk Calculator (Appendix A). The Framingham Risk Calculator can be used to assess the 10-yr absolute risk of CHD and, based on an individual's assigned risk, they can be categorized as either "high," "intermediate," "low," or "optimal" risk (Table 1).

Once patient risk has been determined, patients can be further stratified into risk strata, and therapies can be tailored accordingly. The authors provide specific lifestyle interventions, major risk-factor interventions, preventive therapies, atrial fibrillation/stroke prevention interventions, and Class III (harmful) interventions, according to a woman's risk level.

RISK FACTOR MODIFICATION IN WOMEN

Modification of Blood Lipids

Primary Prevention

The majority of primary prevention trials have focused on middle-aged men. Limited data are available in women, and this provides a barrier to the implementation of strategies to reduce risk in women. The Air Force/Texas Coronary Atherosclerosis Prevention Study (47) is the first primary prevention statin study to include a large number of women (997/6605). Therapy with the cholesterol-lowering drug, lovastatin (Mevacor), reduced the risk of first acute major coronary events in healthy adults with average-to-mildly elevated cholesterol levels and lowered HDL by 36%. The trial included 6605 healthy adults aged 45 to 73 yr (997 women, 487 Hispanic Americans, and 206 African Americans). Inclusion criteria for the study included no evidence of CAD, an LDL-C between 130 and 190 mg/dL, HDL less than 45 mg/dL (<47 mg/dL for women), and TG levels less than 400 mg/dL. None of the participants had evidence of heart disease; 22%

Table 1
Risk Group Based on Framingham Global Risk and Clinical Disease

Risk group	Framingham global risk (10-yr absolute CHD risk)	Clinical examples
High risk	>20%	• Established CHD • Cerebrovascular disease • Abdominal aortic aneurysm • Diabetes mellitus • Chronic kedney disease
Intermediate risk	10–20%	• Subclinical DVBD (e.g., coronary calcification) • Medatoblic syndrome • Multiple risk factors • Markedly elevated levels of a single risk factor • First-degree relative (s) with early-onset (age: <55 yr in men and <65 yr in women) atherosclerotic CVD
Lower risk	<10%	• May include women with multiple risk factors, metabolic syndrome, or 1 or no risk factors
Optimal risk	<10%	• Optimal levels of risk factors and heart-healthy lifestyle

had hypertension, 2% had diabetes, and 12% were smokers. Preliminary results indicate that patients taking lovastatin had reduced risk for coronary events. Their risk of first acute coronary event (sudden death, MI, unstable angina) was reduced by 36%, risk of first coronary events was reduced by 54% in women, 34% in men, 43% in hypertensive and diabetic patients, and 29% in the elderly. Patients in the lovastatin group also had a 33% reduction in procedures such as angioplasty and bypass, and a 34% reduction in hospitalization because of unstable angina.

These results are significant for several reasons. The study included a large number of minorities, and, in general, included patients that would not ordinarily have been considered candidates for cholesterol-lowering therapy based on precious NCEP guidelines. This group, however, represents the majority of people who eventually develop heart disease. This study represents a significant advance in our understanding of the role of reducing cholesterol in preventing new onset of heart disease in apparently healthy persons. The West of Scotland Coronary Prevention Study (WOSCOPS) *(48)* demonstrated that treatment of relatively high-risk men with clearly elevated cholesterol levels significantly reduced their risk of heart attack and death from heart disease. The Air Force/Texas Coronary Atherosclerosis Prevention Study dramatically expands the number of people who are possibly candidates for drug therapy for their cholesterol levels to include women, patients with diabetes, and minorities.

SECONDARY PREVENTION

Recent trials have demonstrated that the most significant benefit for lipid lowering in women is in women with existing CAD. Although few studies include women, and very

few analyze women in a separate group, recent data suggest a significant decrease in coronary morbidity and mortality with the aggressive lowering of cholesterol levels in women. The impact of drug therapy seems comparable or even more effective in altering lipid levels in women, compared with men in both primary and secondary prevention. A consistent, albeit limited, set of data exists in women. Recent data from the Scandinavian Simvastatin Survival Study (4S) *(49)*, Cholesterol and Recurrent Events (CARE) *(50)*, and Long-Term Intervention with Pravastatin in Ischaemic Disease (LIPID) studies have expanded our knowledge regarding the importance of lipid lowering with statins in women.

In the 4S trial *(49)* of 4444 patients, 18% of whom were women, simvastatin produced mean changes in TC, LDL-C, and HDL-C of –25%, –35%, and +8%, respectively. The probability that a woman avoided a major coronary event was 77.5% in the placebo group and 85.1% in the treatment group. Total mortality and risk for a major coronary event were similar for both genders. Other benefits of treatment included a 37% reduction ($p < 0.00001$) in the risk of undergoing myocardial revascularization procedures.

In the CARE study *(50)*, designed to address the question of whether LDL-C lowering with pravastatin in patients with CHD and normal or only mildly elevated LDL-C concentrations provided clinical benefit, a greater reduction in CHD death and nonfatal MI was observed in the subset of women in this study as compared with men. These data corroborate the findings from other trials that the benefits of lipid-lowering therapy start to appear relatively soon after the initiation of therapy. Women may have a greater benefit from cholesterol-reduction interventions.

The LIPID study, performed in New Zealand and Australia, was a double-blind, random, placebo-control study on 9014 subjects (1511 of whom were women, one-third older than age 65 yr, and 777 had diabetes) using 40 mg/d pravastatin. Subjects age 31 to 75 yr, who experienced an acute MI or unstable angina within the previous 3 mo to 3 yr and had TC values from 155 to 270 mg/dL, and TG levels less than 445 mg/dL, were eligible for participation. The primary endpoint, coronary mortality, was reduced by 24% ($p < 0.0005$). Secondary objectives, total mortality (reduced by 23%; $p < 0.0001$), and overall cardiac events (23% reduction; $p < 0.0001$) were also met, with demonstrated positive results. The risk reduction in MI incidence was 29%; $p < 0.00001$. Procedure rates of coronary artery bypass graft and percutaneous transluminal coronary angioplasty were also reduced by 24 and 18%, respectively. Stroke incidence was reduced by 20% ($p = 0.022$).

Although the 4S trial was the first secondary prevention trial to clearly demonstrated a reduction in total mortality, the LIPID trial has significant differences in design and hypotheses. Important differences exist between the LIPID study and 4S cohort. Fully 80% of the LIPID enrollees were not candidates for 4S, based on their cholesterol level, age, or history of CAD. LIPID is the first study to examine the use of a hydroxy-methylglutaryl–coenzyme A reductase inhibitor in patients with a history of unstable angina. The LIPID study provides important data on noncoronary mortality and on other groups, such as women and patients with diabetes who, to date, were underrepresented in clinical trials.

Postmenopausal women with a history of CHD may need more aggressive treatment for elevated cholesterol, according to a recent study. The Heart and Estrogen/Progestin Replacement Study (HERS) *(51,52)*, involving 2763 women with a known history of CAD, found that although 47% of the HERS participants were currently receiving some

form of cholesterol-lowering medication, 63% had LDL-C levels that exceeded the NCEP guidelines. Therefore, many of the women who were eligible to receive cholesterol-lowering drug therapy based on their elevated cholesterol levels either were not receiving drug treatment, or were not treated aggressively enough. Of the study's participants, 91% had LDL-C levels that exceeded the 1993 Adult Treatment Panel goal of less than 100 mg/dL.

Most of the women were white (88.7% white, 7.9% African American, and 2% Hispanic) and most were generally inactive and overweight. Many were ex-smokers (49%) and more than 13% still smoked. More than half (59.5%) had high blood pressure and 23% had diabetes. The researchers found that women with one or more of the following conditions were less likely to be taking a cholesterol-lowering agent: were African American, Hispanic, or of other ethnic identity; had a higher BMI; were sedentary; were a consumer of alcohol or tobacco; or had a diagnosis of CAD that preceded 1985. Women with lower LDL-C levels tended to have postgraduate education, participated in an exercise program, and were never married.

Cholesterol should be treated in women, as in men, and women may benefit more. The fact that premenopausal women are at lower risk of heart disease than men of the same age has been misinterpreted by many to mean that risk factors are not as important to treat in women as in men.

Despite ample data on the benefits of lipid lowering, data from the HERS study in women with heart disease indicate less than half (47%) of women were being treated with lipid-lowering therapy and, of these, less than 1 in 10 women (8%) reached the goal LDL-C of 100 mg/dL.

Dietary Modification and Weight Loss in Women

Efforts to prevent or treat obesity have had only limited success. Striking excesses in morbidity and mortality from CHD attributable to obesity in middle-aged women have stimulated greater efforts to understand and treat the problem of obesity in women. The presence of excess truncal fat in both men and women correlates with increases in LDL-C and decreases in HDL-C, accounting for the increase risk of CHD observed in central obesity. Adipose tissue in postmenopausal women can serve as a source of estrogen synthesis. Thus, the benefits of weight reduction in older women may be offset by the loss of estrogen-producing adipose tissue. As an additional consequence, the expected increases in HDL-C and decline in LDL-C with weight loss may be less evident than in men.

The NCEP dietary intervention recommends that dietary changes should be made in two steps. Step I involves an intake of saturated fat of 8 to 10% of total calories, 30% or less of the total calories should be derived from fat, and less than 300 mg of cholesterol per day. If this diet proves inadequate to achieve the goals, the patient should proceed to the Step II diet. Step II calls for further reductions in saturated fat intake, to less than 7% of calories and reductions in cholesterol to less than 200 mg/d. The polyunsaturated/saturated fat ratio should, thus, be increased.

All reduced-fat diets have a beneficial effect on LDL-C, but they consistently also reduce HDL-C, which is disadvantageous for women. Furthermore, the literature observes specific gender differences for diet responsiveness. Furthermore, menopausal status may affect dietary responsiveness. Men have a greater decline in LDL-C and TG levels than in postmenopausal women, whereas postmenopausal women have a greater decline in HDL-C levels than in men when following a low-fat diet.

From the woman's perspective, the most important problem with diet therapy seems to be the accompanying decrease of HDL-C. The decrease is more severe in women, and even more extreme in postmenopausal women. Given that the inverse relationship of HDL-C to cardiac events may be more emphatic in women than the adverse risk imparted by LDL-C, the conclusion is that diet may have the opposite of the desired effect. As suggested, for women with a very high LDL-C who are at risk for CHD, all available techniques must be used to lower LDL-C. For low-risk women, unless they have a weight problem, the benefits of a low-fat diet are far from clear.

In addition to caloric restriction and behavior modification, exercise is one of the most effective methods of weight loss for the obese patient. The greatest weight losses have been reported in a combined regime of diet and exercise rather than diet or exercise alone. Two issues important to weight loss effectiveness are degree of loss and duration of loss. Even if weight is lost, studies indicate that, in the vast majority of cases, weight loss maintenance frequently fails because of the many physiological factors that contribute to obesity. Approximately two-thirds of persons who lose weight will regain it within 1 yr, and almost all persons who lose weight will regain it within 5 yr. As evidenced by a substantial research, this short-term weight loss is ineffective in modifying coronary risk factors. Additional health risks that accompany weight cycling are increased cardiovascular morbidity and mortality, as well as increased abdominal fat, blood pressure, and insulin resistance.

Exercise

Exercise is generally accepted as a mechanism to increase HDL-C and to lower LDL-C levels in men. Although a number of studies have been performed in women, they unfortunately fail to consider potential confounders, such as hormonal status and body composition. Cross-sectional studies comparing active and sedentary women report a positive association between exercise and HDL-C in both premenopausal and postmenopausal women. Results from longitudinal training studies are more difficult to interpret because of experimental design, inadequate type, duration, and intensity of the exercise interventions or lipid measurements made without regard for the phase of the menstrual cycle or if the studies were performed in women with high baseline HDL-C levels. Because lipids vary approx 10 to 25% through the course of the menstrual cycle, menstrual phase should be controlled in premenopausal women when determining lipid changes after an exercise intervention.

Generally, intervention studies suggest that exercise training programs in the absence of other interventions attenuate the age-related increase in TC level but do not cause HDL-C levels to rise appreciably in older women. In younger women, high volumes of exercise (accompanied by decreased body fat) may increase HDL-C.

In conclusion, exercise improves the lipid profile but probably less strongly for women than for men. Again, hormonal status may influence the response. Postmenopausal women seem to exhibit a greater response to exercise, even if some training studies are controversial. Exercise at least seems to attenuate the age-related modifications in the lipid profile.

Antioxidant Therapy

Antioxidants may suppress the formation of oxidized LDL and, thereby, influence the formation of atherosclerotic plaque. Both epidemiological and laboratory studies suggest that antioxidants can provide a protective effect on coronary arteries.

The Nurses' Health Study assessed the relative risk of a major CAD event in 87,245 female nurses followed for up to 8 yr. Relative risk of major coronary disease of nurses in the lowest quintile of vitamin E intake was compared with risk in the highest quintile (relative risk, 0.66 after adjustment for age and smoking). Adjustment for a variety of other coronary risk factors and nutrients, including other antioxidants, had little effect on the results. As the authors point out: "Although these prospective data do not prove a cause-and-effect relation, they suggest that among middle-aged women the use of vitamin E supplements is associated with a reduced risk of coronary heart disease." No large randomized clinical trials of antioxidants have yet been reported, albeit two such trials, the Women's Health Initiative and an ancillary Trial of Antioxidant Therapy, are in progress.

Smoking Cessation

Significant gender differences exist in smoking-cessation behavior. Some are ascribed to chemistry, others to a lack of confidence in the ability to quit, and still others are concerns regarding after cessation weight gain. In addition, nicotine may have different effects on women and men.

Cigarette smoking carries an especially increased hazard for young women because it is often accompanied by oral contraceptive use, a combination that promotes thrombogenesis. In general, women are less likely to contemplate smoking cessation than men, and are likely to smoke to reduce tension and control weight. Although women quit smoking at the same rate as men, they are less able to maintain cessation during the long term. Women's anxiety about after cessation weight gain is a major impediment to their attempting to quit smoking. Smoking cessation has also been suggested as a possible contributing factor to the increase in prevalence of overweight in the United States. After cessation weight gain, an average of 10 lb during a 10-yr period, seems to be caused both by increased eating and the metabolic changes produced by nicotine withdrawal. Nicotine gum has been shown to partially reduce or delay weight gain.

The clinical implications are that smoking-cessation programs for women may have to emphasize strategies to help them develop confidence to stop smoking, to make a commitment to quitting, and to develop strategies for maintaining cessation for extended periods of time. Smoking-cessation programs for women should emphasize techniques for reducing tension and for weight control.

Former smokers live longer than continuing smokers and a person 50 yr or younger who quits smoking has a 50% reduction in mortality during the next 15 yr vs a smoker. In the Nurse's Health Study, the CHD risk is decreased by 30% within only 2 yr after cessation. These benefits extend to the population with diagnosed CAD. Overall, the bulk of studies in indicate a 30 to 50% reduction in CHD mortality in the first 2 yr, and a more gradual decline in the next 10 to 20 yr, before the smoker mirrors the CHD mortality risk of a never smoker.

Twelve-year follow-up data from the Nurse' Health Study examined the relationship of time since smoking with reduction in CHD incidence and mortality in middle-aged women. On stopping smoking, one-third of the excess risk of CHD was eliminated within 2 yr of cessation. Thereafter, the excess risk returned to the level of those who had never smoked during the interval 10 to 14 yr after cessation.

ROLE OF HRT IN THE PREVENTION OF CVD

Much controversy surrounds the role of HRT in CVD. Although pathophysiological and epidemiological data suggest the beneficial cardiovascular effects of estrogen, more

recent data from large, randomized controlled trials demonstrate no benefit and potential harm of HRT when used for the primary or secondary prevention of CAD.

The Women's Health Initiative was designed to evaluate the effect of three separate preventive strategies (hormone therapy [HT], diet, and calcium supplements) on disease outcomes in healthy postmenopausal women aged 50 to 79 yr *(53,54)*. In one arm of the trial, 16,608 women were randomized to either combined 0.625 mg esterified estrogens and 2.5 mg medroxyprogesterone (MPA) or placebo. The trial was halted early because of an increased hazard ratio (HR) for breast cancer (HR, 1.26; range, 1.00–1.59). Cardiovascular events were also increased during the study (HR, 1.29; 1.02–1.63), as were the risks of stroke (HR, 1.41; 1.07–1.85) and pulmonary emboli (HR, 2.13; 1.39–3.25). Similarly, the Postmenopausal Estrogen/Progestin Interventions *(55)* trial of 875 women demonstrated a higher, albeit nonsignificant, incidence of cardiovascular and thrombotic events among women assigned to HRT. In a pooled analysis of 22 published small, randomized trials of HRT encompassing 4124 women, the calculated odds ratio for cardiovascular events in women assigned to hormones vs those not assigned to hormones was 1.39 (95% confidence interval [CI], 0.48–3.95) *(56)*.

Whether HRT would reduce subsequent cardiovascular events in women with existing CAD has been investigated in several trials. The first large-scale clinical trial to examine the cardioprotective effect of estrogen in postmenopausal women was HERS. HERS was a multicenter, randomized, double-blind, placebo-controlled trial that enrolled 2763 postmenopausal women (mean age, 67 yr); randomized to MPA plus 0.625 mg conjugated esterified estrogen (CEE) or placebo *(51)*. There was no overall difference in the primary CAD outcome (nonfatal MI and CAD death combined) between the treatment and placebo groups. Nonfatal MI or CAD death occurred in 179 women in the hormone group and 182 women in the placebo group (relative hazard, 0.99; 95% CI, 0.81–1.22). During the first year, there was a statistically significant 52% excess risk of CAD events in the HT group *(57)*. An additional 6.8 yr of follow-up (with approximately half of the original cohort continuing HT) also failed to show any evidence of long-term cardiovascular benefit *(52)*.

In the Estrogen in the Prevention of Reinfarction Trial *(58)*, investigators randomized 1017 women (mean age, 63 yr) with previous MI to either estradiol valerate daily or placebo. After 2 yr, the frequency of reinfarction or cardiac death did not differ by treatment assignment (rate ratio, 0.99; 95% CI, 0.70–1.41), and there was also no difference in all-cause mortality. Similarly, the Estrogen Replacement and Atherosclerosis trial randomized 309 postmenopausal women (mean age, 66 yr) to receive 0.625 mg CEE alone (for women without a uterus), 0.625 mg CEE with 2.5 mg of MPA daily (for women with a uterus), or placebo. After an average follow-up of 3.2 yr, the mean minimal coronary artery diameters did not differ significantly by treatment group, despite significant reductions in LDL-C and increases in HDL-C levels in the women assigned to HT *(59,60)*. Finally, the Women's Angiographic Vitamin and Estrogen trial *(61)* randomized 423 postmenopausal women (mean age, 66 yr) to daily oral 0.625 mg CEE plus 2.5 mg MPA with or without vitamins E and C. At follow-up, there was greater progression of coronary atherosclerosis in the treatment groups. Other studies investigating the role of estrogen in the secondary prevention of cerebrovascular disease also failed to show benefit *(62)*. In the Women's Estrogen for Stroke Trial, women receiving estradiol had an increase in risk for CAD *(63)*. In this randomized, double-blind, placebo-controlled trial of estrogen therapy (1 mg/d of estradiol-17β) in 664 postmenopausal women (mean age, 71 yr) with recent cerebrovascular events, estrogen therapy did not reduce the risk

of death or nonfatal stroke, and women randomized to estrogen therapy had a higher risk of fatal stroke and their nonfatal strokes were associated with slightly worse neurological and functional deficits.

In summary, HRT does not decrease, and may in fact increase, the incidence of CAD. Currently, long-term HRT is not recommended for either primary or secondary prevention of CAD. The AHA Science Advisory: Hormone Replacement Therapy and Cardiovascular Disease states the following: "For women who already have CAD: Hormone Replacement Therapy (HRT) should not be initiated for the secondary prevention of CAD. The decision to continue or stop HRT in women with CAD who have been undergoing long-term HRT should be based on established non-CAD benefits and risks and patient preference. Reinstitution of HRT should be based on established non-CAD benefits and risks, as well as patient preference. For women who do not have CAD: There is insufficient data to suggest that HRT should be initiated for the sole purpose of primary prevention of CAD. Initiation and continuation of HRT should be based on established non-CAD benefits and risks, possible CAD benefits and risks, and patient preference" (64).

CONCLUSION

CVD is the leading cause of morbidity and mortality in women, with the vast majority of cardiovascular events occurring in the postmenopausal years. Most of our knowledge of CVD comes from studies in middle-aged men. Recent emphasis on women's health in general, and in cardiovascular health in particular, has lead to increasing evidence that significant gender differences do exist in CAD incidence, in risk factors, and in the modification of cardiovascular risk in women.

Health care providers must coordinate their efforts to effectively treat and prevent CVD in women in such a way as to take into account the unique biology, physiology, and epidemiology of CVD in women. There is increasing evidence of the roles of traditional and nontraditional risk factors in the development of CVD in women and in developing new strategies to incorporate this evidence into programs of prevention.

KEY POINTS

1. CVD is the leading cause of mortality among women in the United States—500,000 women each year die of CHD.
2. Deaths in women from CVD are almost twice the number of deaths caused by cancer.
3. Approximately one of every two women in the United States will die from some cardiovascular event—most likely, MI, hypertensive heart disease, or stroke.
4. Special emphasis must also be placed on those uniquely female attributes that modify coronary risk; specifically, oral contraceptives, pregnancy, menopausal status, and the use of postmenopausal HT.
5. Most of our knowledge of CVD comes from studies in middle-aged men.
6. Recent emphasis on women's health in general, and in cardiovascular health in particular, has lead to increasing evidence that significant gender differences do exist in CAD incidence, in risk factors, and in the modification of cardiovascular risk in women.
7. Health care providers must coordinate their efforts to effectively treat and prevent CVD in women in such a way as to take into account the unique biology, physiology, and epidemiology of CVD in women.
8. There is increasing evidence of the roles of traditional and nontraditional risk factors in the development of CVD in women and in developing new strategies to incorporate this evidence into programs of prevention.

Appendix A
Framingham Point Score Estimate of 10-Yr Risk for Women

Age	Points
20–34	−7
35–39	−3
40–44	0
45–49	3
50–54	6
55–59	8
60–64	10
65–69	12
70–74	14
75–79	16

Total cholesterol (mg/dL)	Points				
	Age 20–39	Age 40–49	Age 50–59	Age 60–60	Age 70–79
<160	0	0	0	0	0
160–199	4	3	2	1	1
200–239	8	6	4	2	1
240–279	11	8	5	3	2
≥280	13	10	7	4	2

Smoking	Points				
	Age 20–39	Age 40–49	Age 50–59	Age 60–60	Age 70–79
Nonsmoker	0	0	0	0	0
Smoker	9	7	4	2	1

HDL (mg/dL)	Points
≥60	−1
50–59	0
40–49	1
<40	2

Systolic BP (mmHg)	If untreated	If treated
<120	0	0
120–129	1	3
130–139	2	4
140–159	3	5
≥160	4	6

Point total	10-Yr risk (%)
<9	<1
9	1
10	1
11	1
12	1
13	2
14	2
15	3
16	4
17	5
18	6
19	8
20	11
21	14
22	17
23	22
24	27
≥25	≥30

10-Yr Risk_____%

233

REFERENCES

1. Anonymous. Major cardiovascular disease (CVD) during 1997–1999 and major CVD hospital discharge rates in 1997 among women with diabetes—United States. MMWR—Morbidity & Mortality Weekly Report. 2001;50(43):948–954.
2. Kuster GM, Buser P, Osswald S, et al. Comparison of presentation, perception, and six-month outcome between women and men > or = 75 years of age with angina pectoris. Am J Cardiol 2003;91(4):436–439.
3. Lewis SJ. Cardiovascular disease in postmenopausal women: myths and reality. Am J Cardiol 2002;89(12A):5E–10E; discussion 10E–11E.
4. Knopp RH. Risk factors for coronary artery disease in women. Am J Cardiol 2002;89(12A):28E–34E; discussion 34E–35E.
5. Kannel WB. The Framingham Study: historical insight on the impact of cardiovascular risk factors in men versus women. J Gend Specif Med 2002;5(2):27–37.
6. Bertsias G, Mammas I, Linardakis M, Kafatos A. Overweight and obesity in relation to cardiovascular disease risk factors among medical students in Crete, Greece. BMC Public Health 2003;3(1):3.
7. Anonymous. Prevalence of selected cardiovascular disease risk factors among American Indians and Alaska Natives—United States, 1997. MMWR—Morbidity & Mortality Weekly Report 2000;49(21):461–465.
8. Vaccarino V. Women and outcomes of coronary artery bypass surgery: do we have an answer? [comment]. Am Heart J 2003;146(6):935–937.
9. Gorman Koch C, Mora Mangano C, Schwann N, Vaccarino V. Is it gender, methodology, or something else? J Thorac Cardiovasc Surg 2003;126(4):932–935.
10. Abramson JL, Veledar E, Weintraub WS, Vaccarino V. Association between gender and in-hospital mortality after percutaneous coronary intervention according to age. Am J Cardiol 2003;91(8):968–971, A964.
11. Smith GL, Masoudi FA, Vaccarino V, Radford MJ, Krumholz HM. Outcomes in heart failure patients with preserved ejection fraction: mortality, readmission, and functional decline [see comment]. J Am Coll Cardiol 2003;41(9):1510–1518.
12. Vaccarino V, Abramson JL, Veledar E, Weintraub WS. Sex differences in hospital mortality after coronary artery bypass surgery: evidence for a higher mortality in younger women. Circulation 2002;105(10):1176–1181.
13. Vaccarino V, Parsons L, Every NR, Barron HV, Krumholz HM. Sex-based differences in early mortality after myocardial infarction. National Registry of Myocardial Infarction 2 Participants. [see comment]. N Engl J Med 1999;341(4):217–225.
14. Vaccarino V, Chen YT, Wang Y, Radford MJ, Krumholz HM. Sex differences in the clinical care and outcomes of congestive heart failure in the elderly. Am Heart J 1999;138(5 Pt 1):835–842.
15. Krumholz HM, Philbin DM Jr, Wang Y, et al. Trends in the quality of care for Medicare beneficiaries admitted to the hospital with unstable angina. [see comment]. J Am Coll Cardiol 1998;31(5):957–963.
16. Nohria A, Vaccarino V, Krumholz HM. Gender differences in mortality after myocardial infarction. Why women fare worse than men. Cardiol Clin 1998;16(1):45–57.
17. Vaccarino V, Krumholz HM, Mendes de Leon CF, et al. Sex differences in survival after myocardial infarction in older adults: a community-based approach. [see comment]. J Am Geriatr Soc 1996;44(10):1174–1182.
18. Wenger NK. Coronary risk reduction in the menopausal woman. Rev Port Cardiol 1999;18(Suppl 3):III39–47.
19. Mukherjee D, Hsu A, Moliterno DJ, Lincoff AM, Goormastic M, Topol EJ. Risk factors for premature coronary artery disease and determinants of adverse outcomes after revascularization in patients < or = 40 years old. Am J Cardiol 2003;92(12):1465–1467.
20. Cole JH, Miller JI 3rd, Sperling LS, Weintraub WS. Long-term follow-up of coronary artery disease presenting in young adults. [see comment]. J Am Coll Cardiol 2003;41(4):521–528.
21. Lee PY, Alexander KP, Hammill BG, Pasquali SK, Peterson ED. Representation of elderly persons and women in published randomized trials of acute coronary syndromes. JAMA 2001;286(6):708–713.
22. Hulley SB. The US National Cholesterol Education Program. Adult treatment guidelines. Drugs 1988;36(Suppl 3):100–104.
23. Greenlund KJ, Giles WH, Keenan NL, Croft JB, Casper ML, Matson-Koffman D. Prevalence of multiple cardiovascular disease risk factors among women in the United States, 1992 and 1995: the Behavioral Risk Factor Surveillance System. J Womens Health 1998;7(9):1125–1133.
24. Rifkind BM, Tamir I, Heiss G, Wallace RB, Tyroler HA. Distribution of high density and other lipoproteins in selected LRC prevalence study populations: a brief survey. Lipids 1979;14(1):105–112.

25. Bittner V. Lipoprotein abnormalities related to women's health. Am J Cardiol 2002;90(8A):77i–84i.
26. Stensvold I, Urdal P, Thurmer H, Tverdal A, Lund-Larsen PG, Foss OP. High-density lipoprotein cholesterol and coronary, cardiovascular and all cause mortality among middle-aged Norwegian men and women. Eur Heart J 1992;13(9):1155–1163.
27. Kannel WB, McGee D, Gordon T. A general cardiovascular risk profile: the Framingham Study. Am J Cardiol 1976;38(1):46–51.
28. Wilson PW, Garrison RJ, Castelli WP, Feinleib M, McNamara PM, Kannel WB. Prevalence of coronary heart disease in the Framingham Offspring Study: role of lipoprotein cholesterols. Am J Cardiol 1980;46(4):649–654.
29. Wilson PW, D'Agostino RB, Levy D, Belanger AM, Silbershatz H, Kannel WB. Prediction of coronary heart disease using risk factor categories. [see comment]. Circulation 1998;97(18):1837–1847.
30. Livshits G, Weisbort J, Meshulam N, Brunner D. Multivariate analysis of the twenty-year follow-up of the Donolo–Tel Aviv Prospective Coronary Artery Disease Study and the usefulness of high density lipoprotein cholesterol percentage. Am J Cardiol 1989;63(11):676–681.
31. Brunner D, Weisbort J, Meshulam N, et al. Relation of serum total cholesterol and high-density lipoprotein cholesterol percentage to the incidence of definite coronary events: twenty-year follow-up of the Donolo–Tel Aviv Prospective Coronary Artery Disease Study. Am J Cardiol 1987;59(15):1271–1276.
32. Walden CE, Knopp RH, Wahl PW, Beach KW, Strandness E Jr. Sex differences in the effect of diabetes mellitus on lipoprotein triglyceride and cholesterol concentrations. N Engl J Med 1984;311(15):953–959.
33. Colditz GA, Manson JE, Hankinson SE. The Nurses' Health Study: 20-year contribution to the understanding of health among women. J Womens Health 1997;6:49–62.
34. Dubbert PM, Carithers T, Sumner AE, et al. Obesity, physical inactivity, and risk for cardiovascular disease. Am J Med Sci 2002;324(3):116–126.
35. Kohl HW 3rd. Physical activity and cardiovascular disease: evidence for a dose response. Med Sci Sports Exerc 2001;33(6 Suppl):S472–483; discussion S493–474.
36. Lawler JM, Hu Z, Green JS, Crouse SF, Grandjean PW, Bounds RG. Combination of estrogen replacement and exercise protects against HDL oxidation in post-menopausal women. Int J Sports Med 2002;23(7):477–483.
37. Lowensteyn I, Coupal L, Zowall H, Grover SA. The cost-effectiveness of exercise training for the primary and secondary prevention of cardiovascular disease. J Cardiopulm Rehabil 2000;20(3):147–155.
38. Smith SC Jr, Amsterdam E, Balady GJ, et al. Prevention Conference V: Beyond secondary prevention: identifying the high-risk patient for primary prevention: tests for silent and inducible ischemia: Writing Group II. Circulation 2000;101(1):E12–16.
39. Thompson PD, Buchner D, Pina IL, et al. Exercise and physical activity in the prevention and treatment of atherosclerotic cardiovascular disease: a statement from the Council on Clinical Cardiology (Subcommittee on Exercise, Rehabilitation, and Prevention) and the Council on Nutrition, Physical Activity, and Metabolism (Subcommittee on Physical Activity). [see comment]. Circulation 2003;107(24):3109–3116.
40. Wannamethee SG, Shaper AG. Physical activity in the prevention of cardiovascular disease: an epidemiological perspective. Sports Med 2001;31(2):101–114.
41. Wenger NK. Preventive coronary interventions for women. Med Sci Sports Exerc 1996;28(1):3–6.
42. Whitlock EP, Williams SB. The primary prevention of heart disease in women through health behavior change promotion in primary care. Womens Health Issues 2003;13(4):122–141.
43. Miller TD, Fletcher GF. Exercise and coronary artery disease prevention. Cardiologia 1998;43(1):43–51.
44. Miller TD, Balady GJ, Fletcher GF. Exercise and its role in the prevention and rehabilitation of cardiovascular disease. Ann Behav Med 1997;19(3):220–229.
45. Grundy SM, Bazzarre T, Cleeman J, et al. Prevention Conference V: Beyond secondary prevention: identifying the high-risk patient for primary prevention: medical office assessment: Writing Group I. Circulation 2000;101(1):E3–E11.
46. Mosca L, Appel L, Benjamin E, et al. Evidence-based guidelines for cardiovascular disease prevention in women. Circulation 2004;109:672–693.
47. Downs JR, Clearfield M, Weis S, et al. Primary prevention of acute coronary events with lovastatin in men and women with average cholesterol levels: Results of AFCAPS/TexCAPS. JAMA 1998;279:1615–1622.
48. No authors listed. Influence of Pravastatin and Plasma Lipids on Clinical Events in the West of Scotland Coronary Prevention Study (WOSCOPS). Circulation 1998;97(15):1440–1445.
49. Scandinavian Simvastatin Survival Study Group: randomized trial of cholesterol lowering in 4444 patients with coronary heart disease: the Scandinavian Simvastatin Survival Study (4S). Lancet 1994;344:1383–1389.

50. Sacks FM, Pfeffer MA, Moye LA, et al. The effect of pravastatin on coronary events after myocardial infarction in patients with average cholesterol levels. The Cholesterol and Recurrent Events Trial Investigators. N Engl J Med 1996;335:1001–1009.

51. Grady D, Applegate W, Bush T, Furberg C, Riggs B, Hulley SB. Heart and Estrogen/progestin Replacement Study (HERS): design, methods, and baseline characteristics. Control Clin Trials 1998;19(4):314–335.

52. Grady D, Herrington D, Bittner V, et al. Cardiovascular disease outcomes during 6.8 years of hormone therapy: Heart and Estrogen/Progestin Replacement Study follow-up (HERS II). [see comment] [erratum appears in JAMA 2002;288(9):1064]. JAMA 2002;288(1):49–57.

53. Hays J, Ockene JK, Brunner RL, et al. Effects of estrogen plus progestin on health-related quality of life. [see comment]. N Engl J Med 2003;348(19):1839–1854.

54. Rossouw JE, Anderson GL, Prentice RL, et al. Risks and benefits of estrogen plus progestin in healthy postmenopausal women: principal results From the Women's Health Initiative randomized controlled trial. [see comment] [summary for patients in CMAJ 2002;167(4):377–378]. JAMA 2002;288(3):321–333.

55. Anonymous. Effects of estrogen or estrogen/progestin regimens on heart disease risk factors in postmenopausal women. The Postmenopausal Estrogen/Progestin Interventions (PEPI) Trial. The Writing Group for the PEPI Trial. [see comment] [erratum appears in JAMA 1995;274(21):1676]. JAMA 1995;273(3):199–208.

56. Hemminki E, McPherson K. Impact of postmenopausal hormone therapy on cardiovascular events and cancer: pooled data from clinical trials. [see comment]. BMJ 1997;315(7101):149–153.

57. Hulley S, Grady D, Bush T, et al. Randomized trial of estrogen plus progestin for secondary prevention of coronary heart disease in postmenopausal women. Heart and Estrogen/progestin Replacement Study (HERS) Research Group. [see comment]. JAMA 1998;280(7):605–613.

58. Cherry N, Gilmour K, Hannaford P. Oestrogen therapy for prevention of reinfarction in postmenopausal women: a randomized placebo controlled trial. Lancet Available at: http://image.thelancet.com/extras/02art11268web.pdf.

59. Herrington DM, Reboussin DM, Brosnihan KB, et al. Effects of estrogen replacement on the progression of coronary-artery atherosclerosis. [see comment]. N Engl J Med 2000;343(8):522–529.

60. Herrington DM, Howard TD, Hawkins GA, et al. Estrogen-receptor polymorphisms and effects of estrogen replacement on high-density lipoprotein cholesterol in women with coronary disease. [see comment]. N Engl J Med 2002;346(13):967–974.

61. Waters DD, Alderman EL, Hsia J, et al. Effects of hormone replacement therapy and antioxidant vitamin supplements on coronary atherosclerosis in postmenopausal women: a randomized controlled trial. [see comment]. JAMA 2002;288(19):2432–2440.

62. Hurn PD, Brass LM. Estrogen and stroke: a balanced analysis. Stroke 2003;34(2):338–341.

63. Viscoli CM, Brass LM, Kernan WN, Sarrel PM, Suissa S, Horwitz RI. A clinical trial of estrogen-replacement therapy after ischemic stroke. [see comment]. N Engl J Med 2001;345(17):1243–1249.

64. Mosca L, Collins P, Herrington DM, et al. Hormone replacement therapy and cardiovascular disease: a statement for healthcare professionals from the American Heart Association. [see comment]. Circulation 2001;104(4):499–503.

III STRATEGIES FOR PREVENTION

13   Subclinical Atherosclerosis

Rahman Shah, MD and JoAnne Micale Foody, MD

CONTENTS

INTRODUCTION
SUBCLINICAL ATHEROSCLEROSIS
PRIMORDIAL PREVENTION AND RISK FACTORS FOR ATHEROSCLEROSIS
DIAGNOSIS OF SUBCLINICAL ATHEROSCLEROSIS
TREATMENTS
CONCLUSIONS
REFERENCES

INTRODUCTION

Risk stratification is a key component to recently developed consensus statements and guidelines for the prevention of cardiovascular disease (CVD), including the National Cholesterol Education Program (NCEP) Adult Treatment Panel (ATP) III and American College of Cardiology/American Heart Association (AHA) guidelines. In an effort to provide clinicians with guidance regarding the primary prevention of CVD and the identification of high-risk individuals, various organizations have developed consensus statements and clinical guidelines. Each stresses the centrality of risk stratification in tailoring individualized therapy and identifies high-risk individuals through categorical risk factor counting (categorical method) or continuous risk thresholds (continuous variables method). The NCEP ATP III, for example, varies the cholesterol thresholds for initiation of treatment and goals of therapy based on the presence of vascular disease or coexistent risk factors. Other consensus groups, including the Joint European Societies Expert Panel, recommend that pharmacological therapy be based on assessment of absolute risk.

Although these recommendations are based on the best available evidence, these strategies may lack the sensitivity to identify patients with substantial preclinical atherosclerosis who are at highest risk for future coronary events. In a review of various methods for the prediction of coronary risk, Haq et al. found that risk-factor counting and cholesterol thresholds were not sufficiently accurate for tailoring pharmacological therapy in primary prevention. In this review, a cholesterol threshold of at least 6.5 mmol/L (~260 mg/dL) and the presence of two risk factors had a sensitivity of only 59% and a specificity of 63% for predicting risk *(1)*. Framingham-based methods were highly sensitive but had low specificity; that is, they could identify high-risk patients but often inappropriately

From: *Contemporary Cardiology: Preventive Cardiology:*
Insights Into the Prevention and Treatment of Cardiovascular Disease, Second Edition
Edited by: J. M. Foody © Humana Press Inc., Totowa, NJ

identified patients at low risk. However, in other patient groups, such as those with the metabolic syndrome and a positive family history of coronary disease, the Framingham risk equation may have inadequate sensitivity for identifying risk.

Furthermore, recent insights into the atherosclerotic process have challenged conventional wisdom regarding atherosclerosis and a "high-risk" approach to risk factor modification. Findings from autopsy studies, such as the Bogalusa Heart Study (2) and the Pathobiological Determinants of Atherosclerosis in Youth (PDAY) Research Group (3), have indicated that coronary atherosclerosis begins early in life and that its progression is strongly influenced by conventional risk factors. A recent report of intravascular ultrasound evaluations during routine baseline coronary angiography of newly transplanted hearts from young donors noted the common presence of atherosclerotic plaque, and significant stress-induced perfusion abnormalities are seen in a substantial minority of asymptomatic high-risk populations by radionuclide tomographic myocardial perfusion imaging (MPI). These findings support the concept that atherosclerosis begins early and highlight the magnitude of preclinical atherosclerosis in the general population. They also support the potential for early detection and intervention before the symptomatic clinical presentation of coronary artery disease (CAD), which is often sudden death or myocardial infarction (MI).

Our expanding knowledge of the atherosclerotic process, coupled with the limitations of our current risk stratification constructs, underscores the need to identify preclinical atherosclerosis more aggressively. Most cases of CAD do not occur in traditionally defined "high-risk" groups, but, rather, occur among those with "average" risk. This is reflected by the fact that the majority of patients with CAD have cholesterol levels indistinguishable from patients without CAD, and that current guidelines significantly underestimate the risk of coronary events. Therefore, current reliance on a high-risk approach to risk factor modification may limit our ability to provide the most benefit to the greatest number. Given interindividual variation in risk factors and cardiovascular risk, it is imperative that clinicians develop strategies to adequately assess risk and to match the level of risk with the intensity of treatment. This chapter highlights improving risk stratification in asymptomatic individuals.

SUBCLINICAL ATHEROSCLEROSIS

Atherosclerosis is derived from the Greek word *athere* meaning "gruel" or "porridge" and *sclerosis* meaning "hard." The name defines the mature atherosclerotic plaque, which consists of two components—the lipid-rich (soft) component and the collagen-rich (hard) component, but atherosclerosis is an insidious and chronic progressive fibroinflammatory process. It has been shown to progress in different morphological stages and phases.

The existence of atherosclerosis has been recognized for several centuries and longer than 150 yr as a pathological condition (4). Early in history, two types of intimae lesions, the fatty streak (a thin lipid deposit in thin intima in children) and the fibrous plaque (a thick fibrolipidic lesion in adults) were recognized and associated with atherosclerosis. However, there was controversy regarding whether the two types of lesion were an early and advanced expression of the same disease (5). Ludwig Aschoff was a leading pathologist who recognized that the two lesions are the different stages of the same disease. Aschoff designated the child form atherosis/atheromatosis. The other component, fibrosis (sclerosis, formation of collagen) added to the lipid component later in adult life to complete the mature atherosclerotic plaque.

Nomenclature and main histology	Sequences in progression	Main growth mechanism	Earliest onset	Clinical correlation
Type I (initial) lesion Isolated macrophage foam cells	I	Growth mainly by lipid accumulation	From first decade	Clinically silent
Type II (fatty streak) lesion Mainly intracellular lipid accumulation	II			
Type III (intermediate) lesion Type II changes and small extracellular lipid pools	III		From third decade	
Type IV (atheroma) lesion Type II changes and core of extracellular lipid	IV			
Type V (fibroatheroma) lesion Lipid core and fibrotic layer, or multiple lipid cores and fibrotic layers, or mainly calcific, or mainly fibrotic	V	Accelerated smooth muscle and collagen increase	From fourth decade	Clinically silent or overt
Type VI (complicated) lesion Surface defect, hematoma-hemorrhage, thrombus	VI	Thrombosis, hematoma		

Fig. 1. American Heart Association classiffication of human atherosclerotic lesion. (From ref. 7 with permission.)

In the 1950s, pathologists classified atherosclerosis into progressive stages of fatty streak, fibrous plaque, and complicated lesion *(6)*. The World Health Organization later added the term atheroma (advanced lesion with predominate lipid component). Different investigators continue to use different names, including fibroatheroma, atheromatous plaque, fibrolipid plaque, or fibrofatty plaque *(4)*. In 1995, the AHA classification divided atherosclerotic lesions into six types to provide a standard framework of histological morphologies of lesions and to allow correlation of composition of lesions with clinical manifestations of disease, as summarized in Fig. 1 *(7)*.

Typically, early lesions (type I and II) occur in infants and children, type III lesions evolve soon after puberty (bridge between early and advanced stages), and advanced lesions start after the third decade of life. Clinical manifestation of atherosclerosis is caused by reduction of blood flow and insufficient delivery of oxygen and nutrients to affected organs. Insufficient blood flow to the heart muscle results in ischemia or infarction, leading to angina or MI. Reduced blood flow to the brain causes stroke and intermittent claudication, with restricted blood flow to the lower extremities. Coronary flow begins to decrease with stenosis greater than 50%, and decreases rapidly when stenosis exceeds 70% *(8)*. Thus, the early lesions are clinically silent. In the early stages of atherosclerosis, the sequence is predictable, characteristic, and uniform, but lesions may subsequently progress in different morphogenetic sequences, resulting in several characteristic lesion types and clinical syndromes (Fig. 2).

PRIMORDIAL PREVENTION AND RISK FACTORS FOR ATHEROSCLEROSIS

Atherosclerotic disease remains the leading cause of both death and disability in North America *(9)*. Although considerable energy and progress in the primary and secondary prevention of CVD has occurred in the past 30 yr, it may be appropriate to consider the

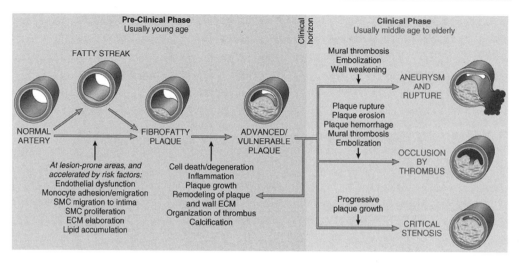

Fig. 2. Schematic summary of the natural history, morphological features, pathogenic events, and clinical complications of atherosclerosis. (From ref. 7 with permission.) SMC, smooth muscle cell; ECM, extracellular matrix.

role of primordial prevention (i.e., the prevention of risk factors) in the maintenance of cardiovascular health. This may be the only viable strategy if our goal is to eliminate these diseases and expand the current achievements of primary and secondary prevention. A predominant focus of the medical community on disease states may inadvertently undervalue health maintenance. Atherosclerosis begins in childhood or adolescence and progresses at a variable rate until it reaches the clinical threshold. Once identified, persons with subclinical atherosclerosis should be considered candidates for intensive efforts to prevent, delay, or mitigate overt clinical disease. Therefore, primary prevention of atherosclerosis, as contrasted with primary prevention of clinically manifest atherosclerotic disease, must begin in childhood or adolescence.

Age

Atherosclerosis has been associated with increasing age. Although some of the early changes of atherosclerosis have been shown to occur early in life, the overall prevalence and the severity of atherosclerotic diseases increases with age. The PDAY, a multi-institutional autopsy study conducted in US medical centers that enrolled 2876 study subjects between 15 and 34 yr old, who were black or white, men or women, who died of external causes and underwent autopsy between June 1, 1987 and August 31, 1994 showed that intimal lesions appeared in all of the aortas and more than half of the right coronary arteries of the youngest age group (15–19 yr) and increased in prevalence and extent with age through the oldest age group (30–34 yr). This age–disease relationship is consistent across genders and ethnic groups in the United States (3). Moreover, 40% of 318 asymptomatic adults and offspring of the Framingham Heart Study participants had subclinical atherosclerosis as assessed by magnetic resonance imaging (MRI), and the plaque prevalence and all measures of plaque burden increased with the age group (10). In the Bogalusa Heart Study, autopsies in 204 individuals aged 2 to 39 yr who died of a variety of causes (predominantly trauma) revealed coronary fatty streaks in 50% of those aged 2 to 15 yr and in 85% of those aged 26 to 39 yr. Coronary atheromas were found

in 8% of those aged 2 to 15 yr, 33% of those aged 16 to 20 yr, 52% of those aged 21 to 25 yr, and 67% of those aged 26 to 39 yr *(2)*.

Dyslipidemia

The connection between cholesterol and atherosclerotic plaques was first reported by Anitschkow in 1912, when he showed atherosclerotic plaques (similar to those occurring in humans) in rabbits fed diets high in cholesterol *(11)*. Later, the Bogalusa Heart Study showed that the severity of the atherosclerotic plaques in aorta correlated positively with the percent of dietary calories from fat in humans *(12)*. The International Atherosclerosis Project showed that mean serum total cholesterol correlated well with severity of atherosclerosis at necropsy of 23,207 persons from 14 countries *(11)*.

Animal studies have shown that increased levels of low-density lipoprotein (LDL) initiate and sustain atherogenesis *(12,13)*. Humans with familial hyperlipidemia with very high LDL exhibit premature atherosclerotic disease *(14)*. There is extensive evidence for the atherogenicity of LDL derived from studies in experimental animals, population surveys, and clinical trials in humans *(11–13)*. Investigators have also shown development of atherosclerosis in animals and human with elevated triglyceride and decreased high-density lipoprotein (HDL) *(13)*. Although high LDL-cholesterol (C) is the primary lipid risk factor, other lipid parameters increase the risk of atherosclerosis in persons with or without an elevated LDL-C. In PDAY, very low-density lipoprotein and LDL-C levels were positively, and HDL-C levels were negatively associated with both fatty streaks and raised lesions in the aorta and right coronary artery, particularly after age 25 yr.

Smoking

Cigarette smoking is a major risk factor for the development of atherosclerosis *(15)*. Reports from PDAY have demonstrated that smoking is strongly associated with the prevalence and extent of grossly visible raised lesions in the abdominal aorta. In addition, it also showed that smokers had more than twice as many advanced lesions, types IV and V, as nonsmokers (32 vs 14%) and fewer early lesions, types I, II, and III, than nonsmokers (38 vs 62%) in coronary arteries. Even passive smoking has been shown to cause atherosclerosis *(16)*. In the Bogalusa Heart Study, cigarette smokers had a significantly increased percentage of coronary artery intimal surface involvement for fatty streaks, and a nonsignificantly greater percentage of involvement for fibrous plaques *(2)*. In the Atherosclerosis Risk in Communities study, both active smoking and exposure to environmental tobacco smoke were associated with the progression of an index of atherosclerosis *(17)*.

Diabetes Mellitus

Diabetes mellitus (DM) has been shown to promote the development and progression of atherosclerotic diseases and to increase the thrombotic complication of atherosclerotic diseases *(18)*. Multiple postmortem studies have documented a distribution of atherosclerotic changes that is more diffuse in patients with diabetes *(17)*. Children with type 1 DM and adults with type 2 DM have more atherosclerotic plaque then their nondiabetic counterparts *(19–21)*. In PDAY, elevated glycohemoglobin levels were associated with raised lesions throughout the 15- to 34-yr age span. The Tromsø Study showed that the level of hemoglobin (Hb) A_{1C} was significantly related to the risk of carotid plaques (predominantly hard plaques), and that the risk increased continuously across increasing HbA_{1C} levels *(22)*.

Hypertension

Most Americans with hypertension die of complications of atherosclerosis. Multiple epidemiological studies have shown the strong relationship of hypertension with atherosclerosis *(23)*. Although the development of risk-factor thresholds (e.g., hypertension being defined as a blood pressure (BP) greater than 140/90 mmHg, systolic and diastolic, respectively) has helped patients and clinicians focus on treatment objectives, such cut points have obscured the continuum of risk. Normal levels in this construct may inappropriately be assumed to be desirable. For instance, BP levels considered by most clinicians and patients to be "normal" (systolic pressure of 130 to 139 mmHg, or diastolic pressure of 85 to 89 mmHg, or both) are associated with a risk factors-adjusted hazard for CVD of 2.5 in women and 1.6 in men.

Obesity and Metabolic Syndrome

Obesity and insulin resistance have been linked to the early development of atheroma in young adults, independent of other cardiovascular risk factors *(24)*. In the PYAD study, body mass index (BMI) was associated with both fatty streaks and raised lesions of the right coronary artery. The Bogalusa Heart Study found a striking increase in the extent of lesions with obesity and an increasing number of metabolic syndrome risk factors. The National Heart, Lung, and Blood Institute Family Heart Study also showed that the metabolic syndrome and most of its components are associated with a higher prevalence of calcified atherosclerotic plaque in the coronary arteries and abdominal aorta in white and African American men and women *(25)*.

Family History/Genetic Factors

Several researchers have shown that atherosclerosis is at least partially genetically determined *(26)*. From 64 to 92% of variation in common carotid artery wall thickness (a commonly used surrogate marker of atherosclerosis in populations) is explained by familial factors *(27)*. Recent evidence from the Framingham Heart Study suggests that up to 50% of the variation in abdominal calcification (another surrogate marker of atherosclerosis) is determined by familial factors *(28)*. A recent study showed an association between a reported family history of early onset (before age 55 yr) coronary heart disease (CHD), with the presence and burden of coronary artery calcium (a marker of subclinical atherosclerosis) in electron beam computed tomography (EBCT) in 8549 asymptomatic men and women referred for testing *(29)*. Unfortunately, a major gene for atherosclerosis has not been detected yet *(26)*.

Male Gender and Postmenopausal Status

Several epidemiological and observational studies have shown that atherosclerotic diseases are more common in men than premenopausal women. This is probably because of the different lipid profile, because premenopausal women usually have higher HDL levels, and because HDL levels decrease after menopause. In experimental and observational studies, estrogen has been shown to decrease LDL levels, increase HDL levels, and to decrease progression and even cause regression of atherosclerosis *(30)*. Therefore, estrogen should decrease clinically manifest atherosclerotic diseases. However, recently completed randomized trials did not show the same effect *(31,32)*. Therefore, the relationship of estrogen with atherosclerotic disease remains complex at this time, as discussed in additional detail in the Treatments section.

Sedentary Lifestyle

Lack of exercise (sedentary lifestyle) has been recognized as a risk factor for atherosclerosis and is generally thought to be in addition to the effects of lack of exercise on body weight, BP, or lipids *(33)*.

Novel Risk Factors

Other potential risk factors are hyperhomocysteinemia, hypercoagulable states, depression, infection, hypothyroidism, and elevated apolipoprotein B *(26,34)*.

DIAGNOSIS OF SUBCLINICAL ATHEROSCLEROSIS

Medical Office Assessment

Office assessment includes basic history, physical examination, basic laboratory tests, and electrocardiogram (ECG). The focus of medical assessment is to detect risk factors. The risk factors for adult CHD have been associated with the prevalence and severity of atherosclerosis in autopsied young people decades before the occurrence of CHD. The same risk factors were associated with atherosclerosis in living young people whose arteries were evaluated by noninvasive imaging. INTERHEART was a standardized case–control study with 15,152 cases and 14,820 controls at 262 participating centers in 52 countries throughout Africa, Asia, Australia, Europe, the Middle East, and North and South America. INTERHEART identified nine easily measured risk factors (smoking, lipids, hypertension, diabetes, obesity, diet, physical activity, alcohol consumption, and psychosocial factors) that account for more than 90% of the risk of acute MI *(35)*.

Several methods have been used to sum risks. A number of multivariate risk models have been developed for estimating the risk of cardiovascular events based on assessment of multiple variables *(36)*. The AHA favored a method proposed by the Framingham researchers *(36)*. Framingham scoring uses only the "standard" risk factors (smoking, BP, serum cholesterol, HDL-C, blood glucose, and age). These equations calculate the absolute risk of CHD events for patients with no known previous history of CHD, stroke, or peripheral vascular disease (primary prevention). The Framingham risk factors were developed in a large prospective cohort of men and women from the United States aged 30 to 74 yr, and have been subsequently validated in multiple diverse populations *(37)*.

The Framingham equations predict the degree of risk well in white and African-American men and women (between the ages of 30 and 65 yr), with the exception that Framingham equations underpredict BP-associated risk in black women *(37–41)*. However, it does not predict the degree of risk as well in populations outside of the United States, in certain US ethnic groups (Japanese men, Hispanic men, and Native American women), in men and women younger than 30 yr or older than 65 yr, and in persons with diabetes *(37–41)*. The Framingham equations also are less precise in patients with severe hypertension or left ventricular hypertrophy because fewer numbers of participants in the original Framingham cohort had these risk factors. Another limitation is that this risk model identifies patients who are more or less likely to develop CVD within a defined period (e.g., 10 yr). Patients with less than a 10% likelihood are considered at low risk. However, this approach does not consider lifetime risk. In addition, conditional and predisposing risk factors such as blood glucose level, HbA_{1C}, triglycerides, lipoprotein A, small, dense LDL particles, homocysteine, C-reactive protein (CRP), microalbuminuria, coagulation factors, weight or BMI, physical activity, and family history of premature CVD are not used in the Framingham risk equation *(37)*. However, the AHA nonetheless

stressed that several of the conditional and predisposing risk factors undoubtedly contribute to the development of CHD *(36)*. Thus, the detection and even therapeutic modification of these risk factors may be appropriate in some patients.

Framingham formulas predict the risk of CHD events in people older than the age of 30 yr. Recently, the PDAY developed risk scores that use traditional CHD risk factors to predict the probability of advanced atherosclerotic lesions in young persons, 15 to 34 yr of age. PDAY formulas predict the risk of advanced preclinical atherosclerosis in young people years before CHD, just as the Framingham formulas predict the risk of CHD events in older people. The PDAY study result has been strongly supported by findings from other recent cohort studies *(42)*.

The risk scores are calculated by adding the points for each risk factor given in Table 1. For example, a man (0 points) aged 25 to 29 yr (10 points) with a non-HDL-C concentration of 160 to 189 mg/dL (4 points) who smokes (1 point), is obese (6 points), and has no other risk factors has a coronary artery risk score of 21, with 11 of the points caused by modifiable risk factors. Figure 3 indicates that this individual has an approx 25% probability of having a target coronary artery lesion.

Tests for Silent Ischemia

Silent ischemia is defined as the presence of objective evidence of myocardial ischemia in the absence of chest discomfort or other anginal equivalents. The prevalence of silent ischemia in healthy middle age men is approx 2.5% in large-scale screening studies. The prevalence of silent ischemia increases with increasing coronary risk factors. The prevalence of exercise-induced silent ischemia in apparently healthy individuals from one decade to the next in the Baltimore Longitudinal Aging Study were 2.5% for those younger than age 60 yr and greater than 10% for those older than age 70 yr *(43)*. In the Detection of Silent Myocardial Ischemia in Asymptomatic Diabetic Subjects study, the prevalence of silent myocardial ischemia was 22% in asymptomatic diabetic population *(44)*.

Potential tests to detect silent and inducible ischemia are exercise ECG, exercise and pharmacological echocardiogram, exercise and pharmacological MPI, ambulatory ECG monitoring, and positron emission tomography (PET).

EXERCISE ECG TESTING

Exercise testing is frequently used to screen high-risk, asymptomatic persons to detect silent myocardial ischemia. Among asymptomatic individuals, there is evidence that development of an ischemic ECG response at low workloads of exercise testing is associated with a higher incidence of future events, such as angina pectoris, MI, and sudden death. However, use of the exercise ECG to screen subjects who are asymptomatic for CAD is a complex issue because it has low specificity (particularly in asymptomatic persons and especially in women). Therefore, high false-positive results may lead to psychological and work disability as well as unnecessary medical expense. Therefore, according to AHA guidelines, routine use of the exercise ECG in completely unselected asymptomatic populations before office screening for risk cannot be recommended *(36)*. In asymptomatic men older than 40 yr with at least one risk factor, exercise testing may provide useful information as a guide to aggressive risk factor intervention or the need to further evaluate the cause of myocardial ischemia. The role of exercise testing in women and the elderly (>75 yr of age) as a guide to identifying the high-risk patient for primary prevention requires further study *(36)*.

Table 1
Framingham Risk Score for Predicting Target Lesions in Coronary Arteries

Risk factor	Coronary arteries	Abdominal aorta
Age, y		
15–19	0	0
20–24	5	5
25–29	10	10
30–24	15	15
Sex		
M[a]	0	0
F	−1	1
Non-HDL cholesterol, mg/dL[b]		
<130[a]	0	0
130–159	2	1
160–189	4	2
≥220	8	4
HDL cholesterol, mg/dL		
<40	1	0
40–59[a]	0	0
≥60	−1	0
Smoking		
Nonsmoker[a]	0	0
Smoker	1	4
Blood pressure		
Normotensive[a]	0	0
Hypertensive	4	3
Obesity (BMI, kg/m^2)		
Men		
≤30[a]	0	0
>30	6	0
Women		
≤30[a]	0	0
>30	0	0
Hyperglycemia		
(glycohemoglobin, %)		
<8[a]	0	0
≥8	5	3

[a]Reference category.
[b]SI conversion factor: to convert HDL cholesterol and non-HDL cholesterol to millimoles per liter, multiply by 0.0259.

STRESS ECHOCARDIOGRAPHY

The diagnosis of myocardial ischemia during stress echocardiography (either exercise or pharmacological) is based on the detection of new or worsening wall-motion abnormalities. The extent of these abnormalities is a powerful predictor of adverse outcome. However, few truly asymptomatic individuals have been evaluated for long-term prognosis. In addition, stress echocardiography is costly and has limitations. Therefore, according to AHA guidelines, only limited data exist to support the use of stress echocardiography as a screening tool or in combination with noninvasive risk factors to evaluate asymptom-

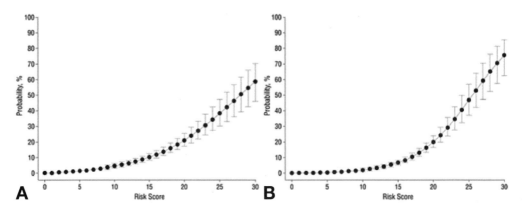

Fig. 3. Estimated probability of target lesions in the coronary arteries (**A**) and the abdominnal aorta (**B**) by risk score. Error bars represent 95% confidence intervals. (From ref. *42* with permission.)

atic populations *(36)*. Although stress echocardiography may be of value in assessing women and the elderly with increased risk factors, further studies are needed to define its role in identifying the high-risk patient for primary prevention *(36)*.

Exercise and Pharmacological MPI

Stress MPI (e.g., planar imaging and single-photon emission computed tomography [SPECT] with 201-thallium or 99m-technetium) can, by the presence and extent of perfusion defects, be used to demonstrate the presence of coronary disease and to risk-stratify and guide management of patients with known or suspected disease. However, development of perfusion defects with exercise or pharmacological stress is dependent on abnormal coronary vasodilator reserve and helpful in flow-limiting coronary artery stenosis; thus, perfusion imaging would be expected to have little value in the detection of patients with early coronary atherosclerotic disease. Therefore, according to AHA guidelines, MPI should not be used broadly in screening unselected asymptomatic populations, but may be valuable in selected populations considered at particularly high risk for CHD *(36)*.

Ambulatory ECG Monitoring (Holter Monitoring)

Holter monitoring has the advantage of providing long-term ECG recording of ischemia during routine daily activities. However, it has low sensitivity and specificity for detection silent ischemia *(36)*. Therefore, according to the American College of Cardiology guidelines, it is considered a class III indication for detecting myocardial ischemia in asymptomatic individuals *(36)*.

Ankle/Brachial BP Index

The ankle–brachial BP index (ABI) is a simple and inexpensive diagnostic test to detect peripheral arterial disease. Abnormal ABI is indicative of significant atherosclerotic burden on vascular bed. Asymptomatic patients with peripheral vascular disease can easily be detected by the ABI (<0.9) which has a sensitivity of 97% and a specificity of 100% for angiographically defined stenosis. In addition, several epidemiological studies in diverse populations have consistently shown that low ABI (<0.90) is a potent predictor of CVD and mortality, and that the ability of the ABI to predict these events is independent of other CVD risk factors *(45)*.

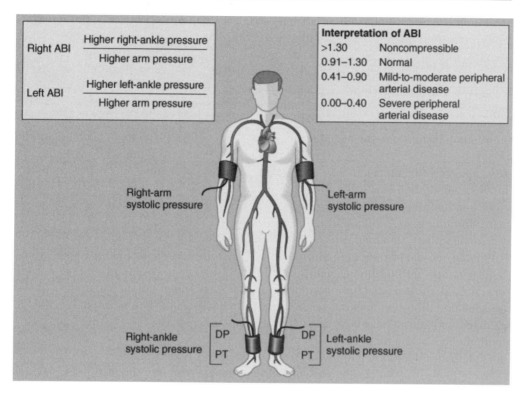

Fig. 4. Measurement and interpretation of the ankle-brachial index. (From ref. *46* with permission.)

Calculation of the ABI is performed by measuring the systolic BP (by Doppler probe) in each arm and in the dorsalis pedis and posterior tibial arteries in each ankle. The higher of the two arm pressures is selected, as is the higher of the two pressures in each ankle. The right and left ABI values are determined by dividing the higher ankle pressure in each leg by the higher arm pressure. An index of 0.9 to 1.3 is normal, 0.7 to 0.9 indicates mild disease, 0.4 to 0.6 reflects moderate disease, less than 0.4 indicates severe disease, and greater than 1.30 suggests a noncompressible calcified vessel (Fig. 4) *(46)*.

AHA recommendations are that the ABI might be a useful addition to the assessment of CHD risk in selected populations, especially in people aged 50 yr and older or those who seem to be at intermediate or higher risk for CVD on the basis of traditional risk factor assessment, such as cigarette smokers or individuals with DM, who have a particularly high risk for peripheral arterial disease. If a patient is found to have an abnormal ABI, this patient can be elevated to a higher risk category. The high relative risk in patients with abnormal ABIs is similar to that of patients who qualify for the AHA secondary-prevention regimens *(36)*.

Imaging Studies

In the last decade, there has been much interest and investigation in detecting subclinical atherosclerosis using imaging studies. These tests include carotid artery duplex scanning, coronary computed tomography (CT) scans (i.e., EBCT), and MRI.

Positron Emission Tomography

In the past few decades, there has been tremendous progress and innovations in cardiac diagnostic testing modalities. Nuclear cardiology techniques to assess CVD have evolved significantly to provide reliable and accurate assessment of the cardiac status of a patient to assist the physician in making beneficial management decisions. Historically, nuclear cardiology techniques primarily involved planar and SPECT myocardial imaging. The relative ease and the cost-effectiveness of cardiac SPECT made it immensely popular and successful. The development of PET has further improved the use of nuclear cardiology in evaluating CVD. In comparison with conventional techniques, PET has the benefit of permitting a true resting scan, allows accurate measurement of the extent of ischemia, and is highly specific for the diagnosis of coronary disease. However, PET scanning is more expensive and of limited availability when compared with conventional techniques. Because PET is insensitive for the detection of coronary stenoses of less than 50%, according to AHA guidelines, its use as a screening test for CHD and risk stratification of asymptomatic patients is not cost-effective (36).

Measurement of Carotid Intima–Media Thickness

Measurement of carotid intima–media thickness (cIMT) with B-mode ultrasound is a noninvasive, highly reproducible, and relatively inexpensive technique for identifying and quantifying preclinical atherosclerosis. Several large, prospective epidemiological studies have shown that cIMT measurements accurately identify prevalent CVD and predict future cardiovascular events independent of traditional CAD risk factors.

Because atherosclerosis is a systemic process and cerebrovascular disease is influenced by the same risk factors as CAD, the carotid arteries can serve as a "window" to the coronary arteries. It has been established that extracranial carotid stenosis predicts future coronary events, and pathology studies have demonstrated that the relationship between the severity of atherosclerosis in the carotid and coronary arteries is as strong as the relationship between any two coronary arteries. Epidemiologically, a 0.1-mm increase in cIMT is associated with an 11% increased risk of an acute MI. In middle-aged and older adults, cIMT consistently is greater in individuals with clinical CVD than in disease-free subjects.

In the Cardiovascular Health Study, cIMT predicted future MI and stroke in individuals older than 65 yr old without a history of CVD. The relationship between cIMT and future cardiovascular events remained significant after adjusting for risk factors, such as age, sex, BP, smoking, lipid levels, presence or absence of DM, and presence or absence of atrial fibrillation, with a composite relative risk per one standard deviation increase of cIMT of 1.44 (95% confidence interval, 1.33–1.55) (36).

Measurement of cIMT by B-mode ultrasound has been validated as a surrogate for atherosclerotic burden more extensively than any other noninvasive modality, and it has been proven to be an independent predictor of future cardiovascular events. As a result, the AHA Prevention Conference V concluded that "in asymptomatic persons >45 yr old a carefully performed carotid ultrasound examination with IMT measurement can provide incremental information to traditional risk factor assessment. In experienced laboratories, this test can now be considered for further verification of CHD risk assessment at the request of a physician" (9). The feasibility of using cIMT in clinical settings has been demonstrated, and strategies for incorporating this noninvasive estimate of atherosclerotic burden into existing CHD risk assessment models also have been described (36).

MAGNETIC RESONANCE IMAGING

MRI is an emerging noninvasive imaging tool with high spatial resolution that continues to prove its value in determining atherosclerotic plaque size, volume, and tissue components. Recent advances have validated MRI measures of plaque location and volume in the vessel wall in the aorta, carotid arteries, and even coronary arteries, and the ability to follow plaque volume serially. MRI has also shown to be useful in serial studies of atherosclerotic plaque progression and regression in the face of therapeutic intervention *(47)*.

According to AHA guidelines, MRI is a promising research tool, but its use seems limited to only a small number of research laboratories at this time and is not ready for application in the identification of patients at high risk for CAD *(36)*.

CORONARY CT

Calcification within the coronary arterial wall is a recognized marker of atherosclerosis. Physicians recognized the association of calcified coronary arteries and the development of symptomatic CAD nearly 200 yr ago *(48)*. Radiographic techniques can detect and quantify the presence of coronary artery calcium deposits with ECG gate images obtained with either helical CT scanning or EBCT. EBCT and helical CT are highly sensitive methods of detecting coronary calcium and are being intensively evaluated as noninvasive means of defining coronary atherosclerotic disease and identifying the asymptomatic but high-risk CAD patient.

The helical CT uses a continuously rotating X-ray source. EBCT uses a fourth-generation CT imaging process and uses a unique electron beam configuration with no moving parts to the imaging chain and inherently defines the heart via three-dimensional acquisition of multiple, high spatial and/or temporal resolution, parallel tomograms. True "snap shot" images (50 or 100 ms) are acquired by timing scan acquisition to the cardiac cycle. Rapid image acquisition allows accurate measurement of calcium deposits in the coronary arteries that are above a prespecified threshold. The speed of acquisition (temporal resolution) is faster for EBCT than it is for helical CT. Coronary calcium is defined as a hyperattenuating lesion above a threshold of 130 Hounsfield units, with an area of at least three adjacent pixels (at least 1 mm^2). The scanner software also allows quantification of coronary calcium area and density.

In 1990, Agatston and colleagues developed a calcium-scoring algorithm based on the X-ray attenuation coefficient (or CT number measured in Hounsfield units) and the area of calcium deposits *(49)*. Thus, coronary artery calcification is traditionally quantitated with Agatston score (Table 2).

Because of the use of the density coefficient, the score shows limited reproducibility and, therefore, is not suitable for sequential scanning to follow progression of disease, thus, the Agatston score has been criticized as not reproducible enough for clinical use. To perform sequential scanning, Callister and associates have described an alternative method of determining the EBCT calcium score that has less variability and, hence, better reproducibility, by quantifying the actual volume of coronary plaque (calcium volume score) *(50)*.

More recently, Raggi and associates have published nomogram tables of the calcium score distribution (Agatston score) by age and sex in a predominantly asymptomatic white population of 9728 people (Table 3) *(51)*. There is a rapid increase in the prevalence and the extent of coronary calcification in men older than 40 yr of age; in women this increase is delayed for 10 to 15 yr.

Table 2
Agatston Method of Calcium Scoring[a]

Lesion peak density (in Hounsfield units)	Density score
<130	0
130–199	1
200–299	2
300–399	3
≥400	4

[a]Agatston Score = area (mm^2) × density score. Total calcium score = Σ score of all 20 slices (left main + left circumflex + left anterior descending + right coronary artery).

Table 3
Calcium Score Nomogram in 9728 Asymptomatic Patients

	35–39 yr	40–44 yr	45–49 yr	50–54 yr	55–59 yr	60–64 yr	65–70 yr
5433 men (n)	479	859	1066	1085	853	613	478
25th percentile	0	0	0	0	3	14	28
50th percentile	0	0	3	16	41	118	151
75th percentile	2	11	44	101	187	434	569
90th percentile	21	64	176	320	502	804	1178
4297 women (n)	288	589	822	903	693	515	485
25th percentile	0	0	0	0	0	0	0
50th percentile	0	0	0	0	0	4	24
75th percentile	0	0	0	10	33	87	123
90th percentile	4	9	23	66	140	310	362

These nomogram tables can be used to classify patients on the basis of the extent of their atherosclerotic disease compared with the expected norm. Investigators have suggested modifying the Framingham Global Risk Score by using a weighted factor based on the patient's individual calcium score percentile. According to the proposed modification, the Framingham Risk Score assigned to a subject undergoing EBCT screening for asymptomatic CAD should be increased if the person's calcium score is in a high percentile and decreased if the person's calcium score is in a low percentile (51).

The presence of coronary calcium correlates strongly with coronary atherosclerosis. Direct relationships have been established between EBCT calcium scores and histological, ultrasonic, and angiographic measures of CHD on a heart-by-heart, vessel-by-vessel, and segment-by-segment basis. Because the severity of coronary atherosclerosis is well-known (from pathological or angiographic studies) to be associated with risk of coronary events, coronary calcium scores, likewise, should correlate with risk for coronary events. However, the extent to which coronary calcium scores predict coronary events independent of the traditional coronary risk factors is not well-studied. Therefore, the AHA recommends "that until there is more definitive information about the additive value of calcium scores in asymptomatic persons, coronary calcium measurement should not be recommended for routine risk assessment in asymptomatic populations. Selected use of the coronary calcium scores in a patient with intermediate coronary disease risk may be appropriate. The AHA looks forward to further research on coronary calcium screening" (36).

The ongoing Multi-Ethnic Study of Atherosclerosis study of the National Heart, Lung, and Blood, is a population-based study to assess the long-term outcome of 6500 asymptomatic individuals undergoing EBCT, as well as other imaging and nonimaging tests *(52)*. It is hoped that this study will provide a final answer on the role of coronary artery calcium in primary prevention.

Assessment of Endothelial Dysfunction

The endothelium has been recognized as playing a central role in vascular homeostasis by controlling the vascular tone, growth, and interaction of the vessel wall with platelets and leukocytes. The healthy endothelium secretes powerful vasodilating (e.g., endothelium-derived relaxing factor) and vasoconstricting substances (e.g., endothelin-1). Endothelial dysfunction is defined as the functional impairment of the endothelium characterized by vasospasm, vasoconstriction, abnormal coagulation and fibrinolysis, and increased vascular proliferation *(53)*. Usually, endothelial dysfunction is combined with cardiovascular risk factors and represents an early, functional stage of atherosclerosis. Endothelial dysfunction is an important early event in the pathogenesis of atherosclerosis, contributing to plaque initiation and progression. Thus, abnormalities in endothelium-dependent vasodilatation may be detected in arteries before the development of overt atherosclerosis *(53)*.

A variety of techniques exist for the assessment of the magnitude of endothelial dysfunction as discussed next *(54)*.

INTRACORONARY ACETYLCHOLINE ADMINISTRATION

This has been the gold standard assessment tool for endothelial function testing for the last decade. Vasoconstriction—rather than vasodilation—in response to intracoronary acetylcholine administration is one of the earliest manifestations of endothelial dysfunction. Response to the effects of acetylcholine on coronary vessels can be assessed with either intracoronary Doppler studies or coronary sinus thermodilution techniques. The measure of endothelial function determined by this method is the change in coronary blood flow.

QUANTITATIVE ASSESSMENT OF CORONARY BLOOD FLOW

The quantitative assessment of the blood flow through a coronary artery, in addition to an assessment of the metabolic activity in the endothelium of the coronary arteries, can be made with PET. The baseline response and response to vasodilatation (usually to intravenous dipyridamole) are determined as the measure of endothelial function. Because the increase in myocardial flow is related to adenosine-induced increases and flow-mediated vasodilation, it is, in part, a measure of endothelial function.

IMPEDANCE PLETHYSMOGRAPHY

In this technique, electrically calibrated plethysmography is used to measure the response of the forearm vasculature to intraarterial infusions of acetylcholine (an endothelium-dependent vasodilator) or methacholine.

PERIPHERAL ARTERIAL TONOMETRY

Reactive hyperemia (RH)–peripheral arterial tonometry (PAT) is a new noninvasive test under investigation to identify individuals with endothelial dysfunction. RH-PAT measures digital pulse volume at rest and during RH (using an occlusion/reperfusion technique). The PAT signal is obtained from a probe that consists of a multicell plethysmograph at the fingertip *(55)*.

Brachial Ultrasound

PET scanning is noninvasive but very expensive compared with intracoronary studies, which are invasive and require a cardiac catheterization laboratory. Because of this, only selected centers have the ability to perform these testing. However, impedance plethysmography has not been extensively used for long-term intervention studies and there is some concern regarding day-to-day variability. Therefore, there is a need for a noninvasive simple method to test endothelial dysfunction.

Brachial artery ultrasound imaging during reactive hyperemia is a tool for quantifying endothelium-dependent vasomotion and establishing the presence of endothelial dysfunction (56). To create a flow stimulus in the brachial artery, a sphygmomanometric (BP) cuff is first placed either above the antecubital fossa or on the forearm. A baseline rest image is acquired, and blood flow is estimated by time averaging the pulsed Doppler velocity signal obtained from a mid-artery sample volume. Thereafter, arterial occlusion is created by cuff inflation to suprasystolic pressure. Typically, the cuff is inflated to at least 50 mmHg above systolic pressure to occlude arterial inflow for a standardized length of time. This causes ischemia and consequent dilation of downstream resistance vessels via autoregulatory mechanisms. Subsequent cuff deflation induces a brief high-flow state through the brachial artery (reactive hyperemia) to accommodate the dilated resistance vessels. The resulting increase in shear stress causes the brachial artery to dilate. The longitudinal image of the artery is recorded continuously from 30 s before to 2 min after cuff deflation. A mid-artery pulsed Doppler signal is obtained on immediate cuff release and no later than 15 s after cuff deflation to assess hyperemic velocity. The variability is acceptable (~2%), and the measurements are reproducible in a good laboratory. Brachial artery flow-mediated vasodilation has been shown to correlate with measures of coronary endothelial function. The main advantages of this approach are the noninvasive nature and the ability to repeat multiple tests in the same patient or the study of large numbers of patients.

A number of studies demonstrate that endothelium-dependent vasomotor function in the brachial arteries predicts long-term cardiovascular risk and supports findings of other clinical and experimental studies, implicating an active role for the endothelium in atherosclerosis. However, these studies demonstrating the prognostic value of endothelial function involved selected high-risk populations; data are lacking on the prognostic value in low-risk populations. Therefore, after reviewing current evidence, an AHA working group concluded that, although the assessment of endothelial function, as measured most typically by flow-mediated brachial artery vasodilatation, is a promising technique that may reflect an independent measure of CVD risk, additional prospective research is needed to demonstrate that this technique can truly add to standard CVD risk prediction. In addition, standardization and improvement of the measurement technique are needed before this modality can become a part of routine clinical assessment of CVD risk (35).

Serum Markers

Inflammatory Markers

It is becoming apparent that inflammation is associated with atherosclerosis and the resulting thrombosis (atherothrombosis). Circulating levels of several inflammatory markers rise in individuals at risk for atherosclerotic events. In particular, elevation of plasma CRP, a nonspecific acute-phase reactant that is easily and reliably measured, has a strong predictive power for cardiovascular events. In addition, levels of CRP also seem

to have strong associations with other inflammation-sensitive proteins (e.g., fibrinogen) as well as BMI, fibrinolytic activity, glucose tolerance status, lifetime exposure to smoking, and some measures of subclinical atherosclerosis *(57)*.

Although such data suggest that elevated CRP plasma levels define risk that warrants therapy among individuals who do not meet current criteria, definitive prospective evidence for a broader application in event reduction remains undetermined.

Because its role and cost-effectiveness in the primary prevention of CVD has not been firmly established by large trials, the AHA has not recommended the implementation of CRP monitoring on a population-wide basis *(58,59)*. At the discretion of the physician, the measurement is considered optional, based on the moderate level of evidence (evidence level C). In this role, high sensitivity (hs)-CRP measurement seems to be best used to detect enhanced absolute risk in persons in whom multiple risk factor scoring projects a 10-yr CHD risk in the range of 10–20% (evidence level B). However, the benefits of this strategy or any treatment based on this strategy remain uncertain. The finding of a high relative risk level of hs-CRP (>3.0 mg/L) may allow for intensification of medical therapy to further reduce risk and to motivate some patients to improve their lifestyle or comply with medications prescribed to reduce their risk. Individuals at low risk (<10% per 10 yr) will be unlikely to have a high risk (>20%) identified through hs-CRP testing *(59)*.

Other potential novel markers under investigation are fibrinogen, plasminogen activator inhibitor-1, cytokines (e.g., interleukin-6 and tumor necrosis factor-α), chemokines (e.g., monocyte chemoattractant protein-1), intercellular adhesion molecules (e.g., inter-cellular cellular adhesion molecule-1), vascular cell adhesion molecule-1, and E-selectin. However, their role in everyday clinical practice remains to be established *(59)*.

Homocysteine

In several cross-section studies, elevated serum homocysteine levels have been shown to correlate with CHD risk, although data are conflicting in prospective studies. As a result, routine general population screening for homocysteine levels is not recommended according to AHA guidelines. However, homocysteine testing should be considered in CHD patients who have no CHD risk factors and in asymptomatic patients with a strong family history of premature CHD *(60)*.

TREATMENTS

Therapeutic Lifestyle Changes

Therapeutic lifestyle changes (TLCs) have been shown to reverse the pathophysiology of the metabolic syndrome, and to improve the other modifiable risk factors of atherosclerosis. Multifactor risk intervention studies have shown significant retardation of disease progression *(61)*. The two major component of TLCs are diet and exercise as discussed next in detail.

DIET

Several well-designed epidemiological studies and dietary intervention trails have established a strong correlation between diet and CHD. The St. Thomas Atherosclerosis Regression Study and other secondary prevention studies have showed that a low-fat diet alone slowed the progression of atherosclerosis and, when combined with lipid-lowering drugs, induced regression of atherosclerosis *(62)*. The Cholesterol Lowering Atherosclerosis Study showed that each quartile of increased consumption of total fat and polyun-

Table 4
Adult Treatment Panel III Dietary Recommendations

Nutrient	Recommended intake
Saturated fat	<7% of total calories
Polyunsaturated fat	Up to 10% of total calories
Monounsaturated fat	Up to 20% of total calories
Total fat	25–35% of total calories
Carbohydrate	50–60% of total calories
Fiber	20–30 g/d
Protein	~15% of total calories
Cholesterol	<200 mg/d
Total calories	Balance energy intake and expenditure to maintain ideal body weight

saturated fat was associated with a significant increase in risk of new atherosclerotic lesions documented by angiogram (63).

AHA dietary guidelines have placed a greater emphasis on an overall eating pattern that achieves a healthy body weight to decrease the risks of atherosclerotic disease. Healthy eating is recommended for the entire population, which includes a variety of fruits, vegetables, grains, low-fat or nonfat dairy products, fish, legumes, poultry, and lean meat, matching energy intake to energy needs (with appropriate changes to achieve weight loss when indicated); and fat intake less than 30% of total calorie intake, with a limitation of saturated fat to less than 10% of energy and cholesterol to less than 300 mg/d. For high-risk groups, the ATP III recommendation is summarized in Table 4.

EXERCISE

There is a consensus that virtually all individuals can benefit from regular physical activity, and the beneficial effect of physical activity on cardiovascular morbidity and mortality and all-cause mortality is widely acknowledged (64). Multiple studies have shown strong inverse associations between long-duration physical activity and the prevalence and degree of subclinical atherosclerosis in an asymptomatic population with multiple metabolic risk factors (65).

The Surgeon General, the Centers for Disease Control and Prevention, the American College of Sports Medicine, and the National Institutes of Health Consensus Development Panel on Physical Activity and Cardiovascular Health recommend that every adult should engage in at least 30 min of moderate-intensity exercise on most, if not all, days of the week to prevent CHD (66).

Lipid-Lowering Agents

Several placebo-controlled studies evaluated changes in coronary artery plaque with statin administration, and have shown that statin-treated subjects were less likely to have atherosclerosis progression and more likely to have stable lesions or even regression (66). Multiple studies also found that, compared with placebo, treatment with statins resulted in either a slower progression of, or a decrease in, intima–media thickness of carotid arteries (67).

Studies have also shown that when nicotinic acid is added to a statin, atherosclerosis is retarded more then with a statin alone (68). Multiple angiographic trials with fibrate

therapy have demonstrated the ability of fibrates to reduce rates of atheromatous plaque progression *(69)*. Statins have been shown to decrease morbidity and mortality in multiple primary prevention trials. Similarly, the Helsinki Heart Study was a primary prevention trial in 4081 men, 40 to 55 yr old, with a non-HDL-C level greater than 200 mg/dL, and compared 600 mg gemfibrozil therapy (orally, twice daily) with placebo. The treated group experienced an overall 34% ($p < 0.02$) reduction in risk for first-time CAD-related events *(70)*.

According to ATP III of the NCEP, LDL-C level is the primary target of therapy. In high-risk people (known CAD or CAD equivalent, including DM), the recommended LDL-C goal is less than 100 mg/dL, but when risk is very high, an LDL-C goal of less than 70 mg/dL is a therapeutic option. This therapeutic option extends also to patients at very high risk who have a baseline LDL-C of less than 100 mg/dL. Moreover, when a high-risk patient has high triglycerides or low HDL-C, consideration can be given to combining a fibrate or nicotinic acid with an LDL-lowering drug. For moderately high-risk persons (two or more risk factors and 10-yr risk of 10–20%), the recommended LDL-C goal is less than 130 mg/dL, but an LDL-C goal of less than 100 mg/dL is a therapeutic option based on recent trial evidence. The latter option extends also to moderately high-risk people who have a baseline LDL-C level of 100 to 129 mg/dL. When LDL-lowering drug therapy is used in high-risk or moderately high-risk persons, it is advised that intensity of therapy be sufficient to achieve at least a 30 to 40% reduction in LDL-C levels. Once the LDL-C target has been reached, if the TG level is greater than 200 mg/dL, the secondary target is the non–HDL-C level, which is a calculated value of TC minus HDL-C. Non–HDL-C is an easily obtainable indirect measure of triglyceride-rich lipoprotein remnants. Goals for non–HDL-C are 30 mg/dL higher than goals for LDL-C. By establishing non–HDL-C goals, NCEP chose to focus on TG instead of HDL as a secondary target of therapy. Low HDL was defined by ATP III as less than 40 mg/dL, although no specific treatment goals for HDL-C were established. Moreover, any person at high risk or moderately high risk who has lifestyle-related risk factors (e.g., obesity, physical inactivity, elevated triglycerides, low HDL-C, or metabolic syndrome) is a candidate for therapeutic life counseling to modify these risk factors, regardless of LDL-C level *(71)*.

Smoking Cessation Counseling

In addition to being a strong risk factor for atherosclerotic disease, smoking affects several other organ system, thus, cigarette smoking remains the primary cause of preventable death and morbidity in the United States. Therefore, smoking cession counseling should be part of all preventive care. Physician counseling in the office, with or without supplemental follow-up, has been associated with a small but significant increase in overall cessation.

Glycemic Control in DM

In the Epidemiology of Diabetes Interventions and Complications study (the long-term follow-up of the Diabetes Control and Complications Trial), mean progression of intima–media thickness was significantly less in those who had received intensive therapy during the Diabetes Control and Complications Trial compared with those who had received conventional therapy (progression of intima–media thickness of the common carotid artery of 0.032 vs 0.046 mm) *(72)*. Progression of carotid intima–media thickness was associated with age, systolic BP, smoking, the ratio of LDL-C to HDL-C, urinary

albumin excretion rate, and the mean glycosylated Hb value during the mean duration. Therefore, the goal should be multifactor risk reduction in addition to attempted glycemic control. The benefits of target-driven, long-term, intensified intervention aimed at multiple risk factors were shown in the Steno-2 study *(73)*.

Thiazolidinediones, such as rosiglitazone or pioglitazone, have been shown to improve endothelial function and inflammatory biomarkers of arteriosclerosis in patients with type II diabetes or metabolic syndrome *(74)*. It seems that their protective effects on the vessel wall are independent of their metabolic action. Therefore, in the absence of contraindication, thiazolidinediones should be a part of treatment regimens of all patients with type 2 diabetes.

Control of Hypertension

In addition to being a major risk factor for atherosclerosis, hypertension is associated with a number of other serious adverse effects. In clinical trials, antihypertensive therapy has been associated with 35 to 40% mean reductions in stroke incidence; 20 to 25% reductions in MI; and greater than 50% reductions in heart failure *(75)*.

There is still debate whether any class of antihypertensive therapy is more cardioprotective than others. Experimental evidence has demonstrated antiatherogenic potential of angiotensin-converting enzyme inhibitors *(76)*. Some clinical trials (Heart Outcomes Prevention Evaluation and European Trial on Reduction of Cardiac Events [EUROPA]) with angiotensin-converting enzyme inhibitors and angiotensin-receptor blockers in high-risk patients led some experts to conclude that these agents have a unique benefit in this setting *(77)*. However, others think the benefit is caused by a decrease in BP. Therefore, at this time, it seems that the available evidence suggests that the attained BP, not the drug used, is of primary importance in such patients.

Moderate Alcohol Intake

Epidemiological studies, as well as growing insights into the mechanisms of alcohol's effects on reducing atherogenesis and thrombosis, suggest a causal cardioprotective effect of alcohol *(78)*. Most of the benefit of alcohol seems to be mediated by an elevation in serum HDL-C, although antioxidant, antithrombotic, and anti-inflammatory effects have also been reported *(78)*. However, there are also several potential deleterious effects of moderate alcohol consumption. Therefore, AHA recommendations are *(79)*: "Moderate intake of alcoholic beverages (one to two drinks per day) is associated with a reduced risk of CHD in populations. There is no clear evidence that wine is more beneficial than other forms of alcohol, although further research is needed. If wine does have additional effects, it seems that many of the same additional biological effects may be achieved with grape juice. Despite the biological plausibility and observational data in this regard, it should be kept in mind that these are insufficient to prove causality. Although moderate use of wine and other alcohol-containing beverages does not seem to lead to significant morbidity, alcohol ingestion, unlike other dietary modifications, poses a number of health hazards. Without a large-scale, randomized, clinical endpoint trial of wine intake, there is little current justification to recommend alcohol (or wine specifically) as a cardioprotective strategy. The AHA maintains its recommendation that alcohol use should be an item of discussion between physician and patient."

Estrogen

Many animal and observational studies have shown that estrogen decreases the progression of subclinical atherosclerosis *(30)*. However, in the wake of the reports of the Women's Health Initiative and the Heart and Estrogen/Progestin Replacement Study *(31,32)*, which unexpectedly showed that combination hormone therapy was associated with adverse CVD effects, estrogen is not recommended for primary prevention of atherosclerotic disease.

Fish Oil

A number of investigators have reported on beneficial effects of increased ω-3 fatty acid (contained in fish oil) intake in patients with CAD. In addition, consumption of fish is associated with a significantly reduced progression of coronary artery atherosclerosis *(80)*. However, an AHA working group has concluded that further studies are needed to establish optimal doses of ω-3 fatty acids (including eicosapentaenoic acid, docosahexaenoic acid, and α-linolenic acid) for both primary and secondary prevention of coronary disease at this time *(81)*.

Antioxidants

Rapidly increasing evidence suggests that inflammation and oxidized LDL play an important role in atherogenesis. Therefore, there has been much interest and literature regarding dietary antioxidants, including vitamin E, vitamin C, lycopene, and several different carotenoids. However, currently available evidence is insufficient to recommend any of them for primary prevention *(82)*. Therefore, the AHA recommends against using antioxidant for primary prevention at this time.

Aspirin

Inflammation-related processes play a key role in the current etiological model of atherosclerosis and its acute complications. Animal studies have shown that aspirin decreases atherosclerotic lesions *(83)*. In the US Physicians' Health Study, among 22,071 male physicians, an alternate-day dose of 325 mg of aspirin conferred a statistically significant, 44% reduction in risk of first MI *(84)*. However, a British trial, also among male physicians, found no significant effects of aspirin, although it was far smaller in sample size (5139) than the US trial *(85)*. Recent reports from the Women's Health Study concluded that healthy women 45 yr of age and older who regularly took low-dose aspirin have a significantly reduced risk of stroke, ischemic stroke, and transient ischemic attack, but not MI, cardiovascular mortality, or all-cause mortality *(86)*.

With respect to guidelines in primary prevention, in 2002, the Preventive Services Task Force and the AHA recommended aspirin for adults whose 10-yr risks of a first coronary heart disease event were at least 6 and 10%, respectively *(87)*. According to the American Diabetes Association Clinical Practice Recommendations 2004, aspirin therapy (75–162 mg/d) should be used for primary prevention in men and women with diabetes with increased cardiovascular risk, including those older than 40 yr of age or who have additional risk factors (family history of CVD, hypertension, smoking, dyslipidemia, or albuminuria) *(88)*. Aspirin therapy should not be recommended for patients younger than 21 yr because of the increased risk of Reye's syndrome, and use of aspirin has not been studied in people younger than 30 yr *(88)*.

Folic Acid

Although several epidemiological studies have shown a relationship between plasma homocystine and CVD, it is not known whether reduction of plasma homocystine by diet and/or vitamin therapy will reduce CVD risk. Therefore, until results of controlled clinical trials become available, population-wide screening is not recommended by AHA *(60)*. According to AHA guidelines, if elevated homocysteine levels are found, patients should be advised to consume the recommended dietary allowance of folic acid *(60)*.

CONCLUSION

Atherosclerosis is a chronic progressive fibroinflammatory process. It starts early in life and progress in different morphological stages before manifesting clinically. Traditional risk factors, such as dyslipidemia, smoking, DM, male gender, metabolic syndrome, genetic factors, sedentary lifestyle, and new novel factors have been shown to initiate and cause progression of atherosclerosis. Multiple diagnostic tests are on the horizon to detect subclinical atherosclerosis. Although they may have a role in individual patients, none are recommended for population based screening at this time. Medical office assessments to detect risk factors and to apply different risk models to predict subclinical atherosclerosis remain the most cost-effective method at this time. Treatment includes aggressive therapeutic lifestyle changes and control of risk factors. Use of aspirin in primary prevention should be individualized. The most important point is to realize that primary prevention of atherosclerosis, as contrasted with clinically manifest atherosclerosis disease, must begin in childhood or adolescence.

REFERENCES

1. Hag IU, Ramsay LE, Jackson PR, Wallis EJ. Prediction of coronary risk for primary prevention of coronary heart disease: a comparison of methods. QJ Med 1999;92:379–385.
2. Berenson GS, Srinivasan SR, Bao W, et al. Association between multiple cardiovascular risk factors and atherosclerosis in children and young adults. The Bogalusa Heart Study. [see comment]. N Engl J Med 1998;338(23):1650–1656.
3. McGill HC Jr, McMahan CA. Determinants of atherosclerosis in the young. Pathobiological Determinants of Atherosclerosis in Youth (PDAY) Research Group. Am J Cardiol 1998;82(10B):26.
4. Faxon DP, Fuster V, Libby P, et al. Atherosclerotic Vascular Disease Conference: Writing Group III: pathophysiology. Circulation 2004;109(21):2617–2625.
5. Stary HC, Chandler AB, Dinsmore RE, et al. A definition of advanced types of atherosclerotic lesions and a histological classification of atherosclerosis. A report from the Committee on Vascular Lesions of the Council on Arteriosclerosis, American Heart Association. Arterioscler Thromb 1995;92(15):512–531.
6. Gore I, Tejada C. The quantitative appraisal of atherosclerosis. Am J Pathol 1957;33:875–885.
7. Schoen FJ. Blood vessel. In: Abbas AK, ed. Robbins and Cotran Pathologic Basis of Disease. 7th ed. Elsevier, St. Louis, 2005, pp. 516–517.
8. Gould KL, Lipscomb K. Effects of coronary stenoses on coronary flow reserve and resistance. Am J Cardiol 1974;34(1):48–55.
9. Strong JP, Malcom GT, McMahan CA, et al. Prevalence and extent of atherosclerosis in adolescents and young adults: implications for prevention from the Pathobiological Determinants of Atherosclerosis in Youth Study. JAMA 1999;281(8):727–735.
10. Jaffer FA, O'Donnell CJ, Larson MG, et al. Age and sex distribution of subclinical aortic atherosclerosis: a magnetic resonance imaging examination of the Framingham Heart Study. Arterioscler Thromb 2002;22(5):849–854.
11. Roberts WC. Preventing and arresting coronary atherosclerosis. Am Heart J 1995;130(3 Pt 1):580–600.
12. Newman WP 3rd, Freedman DS, Voors AW, et al. Relation of serum lipoprotein levels and systolic blood pressure to early atherosclerosis. The Bogalusa Heart Study. N Engl J Med 1986;314(3):138–144.
13. Goldstein JL, Kita T, Brown MS. Defective lipoprotein receptors and atherosclerosis. Lessons from an animal counterpart of familial hypercholesterolemia. N Engl J Med 1983;309(5):288–296.

14. Babiak J, Rudel LL. Lipoproteins and atherosclerosis. Baillieres Clinical Endocrinology & Metabolism 1987;1(3):515–550.

15. Celermajer DS, Sorensen KE, Georgakopoulos D, et al. Cigarette smoking is associated with dose-related and potentially reversible impairment of endothelium-dependent dilation in healthy young adults. Circulation 1993;88(5 Pt 1):2149–2155.

16. Zhu BQ, Sun YP, Sievers RE, et al. Passive smoking increases experimental atherosclerosis in cholesterol-fed rabbits.[see comment]. J Am Coll Cardiol 1993;21(1):225–232.

17. Howard G, Wagenknecht LE, Burke GL, et al. Cigarette smoking and progression of atherosclerosis: The Atherosclerosis Risk in Communities (ARIC) Study. [see comment]. JAMA 1998;279(2):119–124.

18. Schoenhagen P, Nissen SE. Coronary atherosclerosis in diabetic subjects: clinical significance, anatomic characteristics, and identification with in vivo imaging. Cardiol Clin 2004;22(4):527–540.

19. Mautner SL, Lin F, Roberts WC. Composition of atherosclerotic plaques in the epicardial coronary arteries in juvenile (type I) diabetes mellitus. Am J Cardiol 1992;70(15):1264–1268.

20. Crall FV Jr, Roberts WC. The extramural and intramural coronary arteries in juvenile diabetes mellitus: analysis of nine necropsy patients aged 19 to 38 years with onset of diabetes before age 15 years. Am J Med 1978;64(2):221–230.

21. Waller BF, Palumbo PJ, Lie JT, et al. Status of the coronary arteries at necropsy in diabetes mellitus with onset after age 30 years. Analysis of 229 diabetic patients with and without clinical evidence of coronary heart disease and comparison to 183 control subjects. Am J Med 1980;69(4):498–506.

22. Jorgensen L, Jenssen T, Joakimsen O, et al. Glycated hemoglobin level is strongly related to the prevalence of carotid artery plaques with high echogenicity in nondiabetic individuals: the Tromso study. Circulation 2004;110(4):466–470.

23. Rajala U, Laakso M, Paivansalo M, et al. Blood pressure and atherosclerotic plaques in carotid, aortic and femoral arteries in elderly Finns with diabetes mellitus or impaired glucose tolerance. J Hum Hypertens 2005;19(1):85–91.

24. McGill HC Jr, McMahan CA, Malcom GT, et al. Relation of glycohemoglobin and adiposity to atherosclerosis in youth. Pathobiological Determinants of Atherosclerosis in Youth (PDAY) Research Group. Arterioscler Thromb 1995;15(4):431–440.

25. Ellison RC, Zhang Y, Wagenknecht LE, et al. Relation of the metabolic syndrome to calcified atherosclerotic plaque in the coronary arteries and aorta. Am J Cardiol 2005;95(10):1180–1186.

26. Smith SC Jr, Milani RV, Arnett DK, et al. Atherosclerotic Vascular Disease Conference: Writing Group II: risk factors. Circulation 2004;109(21):2613–2616.

27. Duggirala R, Gonzalez Villalpando C, O'Leary DH, et al. Genetic basis of variation in carotid artery wall thickness. Stroke 1996;27(5):833–837.

28. O'Donnell CJ, Chazaro I, Wilson PW, et al. Evidence for heritability of abdominal aortic calcific deposits in the Framingham Heart Study. Circulation 2002;106(3):337–341.

29. Nasir K, Michos ED, Rumberger JA, et al. Coronary artery calcification and family history of premature coronary heart disease: sibling history is more strongly associated than parental history. [see comment]. Circulation 2004;110(15):2150–2156.

30. Dubey RK, Imthurn B, Zacharia LC, et al. Hormone replacement therapy and cardiovascular disease: what went wrong and where do we go from here? Hypertension 2004;44(6):789–795.

31. Grady D, Herrington D, Bittner V, et al. Cardiovascular disease outcomes during 6.8 years of hormone therapy: Heart and Estrogen/progestin Replacement Study follow-up (HERS II). [see comment] [erratum appears in JAMA 2002;288(9):1064]. JAMA 2002;288(1):49–57.

32. Rossouw JE, Anderson GL, Prentice RL, et al. Risks and benefits of estrogen plus progestin in healthy postmenopausal women: principal results from the Women's Health Initiative randomized controlled trial. [see comment]. JAMA 2002;288(3):321–333.

33. Vaitkevicius PV, Fleg JL, Engel JH, et al. Effects of age and aerobic capacity on arterial stiffness in healthy adults. Circulation 1456;88(4 Pt 1):1456–1462.

34. Haas DC, Davidson KW, Schwartz DJ, et al. Depressive symptoms are independently predictive of carotid atherosclerosis. Am J Cardiol 2005;95(4):547–550.

35. Yusuf S, Hawken S, Ounpuu S, et al. Effect of potentially modifiable risk factors associated with myocardial infarction in 52 countries (the INTERHEART study): case–control study. [see comment]. Lancet 2004;364(99438):937–952.

36. Greenland P, Abrams J, Aurigemma GP, et al. Prevention Conference V: beyond secondary prevention: identifying the high-risk patient for primary prevention: noninvasive tests of atherosclerotic burden: Writing Group III. Circulation 2000;101(1):4.

37. Sheridan S, Pignone M. Framingham-based tools to calculate the global risk of coronary heart disease. J Gen Intern Med 2003;18(12):1039–1052.

38. Liao Y, McGee DL, Cooper RS. Prediction of coronary heart disease mortality in blacks and whites: pooled data from two national cohorts. Am J Cardiol 1999;84(1):31–36.

39. Liao Y, McGee DL, Cooper RS, et al. How generalizable are coronary risk prediction models? Comparison of Framingham and two national cohorts. Am Heart J 1999;137(5):837–845.

40. Grundy SM, D'Agostino RB Sr, Mosca L, et al. Cardiovascular risk assessment based on US cohort studies: findings from a National Heart, Lung, and Blood institute workshop. Circulation 2001;104(4): 491–496.

41. D'Agostino RB Sr, Grundy S, Sullivan LM, et al. Validation of the Framingham coronary heart disease prediction scores: results of a multiple ethnic groups investigation. [see comment]. JAMA 2001;286(2): 180–187.

42. McMahan CA, Gidding SS, Fayad ZA, et al. Risk scores predict atherosclerotic lesions in young people. Arch Intern Med 2005;165(8):883–890.

43. Cohn PF, Fox KM. Silent myocardial ischemia. Circulation 2003;108:1263–1277.

44. Wackers FJ, Young LH, Inzucchi SE, et al. Detection of silent myocardial ischemia in asymptomatic diabetic subjects: the DIAD study. [see comment] [erratum appears in Diabetes Care 2005;28(2):504]. Diabetes Care 2004;27(8):1954–1961.

45. Resnick HE, Foster GL. Prevalence of elevated ankle-brachial index in the United States 1999 to 2002. Am J Med 2005;118(6):676–679.

46. Hiatt WR. Medical treatment of peripheral arterial disease and claudication. N Engl J Med 2001;344(21):1608–1621.

47. Choi CJ, Kramer CM. MR imaging of atherosclerotic plaque. Radiol Clin North Am 2002;40(4):887–898.

48. Anand DJ, Lahiri A. EBCT coronary calcium imaging for the early detection of coronary artery disease in asymptomatic individuals. Br J Cardiol 2003;10(4):273–280.

49. Agatston AS, Janowitz WR, Hildner FJ, et al. Quantification of coronary artery calcium using ultrafast computed tomography. J Am Coll Cardiol 1990;15(4):827–832.

50. Callister TQ, Cooil B, Raya SP, et al. Coronary artery disease: improved reproducibility of calcium scoring with an electron-beam CT volumetric method. [see comment]. Radiology 1998;208(3):807–814.

51. Salazar HP, Raggi P. Usefulness of electron-beam computed tomography. Am J Cardiol 2002;89(4A):21.

52. Bild DE, Bluemke DA, Burke GL, et al. Multi-ethnic study of atherosclerosis: objectives and design. Am J Epidemiol 2002;156(9):871–881.

53. Davignon J, Ganz P. Role of endothelial dysfunction in atherosclerosis. Circulation 2004;109(23 Suppl 1):15.

54. Anderson TJ. Assessment and treatment of endothelial dysfunction in humans. J Am Coll Cardiol 1999;34(3):631–638.

55. Bonetti PO, Pumper GM, Higano ST, et al. Noninvasive identification of patients with early coronary atherosclerosis by assessment of digital reactive hyperemia. J Am Coll Cardiol 2004;44(11):2137–2141.

56. Celermajer DS, Sorensen KE, Gooch VM. Non-invasive detection of endothelial dysfunction in children and adults at risk of atherosclerosis. Lancet 1992;340:1111–1115.

57. Tracy RP. Inflammation in cardiovascular disease: cart, horse, or both? [see comment]. Circulation 2000;97(20):2000–2002.

58. Loscalzo J, Bonow RO, Jacobs AK. Coronary calcium screening and the American Heart Association news embargo. Circulation 2004;110(23):3504–3505.

59. Pearson TA, Mensah GA, Alexander RW, et al. Markers of inflammation and cardiovascular disease: application to clinical and public health practice: a statement for healthcare professionals from the Centers for Disease Control and Prevention and the American Heart Association. [see comment]. Circulation 2003;107(3):499–511.

60. Malinow MR, Bostom AG, Krauss RM. Homocyst(e)ine, diet, and cardiovascular diseases: a statement for healthcare professionals from the Nutrition Committee, American Heart Association. [see comment]. Circulation 1999;99(1):178–182.

61. Niebauer J, Hambrecht R, Velich T, et al. Attenuated progression of coronary artery disease after 6 years of multifactorial risk intervention: role of physical exercise. Circulation 1997;96(8):2534–2541.

62. Watts GF, Lewis B, Brunt JN, et al. Effects on coronary artery disease of lipid-lowering diet, or diet plus cholestyramine, in the St Thomas' Atherosclerosis Regression Study (STARS) [see comment]. Lancet 1992;339(8793):563–569.

63. Blankenhorn DH, Johnson RL, Mack WJ, et al. The influence of diet on the appearance of new lesions in human coronary arteries. [see comment]. JAMA 1990;263(12):1646–1652.

64. Rothenbacher D, Hoffmeister A, Brenner H, et al. Physical activity, coronary heart disease, and inflammatory response. Arch Intern Med 2003;163(10):1200–1205.

65. Desai MY, Nasir K, Rumberger JA, et al. Relation of degree of physical activity to coronary artery calcium score in asymptomatic individuals with multiple metabolic risk factors. Am J Cardiol 2004;94(6):729–732.

66. Pate RR, Pratt M, Blair SN, et al. Physical activity and public health. A recommendation from the Centers for Disease Control and Prevention and the American College of Sports Medicine. [see comment]. JAMA 1995;273(5):402–407.

67. Balk EM, Karas RH, Jordan HS, et al. Effects of statins on vascular structure and function: a systematic review. Am J Med 2004;117(10):775–790.

68. Taylor AJ, Sullenberger LE, Lee HJ, et al. Arterial Biology for the Investigation of the Treatment Effects of Reducing Cholesterol (ARBITER) 2: a double-blind, placebo-controlled study of extended-release niacin on atherosclerosis progression in secondary prevention patients treated with statins. [see comment]. Circulation 2004;110(23):3512–3517.

69. Ericsson CG, Hamsten A, Nilsson J, et al. Angiographic assessment of effects of bezafibrate on progression of coronary artery disease in young male postinfarction patients. Lancet 1996;347(9005):849–853.

70. Manninen V, Elo MO, Frick MH, et al. Lipid alterations and decline in the incidence of coronary heart disease in the Helsinki Heart Study. JAMA 1988;260(5):641–651.

71. Grundy SM, Cleeman JI, Merz CN, et al. Implications of recent clinical trials for the National Cholesterol Education Program Adult Treatment Panel III guidelines. [erratum appears in Circulation 2004;110(6):763]. Circulation 2004;110(2):227–239.

72. Nathan DM, Lachin J, Cleary P, et al. Intensive diabetes therapy and carotid intima-media thickness in type 1 diabetes mellitus. [see comment]. N Engl J Med 2003;348(23):2294–2303.

73. Gaede P, Vedel P, Larsen N, et al. Multifactorial intervention and cardiovascular disease in patients with type 2 diabetes. [see comment]. N Engl J Med 2003;348(5):383–393.

74. Hetzel J, Balletshofer B, Rittig K, et al. Rapid effects of rosiglitazone treatment on endothelial function and inflammatory biomarkers (early online release). Arterioscler Thromb Vasc Biol 2005;25(9):1804–1809.

75. Neal B, MacMahon S, Chapman N, et al. Effects of ACE inhibitors, calcium antagonists, and other blood-pressure-lowering drugs: results of prospectively designed overviews of randomised trials. Blood Pressure Lowering Treatment Trialists' Collaboration. [see comment]. Lancet 2000;356(9246):1955–1964.

76. Da Cunha V, Tham DM, Martin-McNulty B, et al. Enalapril attenuates angiotensin II-induced atherosclerosis and vascular inflammation. Atherosclerosis 2005;178(1):9–17.

77. Yusuf S, Sleight P, Pogue J, et al. Effects of an angiotensin-converting-enzyme inhibitor, ramipril, on cardiovascular events in high-risk patients. The Heart Outcomes Prevention Evaluation Study Investigators. [see comment] [erratum appears in 2000;342(18):1376]. N Engl J Med 2000;342(3):145–153.

78. Ellison RC. AHA Science Advisory on wine and health: a confusing message about alcohol consumption. [comment]. Circulation 2001;104(13):25.

79. Goldberg IJ, Mosca L, Piano MR, et al. AHA Science Advisory: wine and your heart: a science advisory for healthcare professionals from the Nutrition Committee, Council on Epidemiology and Prevention, and Council on Cardiovascular Nursing of the American Heart Association. [see comment]. Circulation 2001;103(3):472–475.

80. Erkkila AT, Lichtenstein AH, Mozaffarian D, et al. Fish intake is associated with a reduced progression of coronary artery atherosclerosis in postmenopausal women with coronary artery disease. [see comment]. Am J Clin Nutr 2004;80(3):626–632.

81. Krauss RM, Eckel RH, Howard B, et al. AHA Dietary Guidelines: revision 2000: a statement for healthcare professionals from the Nutrition Committee of the American Heart Association. Circulation 2000;102(18):2284–2299.

82. Rimm EB, Stampfer MJ. Antioxidants for vascular disease. Med Clin North Am 2000;84(1):239–249.

83. Kouraklis G, Patapis P, Misiakos E, et al. Effects of acetylsalicylic acid on experimental atherogenesis induced in rabbits. Int Angiol 2004;23(2):139–143.

84. Anonymous. Final report on the aspirin component of the ongoing Physicians' Health Study. Steering Committee of the Physicians' Health Study Research Group. [see comment]. N Engl J Med 1989;321(3):129–135.

85. Peto R, Gray R, Collins R, et al. Randomised trial of prophylactic daily aspirin in British male doctors. Br Med J (Clin Res Ed) 1988;296(6618):313–316.

86. Ridker PM, Cook NR, Lee IM, et al. A randomized trial of low-dose aspirin in the primary prevention of cardiovascular disease in women. [see comment]. N Engl J Med 2005;352(13):1293–1304.

87. Pearson TA, Blair SN, Daniels SR, et al. AHA Guidelines for Primary Prevention of Cardiovascular Disease and Stroke: 2002 Update: Consensus panel guide to comprehensive risk reduction for adult patients without coronary or other atherosclerotic vascular diseases. American Heart Association Science Advisory and Coordinating Committee. Circulation 2002;106(3):388–391.

88. Colwell JA, American Diabetes Association. Aspirin therapy in diabetes. Diabetes Care 2004;27(Suppl 1):S72–73.

14 Exercise Testing and Risk Assessment

Christopher R. Cole, MD and Michael S. Lauer, MD

CONTENTS

INTRODUCTION
STANDARD METHODS OF INTERPRETATION
FUNCTIONAL CAPACITY
ECG DATA
HEART RATE
BLOOD PRESSURE
CONCLUSION
REFERENCES

INTRODUCTON

With the development of advanced imaging modalities, the regular exercise electro-cardiogram (ECG) test has come to be regarded by some as passé. In large part, this is because of the low sensitivity and specificity for the diagnosis of coronary artery disease (CAD). With newer methods of interpretation, however, exercise testing remains a powerful and inexpensive prognostic tool. The use of the exercise test has important implications for risk stratification as a part of prevention strategies and for after myocardial infarction (MI) management. This chapter focuses primarily on the prognostic implications of exercise testing using cardiovascular events and mortality as endpoints. It examines all aspects of the exercise test, including functional capacity, heart rate (HR) changes during exercise, blood pressure (BP) response, and more-recent methods of computerized interpretation of the exercise ECG.

STANDARD METHODS OF INTERPRETATION

Exercise ECGs are interpreted visually at most centers, with a study being considered abnormal if there is at least 1 mm of horizontal or downsloping ST-segment depression at 60 to 80 ms after the J-point *(1)*. This approach has been used for decades. Numerous studies in which patients have undergone both exercise ECG and coronary angiography have demonstrated poor test accuracy with low sensitivity and specificity *(2–6)*. Most of these studies suffer from inherent sequential workup bias, because patients with negative exercise ECGs are less likely to be referred for coronary angiography; this bias results in

From: *Contemporary Cardiology: Preventive Cardiology:*
Insights Into the Prevention and Treatment of Cardiovascular Disease, Second Edition
Edited by: J. M. Foody © Humana Press Inc., Totowa, NJ

inflated sensitivity and deflated specificity *(7–11)*. A recent prospective study of 814 male veterans who agreed to undergo both exercise and coronary angiography demonstrated poor sensitivity (~45%), but reasonably good specificity (~85%) for the diagnosis of coronary disease, defined as the presence of at least one 50% coronary stenosis *(12)*.

The poor diagnostic performance of exercise ECG has led many clinicians to routinely request imaging studies that are more costly, although some groups have argued against this *(13)*. Reasons why the exercise ECG may perform poorly include the following: trying to find the wrong lesion, trying to answer the wrong question, and using the wrong methods:

1. Trying to find the wrong lesion. Exercise ECG relies on the presence of hemodynamically obstructive lesions; a 50% lesion would not be expected to produce stress-induced ischemia.
2. Trying to answer the wrong question. Many, if not most, patients referred for exercise ECG have some degree of coronary disease; the main question for the clinician is whether their disease is severe enough that either myocardial revascularization or aggressive medical therapy are indicated. This requires knowledge of prognosis, rather than diagnosis. Thus, research on exercise testing should focus much more on prediction of events rather than prediction of angiographic findings.
3. Using the wrong methods. Exercise ECG potentially involves much more than looking at visually assessed ECG changes with exercise. Important non-ECG variables to consider include functional capacity *(14)*, HR *(15–18)*, and BP *(19,20)* responses; and arrhythmias *(21)*. Some of these variables have been tightly linked with prognosis. Some researchers have proposed using computerized measures of ST-segment changes adjusted for HR *(22)*.

FUNCTIONAL CAPACITY

A direct relationship between functional capacity and survival has been well-established in a number of prospective, population-based studies *(23–34)*. In the clinical setting, exercise capacity has also proven to be a powerful and independent predictor of cardiac morbidity and mortality and all-cause mortality *(14,35–46)*.

Exercise capacity is usually estimated in the stress lab based on published tables *(1)*. The standard unit is the metabolic equivalent (MET), which is the amount of oxygen consumed at rest. In a typical adult, 1 MET equals 3.5 mL/kg/min of oxygen uptake. Direct measurement of exercise capacity is possible using sophisticated gas exchange analysis, which, in clinical practice, is primarily used in patients with severe heart failure *(47–50)*. Concern has been raised that estimated exercise capacity is inherently inaccurate, particularly when standard treadmill protocols are used, in which case, it tends to be systematically overestimated *(51)*.

A functional classification for an individual may be determined based on the workload achieved. Exercise capacity is strongly correlated with age and gender; therefore, any classification scheme must take these important confounders into account. The classification system in use at the Cleveland Clinic is shown in Table 1. A classification using directly measured oxygen uptake is presented in Table 2 *(52)*.

A number of clinical studies have used exercise capacity as a predictor of mortality. The Seattle Heart Watch Study *(53)* was a prospective study of 1852 men with a known history of CAD. After treadmill testing, the men were followed for 3 yr, during which time, there were 195 deaths. One of the most powerful predictors of death was poor

Table 1
Exercise Capacity Classifications by Age and Sex

| | | | Women | | |
Age	Poor	Fair	Average	Good	High
20–29	<7.5	8–10.3	10.3–12.5	12.5–16	>16
30–39	<7	7–9	9–11	11–15	>15
40–49	<6	6–8	8–10	10–14	>14
50–59	<5	5–7	7–9	9–13	>13
60–69	<4.5	4.5–6	6–8	8–11.5	>11.5
70–79	<3.5	3.5–4.5	4.5–6.5	6.5–8	> 8
≥80	<2.5	2.5–4	4–5.5	5.5–7	> 7
			Men		
Age	Poor	Fair	Average	Good	High
20–29	<8	8–11	11–14	14–17	>17
30–39	<7.5	7.5–10	10–12.5	12.5–16	>16
40–49	<7	7–8.5	8.5–11.5	11.5–15	>15
50–59	<6	6–8	8–11	11–14	>14
60–69	<5.5	5.5–7	7–9.5	9.5–13	>13
70–79	<4.5	4.5–5.5	5.5–8	8–9.5	>9.5
≥80	<3.5	3.5–4.5	4.5–6.5	6.5–7.5	>7.5

For any given age (in years) and workload (in METs) the exercise capacity can be classified into one of five categories.

Table 2
Functional Classification of Patients Based on Measured Gas Exchange

Severity of impairment	Functional class	VO_{2max} (mL/kg/min)
None to mild	A	>20
Mild to moderate	B	16–20
Moderate to severe	C	10–15
Severe	D	<10

Modified from ref. 52.

exercise capacity (as measured by a short duration of exercise). This remained true in both univariate and multivariate analysis of clinical and exercise data.

Subsequently, Bruce and associates (39) prospectively followed 3611 men and 547 women with no known CAD for 10 yr. In asymptomatic men, they found that any clinical risk factor (age >55 yr, hypertension, and tobacco use) when combined with two or more exercise variables (angina on the treadmill, HR <90% of the age-predicted maximum, double product <80% of predicted, or >20% difference between observed VO_{2max} and that expected for a healthy person of similar age) predicted a 33-fold increase in the combined end point of worsened angina, MI, coronary artery bypass surgery, or death.

In a study by Podrid and colleagues *(38)*, 142 men with a history of CAD and a strongly positive exercise test (>2 mm ST-segment depression) were divided into three groups by duration of exercise during a Bruce protocol treadmill test. Men who exercised 1 to 6 min (~6 METs) had a significant increase in mortality when compared with those exercising 6 to 9 min (~8 METs) or greater than 9 min (~11 METs). There were no survival differences between the two groups of higher functional capacity. A low workload is also predictive of cardiac events, as demonstrated by Swada and coworkers *(52)*, who showed an increased cardiac event rate in patients achieving less than 6 METs workload.

Weiner and associates have looked extensively at the Coronary Artery Surgery Study registry regarding exercise capacity *(41–44)*. Most recently, they reported the 16-yr follow-up on 3086 men and 747 women who underwent maximal treadmill testing and coronary angiography *(44)*. The subjects were divided into high-, intermediate-, and low-risk groups on the basis of exercise testing. Men in the high- or intermediate-risk groups had 16-yr survival rates of 61 and 56%, respectively, whereas men in the low-risk group had only a 38% survival rate ($p < 0.0001$). The results for women were similar (79, 73, and 44%, respectively; $p < 0.0001$). Among men, 12-yr survival was improved by coronary artery bypass surgery vs medical therapy in the high-risk subgroup (69 vs 55%, respectively; $p = 0.0025$), but the two therapies were similar in the other two subgroups. Among women, neither medical nor surgical therapy improved 12-yr survival rates in any of the three subgroups.

In the only study to take into account evidence of myocardial perfusion defects, Snader and colleagues *(14)* found that, in 3400 patients with no history of diagnosed CAD undergoing exercise single-photon emission computed tomography thallium testing, patients with average or better functional capacity classifications (Table 1) had a 2.5-yr mortality of less than 2%, compared with 6 and 14%, respectively, in individuals who were in the fair and poor groups (Fig. 1). Of note, more than 81% of the 108 deaths during follow-up occurred in the fair- and poor-capacity groups. The thallium scan was also predictive of mortality in this study. In multivariable analyses including clinical, exercise, and thallium variables, estimated exercise capacity was the strongest predictor of death ($\chi^2 = 34$; $p < 0.0001$), with the only other predictors being age ($\chi^2 = 28$; $p < 0.0001$), male gender ($\chi^2 = 17$; $p < 0.0001$), and abnormal thallium perfusion ($\chi^2 = 5$; $p = 0.03$). Estimated functional capacity and thallium sum score were roughly equivalent predictors of cardiac mortality.

The Duke nomogram (Fig. 2) is a risk stratification tool that incorporates exercise capacity with ST-segment deviation and symptoms on the treadmill to predict 5-yr mortality. The nomogram was derived by regression analysis *(54)* and has been validated prospectively *(55)*, although some researchers have not found a correlation with mortality *(56)*.

To estimate prognosis for an individual patient using the nomogram, a line is first drawn from the maximum amount of ST-segment depression during exercise to the observed degree of angina. A mark is made on the ischemia-reading line where these lines intersect. From this mark, a line is drawn to the workload achieved on the exercise line. The intersection of this line and the prognosis line provides a risk assessment for survival.

ECG DATA

Visual ST-Segment Interpretation

The classic method of interpretation of the exercise ECG test focuses solely on ST-segment depression. An abnormal response is typically defined as ST-segment depression of at least 1 mm that is horizontal or downsloping, or upsloping ST-segment

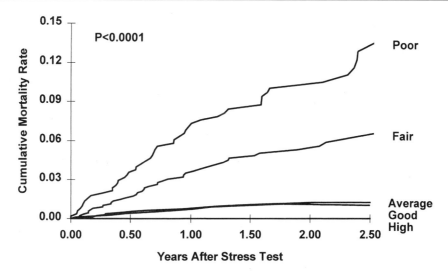

Fig. 1. Kaplan-Meier plot relating age- and gender-specific estimated functional capacity to total all-cause mortality. (From ref. *14.*)

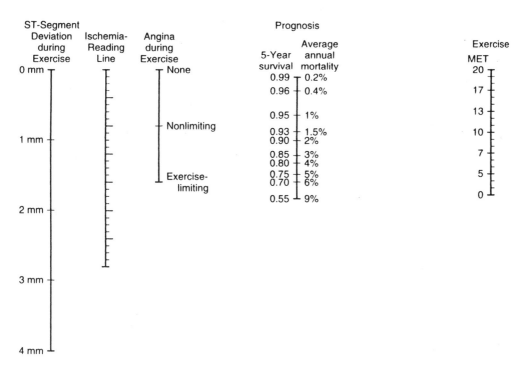

Fig. 2. Duke treadmill exercise score nomogram. *See* text for details. (From ref. *55.*)

depression of at least 1.5 to 2.0 mm. The pathophysiology of the ST-segment change is thought to be caused by a current of ischemia from the affected myocardial cells resulting in a net depression.

Ellestad and Wan *(35)* retrospectively examined the predictive capability of ST-segment depression in 2700 patients who had undergone exercise treadmill testing for cardiovascular morbidity or mortality. There was no association between a positive test and mortality, but there was an association between an early onset of ST-segment depression and mortality in univariate analysis.

In more than 3600 white men enrolled in the Lipid Research Clinic Prevalence Study, a positive exercise test was predictive of cardiac and all-cause mortality in univariate analysis *(57)*. When stratified for age and cardiac risk factors, the test was also predictive. In both this study and the previous study, no adjustments were made for functional capacity. Other investigations have not been able to demonstrate an association between standard visual ST-segment analysis and mortality *(58–61)*.

HR Adjustment of the ST-Segment

Because standard visual ST-segment analysis is imprecise and fails to take workload into account, it has been argued that heart-rate adjusted, computerized ST-segment measurements may improve the diagnostic and prognostic capabilities of exercise ECG *(22)*. Two specific measures have been described, the ST-segment/HR (ST/HR) index and the ST/HR slope.

The ST/HR index is the simplest approach, in which the change in ST-segment depression during exercise is divided by the difference between peak and resting HRs. This index is easy to calculate and can be applied to patients undergoing staggered protocols, such as the Bruce or modified Bruce.

The ST/HR slope is derived by seeking the maximal change in ST-segment depression as a function of HR change during exercise. To be valid, this measure requires a gradual, graded protocol, such as the Cornell protocol.

There is considerable controversy regarding whether computerized ST-segment measurements adjusted for HR changes represent a viable alternative to visually read ST segments. Although some researchers have found that computerized and/or HR-adjusted ST-segment analyses can significantly improve the diagnostic properties of the exercise ECG *(60–64)*, others have been unable to confirm this finding *(12,65,66)*. There have been two major studies relating computerized ST-HR measures to prognosis, one from the Framingham Offspring Study *(58)* and the other from the Multiple Risk Factor Intervention Trial *(59,60)*; both showed that standard visual ST-segment analyses failed to predict events, whereas computerized ST-HR measures did.

Okin and associates *(58)* followed 3168 asymptomatic men and women enrolled in the Framingham Offspring Study for 4 yr. All participants underwent maximum exercise testing at baseline with comparison made between the ST/HR index and standard visual ST-segment analysis. Although visual ST-segment analysis was not effective in predicting coronary events (sudden death, MI, or new-onset angina) the ST/HR index was highly predictive.

The association of the ST/HR index and death was further examined in 6000 men enrolled in the usual care arm of the Multiple Risk Factor Intervention Trial *(59,60)*. All participants underwent maximum exercise testing at enrollment. After 7 yr of follow-up, there were 109 deaths. Visual ST-segment analysis was not predictive of death in this population, whereas the ST/HR index was predictive.

Q-Waves

Although there is an association between Q-waves on the resting ECG and mortality *(67)*, the presence or absence of Q-waves on the resting ECG does not alter the diagnostic accuracy of exercise induced ST-segment depression *(68)*.

QT Dispersion

QT dispersion is defined as the time difference between the shortest QT interval in any lead and the longest QT interval in any other lead. The presence of QT dispersion greater than 60 ms in addition to standard criteria has been proposed as a method of increasing the specificity of the exercise test for diagnosis of CAD *(69)*.

R-Wave Changes

R-waves may change in amplitude during exercise. Leroy *(70)* investigated the prognostic value of these changes in 303 post-MI patients during 4 yr of follow-up. Although there was a significant correlation of increased R-wave amplitude during exercise and three-vessel CAD and with the extent of ST-segment depression during exercise, there was no relation to mortality. There was also an association with angina at follow-up but not with recurrent infarction. Several studies have been published on the diagnostic value of R-wave amplitude changes, with mixed results *(71–76)*.

T-Wave Changes

The T-wave will normally decrease gradually in early exercise and begin to increase in amplitude at maximal exercise. At 1 min into recovery, T-waves have returned to baseline. A T-wave increase of 2.5 mm or greater in lead V2 may increase the sensitivity of the exercise test *(77)*. Although not a common finding, deep T-wave inversion (≤8 mm depression) associated with downsloping ST-segment depression of at least 1 mm is associated with an increased incidence of three-vessel and left-main disease *(78)*. T-wave inversion less than 8 mm is a less-specific finding and may be a normal variant.

T-Wave Alternans

T-wave alternans (TWA) is characterized by microvolt beat-to-beat changes in the T-wave amplitude *(79,80)*. TWA has been demonstrated to have prognostic significance for ventricular tachycardia (VT) for patients with long-QT syndrome *(81–83)* and in patients with ischemic cardiac disease *(84)*.

Recent studies have focused on TWA during exercise testing. Individuals who are at increased risk of ventricular arrhythmias will have a sudden onset of sustained TWA at a HR lower than that of controls (<110 bpm or <70% of maximum predicted HR) *(85)*. Among patients referred for electrophysiology testing, TWA has been demonstrated to be a better predictor than electrophysiology testing of VT or death *(86)*. Other studies of the prognostic capability of TWA in other populations are ongoing *(87)*.

U-Wave Inversion

If they are upright at baseline, U-wave inversions during exercise may be a marker of ischemia, left ventricular (LV) hypertrophy, or diastolic dysfunction *(88–92)*. There are no prognostic studies, to date, of U-wave inversion.

Left Bundle-Branch Block

Approximately 0.5% of patients undergoing exercise testing will develop transient left bundle-branch block (LBBB). Grady and associates (93) examined the prognostic significance of this finding using a control cohort study. They selected 70 patients who developed exercise-induced LBBB and matched them to 70 control subjects based on age, sex, previous history of CAD, and standard risk factors. In 4 yr of follow-up, there were seven deaths, five of which occurred in the exercise-induced LBBB group. There were also higher rates of need for revascularization and implantation of pacemaker or defibrillator in the group that had transient LBBB. The adjusted relative risk (RR) of developing one of these endpoints was 2.78 (95% confidence interval [CI], 1.16–6.65).

Arrhythmias

The occurrence of exercise-induced arrhythmia is generally a marker of worse outcome. Supraventricular arrhythmias have been associated with increased mortality (70), as have VT and fibrillation (94,95). However, not all investigators have found an association between VT and mortality (96,97).

Various groups have reported conflicting results regarding the diagnostic and prognostic significance of exercise-induced ventricular ectopy (e.g., premature ventricular complexes or bigeminy) (21,98–100). Califf and colleagues (98) found that the 236 patients of 1293 consecutive treadmill patients with simple ventricular arrhythmias (at least one premature ventricular complex, but without paired complexes or VT) had a higher incidence of significant CAD (57 vs 44%), three vessel disease (31 vs 17%) and abnormal LV function (43 vs 24%) than did patients without ventricular arrhythmias. In the 620 patients with significant CAD, patients with paired complexes or VT had a higher 3-yr mortality (25%) than did patients with simple ventricular arrhythmias (17%) or patients with no ventricular arrhythmias (10%). In patients with nonsignificant CAD, ventricular ectopy had no prognostic significance.

Schweikert and coworkers (21) demonstrated an association between ventricular ectopy and thallium defects but not severe CAD or 2-yr mortality. Two cohorts consisting of adults without heart failure or known severe resting ventricular ectopic activity were studied. The first cohort consisted of adults ($n = 2743$) who underwent maximal exercise thallium stress testing. The second cohort consisted of adults ($n = 423$) who underwent coronary angiography within 90 ds of treadmill testing. In the thallium cohort, exercise-induced ventricular ectopic activity was associated with a greater frequency of thallium defects (35.2 vs 18.7%; odds ratio [OR], 2.35; 95% CI, 1.62–3.42; $p < 0.001$); after adjusting for possible confounders, this association persisted (for any defect adjusted OR, 1.66; 95% CI, 1.09–2.53; $p = 0.02$). There was no association between exercise-induced ventricular ectopic activity and mortality during 2-yr of follow-up. In the angiographic cohort, there was no association of exercise-induced ventricular ectopy with severe CAD (19 vs 20%; OR, 0.93; 95% CI, 0.41–2.09; p = not significant).

In 1486 patients from the Coronary Artery Surgery Study (99), there was no association between mortality and ventricular ectopy after stratification by severity of CAD. In the 80 patients of 1160 consecutive patients (100) who developed frequent ($\geq 10\%$ of beats in any 1 min) or repetitive (three beats or more in a row) ventricular ectopic beats, there was no difference in mortality when followed during 5 yr.

HEART RATE

HR Rise During Exercise

Maximal exercise HR is related to peak workload in a linear fashion and has been demonstrated to have similar prognostic capabilities to workload achieved *(70)*. Researchers have argued that peak HR is a better prognostic marker than METs because it is a measured value, whereas the workload achieved is usually estimated.

Chronotropic Incompetence

The term chronotropic incompetence refers to an attenuated HR response to exercise. Longer than 20 yr ago, Ellestad performed an exercise test on a 51-yr-old athletic man who had a normal exercise tolerance for age and no symptoms or ST-segment depression during exercise *(101)*. A short time after the exercise test, the man suffered sudden cardiac death; an autopsy revealed severe two-vessel coronary disease with an 80% left anterior descending artery stenosis. Of note, the patient had only reached a maximum HR of 110 bpm during exercise. Later, analyzing follow-up of 2700 patients undergoing exercise testing, Ellestad and his colleagues noted that patients with a slow HR during exercise were more likely to suffer an acute coronary event than patients with ischemic ST-segment depression and a normal HR response *(35)*. Other groups also reported worse prognosis among patients with attenuated exercise heart responses *(102)*, as well as larger burdens of myocardial scar as noted by radionuclide imaging *(103)*.

As imaging modalities such as thallium scintigraphy and stress echocardiography became more popular, interest in the HR response to exercise focused away from prognosis and more toward its impact on test accuracy for the diagnosis of CAD. A number of groups found that an impaired HR response to exercise is associated with reduced test sensitivity *(104–106)*. Indeed, many exercise laboratories will report tests in which patients fail to reach 85% of their age-predicted maximum HR as being "nondiagnostic." Although such a term does at least indirectly imply the need for further testing, it does not carry the ominous connotation as the phrase "evidence of myocardial ischemia."

The physiology behind the HR response to exercise is a complex one that relates to perturbations in resting and exercise sympathetic and parasympathetic tone and neurohormonal milieu. A detailed discussion of the mechanisms underlying normal and abnormal HR responses to exercise is beyond the scope of this review, but can be found elsewhere *(107)*.

The most important determinant of exercise HR response to exercise is age, with decreasing maximal HRs achievable as people get older. The relationship between peak HR and age in a healthy individual has been found to be an inverse linear one; a number of groups have reported on linear equations for estimating peak heart, with 220 minus age in years being one of the more popularly used in clinical exercise laboratories. A commonly used definition of chronotropic incompetence is failure to reach 85% of the age-predicted peak HR.

A major limitation of this approach is that the estimated peak HR has a high standard deviation and, therefore, may be difficult to apply to individuals, as opposed to populations *(108)*. There are other problems with using ability to reach 85% of the age-predicted maximum HR as a measure of chronotropic incompetence. In addition to age, other important predictors of the HR response to exercise are resting HR and physical fitness,

both factors that themselves are predictive of coronary heart disease (CHD) risk *(31,108–111)*. Data from the Framingham Heart Study have shown that ability to reach a target HR is influenced by these two variables and even by age itself *(16)*. Therefore, any effort to relate chronotropic incompetence to prognosis or diagnosis suffers an inherent risk of serious confounding.

To help account for these potential confounding factors, Wilkoff and Miller developed a marker called the chronotropic index *(112)*. The index takes advantage of the linear relation between exercise HR increase and metabolic work. Before exercise, a person has a certain metabolic reserve (MR), which is the difference between their peak oxygen consumption (or exercise capacity) and rest oxygen consumption, which is typically 3.5 mL/kg/min, or 1 MET. As exercise progresses, that MR is used up. Analogously, at rest, there is a potential HR reserve, which is the difference between the peak attainable HR (as estimated, e.g., by 220 minus age) and the resting HR. As exercise progresses, HR reserve, like the MR, is also used up.

During any given stage of exercise, the percent MR used can be expressed as:

$$\%\text{MR used} = [(\text{METs}_{\text{stage}} - \text{METs}_{\text{rest}})/(\text{METs}_{\text{peak}} - \text{METs}_{\text{rest}})] \times 100$$

In an analogous fashion, for the percent HR reserve (HRR) used at any given stage of exercise can be expressed as:

$$\%\text{HRR used} = [(\text{HR}_{\text{stage}} - \text{HR}_{\text{rest}})/(220 - \text{age} - \text{HR}_{\text{rest}})] \times 100$$

Wilkoff and Miller have shown that, in a group of healthy, nonhospitalized adults, a plot of HRR used to MR used during different stages of exercise reveals a tight linear relationship with a slope of approximately one, with a 95% CI of 0.8–1.3 *(112)*. The calculated value of this slope, which has been termed the chronotropic index *(16,113)*, is independent of stage of exercise considered. Thus, chronotropic incompetence can be defined as a ratio of percent HRR used to percent MR used of less than 0.8; this is referred to as a low chronotropic index. The advantage of using this approach to assess chronotropic response is that it accounts for age, functional capacity, and resting HR; *it is not merely a reflection of physical fitness or exercise time*.

One possible problem with this method is that, except for patients undergoing sophisticated gas-exchange analyses, exercise capacity in METs is estimated, and not directly measured. Among patients who undergo symptom-limited testing, one can consider the ratio of HRR used to MR used at peak exercise, when, by definition, the proportion of MR used has a value of 1. Using this approach, the chronotropic index is based entirely on directly measured variables, i.e., resting HR, peak HR, and age *(114)*. Because the value of the chronotropic index is independent of stage of exercise considered, this measure, at least indirectly, takes into account effects of functional capacity as well *(112)*.

A study by Brener and colleagues examined the association of chronotropic response to exercise and angiographic severity of coronary disease *(18)*. Among 475 patients who underwent exercise testing and coronary angiography within 180 d, peak heart, percent target HR achieved, and the chronotropic index were all closely related to the number of diseased coronary arteries. Also of note, despite the anatomic relationship between the right coronary artery and the sinus node, there was no association between isolated disease of the proximal right coronary artery and chronotropic response. In contrast, after adjusting for age and gender, stenosis in the proximal left anterior descending artery was strongly associated with peak HR (for each 10 bpm decrement, OR, 1.23; 95% CI, 1.07–

1.41; $p = 0.03$), percent target HR achieved (for each 10% decrement, OR 1.44; 95% CI, 1.15–1.81; $p = 0.02$), and chronotropic index (for each 0.2 decrement, OR 1.6; 95% CI, 1.03–1.54; $p = 0.02$).

Lauer studied 1575 healthy male participants of the Framingham Heart Study who underwent graded-exercise testing according to the Bruce protocol and were followed for nearly 8 yr. *(16)*. There were 327 who failed to reach 85% of their age-predicted maximum HR; of these, 21 (6%) men died and 44 (14%) men experienced an incident CHD event. In contrast, of the 1248 subjects who reached their target HR, only 34 (3%) men died and only 51 (4%) men experienced CHD events. The chronotropic index also stratified subjects well for prediction of death and CHD events. After adjusting for ST-segment changes and standard cardiovascular risk factors, all-cause mortality was predicted by the change in HR with exercise ($p = 0.04$) and by the chronotropic index as measured during stage 2 of exercise ($p = 0.05$).

Although these studies showed that chronotropic incompetence was predictive of mortality among healthy adults, the possibility that this was merely a manifestation of MI could not be excluded. Therefore, Lauer and associates studied 231 consecutive adults (mean age 57 yr, 146 men) who underwent stress echocardiography at the Cleveland Clinic Foundation and who were not taking β-blockers *(115)*. After 41 mo of follow-up, 41 patients died, had a nonfatal MI, or underwent myocardial revascularization at least 3 mo after the stress test. Failure to reach 85% of the age-predicted maximum HR was predictive of events (RR, 2.47; 95% CI, 1.28–4.79; $p = 0.007$), as was a chronotropic index less than 0.8 (RR, 2.44; 95% CI, 1.31–4.55; $p = 0.005$). Even after adjusting for myocardial ischemia by echocardiography and other possible confounders, failure to reach 85% of the target HR remained predictive (adjusted RR, 2.20; 95% CI, 1.11–4.37; $p = 0.02$), as was a low chronotropic index (adjusted RR, 1.85; 95% CI, 0.98–3.47; $p = 0.06$).

These findings were confirmed in a population of 1877 men and 1076 women who underwent single-photon emission computed tomography thallium exercise testing *(17)*. None were taking β-blockers and none had undergone previous cardiac invasive procedures or had a history of congestive heart failure. Failure to reach 85% of the age-predicted maximum HR was noted in 316 (11%) patients, whereas a low chronotropic index was noted in 762 (26%) patients; thallium perfusion defects were found in 612 (21%) patients. Death during 2 yr of follow-up occurred in 91 patients. Even after adjusting for thallium evidence of ischemia and other possible confounders, failure to reach 85% of the age-predicted maximum HR was predictive of death (adjusted RR, 1.84; 95% CI, 1.13–3.00; $p = 0.01$), as was a low chronotropic index (adjusted RR 2.19; 95% CI, 1.43–3.44; $p = 0.0003$). Of note, a low chronotropic index by itself was as ominous a sign as thallium perfusion defects; the presence of both was associated with a particularly poor prognosis (Fig. 3).

It is unclear why chronotropic incompetence is associated with an adverse outcome. Previous investigators had argued that a slower HR during exercise represents a compensatory mechanism for hearts beset by a heavy ischemic burden, but the ability to predict events many years after testing argues that the mechanism must be more complex *(101)*. Nonetheless, there must be some relation to ischemia, given the association of chronotropic incompetence with angiographic severity of coronary disease *(18)* and with thallium perfusion defects *(103)* and the improvement of chronotropic response with myocardial revascularization *(116)*. Another possible mechanism might be that subtle alterations of autonomic tone are themselves markers, if not outright contributors, to the

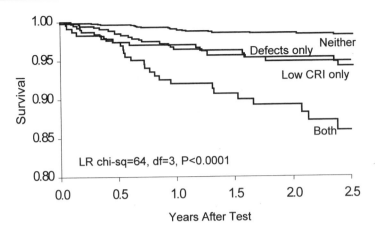

Fig. 3. Kaplan-Meier plot relating chronotropic incompetence (CRI), thallium defects, or both to all-cause mortality. (From ref. *17*.)

severity and activity of atherosclerosis. Investigations in this area have included consideration of the Bezold-Jarish reflex *(117)*, decreased vagal activity at rest *(57)*, and the relation between resting HR and coronary disease risk *(108)*. Investigators have argued that the relationship between chronotropic incompetence and outcome may parallel the associations between exercise HR responses and severity of neurohormonal alterations in patients with congestive heart failure *(118,119)*.

HR Recovery

Not only is the HR increase during exercise important, but the HR decrease after exercise also has important prognostic implications. A recent study examined this association between mortality and HR recovery immediately after exercise *(15)*. Cole and associates followed 2428 consecutive adults who underwent symptom-limited exercise thallium testing for 6 yr. HR recovery was defined as the change in HR from peak exercise to 1 min of recovery. An abnormal HR recovery was defined as at most 12 bpm. The end point of the study was all-cause mortality.

In 6 yr of follow-up, there were 213 deaths. In univariate analysis, a low HR recovery strongly predicted mortality (Fig. 4; mortality at 6 yr, 19 vs 5%; RR, 3.96; 95% CI, 3.02–5.19; $p < 0.0001$). Even after adjusting for age, gender, medications, thallium perfusion defects, hypertension, diabetes, smoking, resting HR, chronotropic response during exercise, and workload achieved, a low HR recovery remained highly predictive of death (adjusted RR, 2.00; 95% CI, 1.49–2.68; $p < 0.001$).

These findings held true if HR recovery was considered as a continuous variable or a log-transformed value and also when stratified by age, gender, history of CAD, thallium perfusion defects, use of β-blockers, or vasodilating drugs. Even in patients with completely normal thallium scans, an abnormal HR recovery was significantly predictive of mortality. Although a minority of patients (26%) had an abnormal HR recovery, the majority of deaths (56%) were among those who had an abnormally low value. This is in marked contrast to most risk factors, which, although they identify high-risk groups, predict only a minority of events.

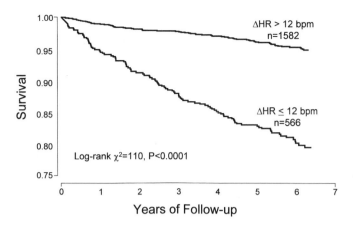

Fig. 4. Kaplan-Meier plot relating HR recovery to all-cause mortality (based on data from ref. *15*).

The prognostic potential of HR recovery also held true in a larger population of healthy young adults undergoing submaximal exercise testing *(120)*. There were 5234 healthy adults with no known heart disease, who were followed for 12 yr after submaximal exercise testing. An abnormal HR recovery was defined as a less than 42-beat decrease in HR, 2 min into recovery. Those with abnormal HR recovery had a 2.5-fold increase in mortality during the study period (10 vs 4%). These findings remained true even after adjustment for multiple confounding risk factors.

The potential mechanisms for why HR recovery predicts mortality may be related to vagal activity. Imai and colleagues studied the HR recovery after maximal and submaximal exercise in normal individuals, athletes, and patients with heart failure *(121)*. In all groups, the decrease in HR immediately after exercise was markedly prolonged after atropine administration, but not with β-blockade, suggesting that HR recovery is primarily a function of the parasympathetic nervous system. This effect was independent of age and exercise intensity but was more pronounced in athletes and attenuated in those with heart failure. These studies would seem to suggest that increased HR recovery is a marker of increased parasympathetic activity that has been associated with a reduction in the risk of death *(122)*.

BLOOD PRESSURE

An exaggerated BP response to exercise (or "exercise hypertension") has been associated with a higher risk of developing hypertension at rest *(123,124)*. Based on exercise test data recording in healthy adults in the Framingham Offspring Study, we defined exercise hypertension as a peak systolic BP of at least 210 mmHg in men and 190 mmHg in women *(125)*. Previous reports regarding its prognostic significance have shown conflicting results *(126–132)*.

A report from a Veteran Administration clinic in which exercise testing had been performed in normotensive subjects found that exercise hypertension was associated with a greater likelihood of echocardiographic LV hypertrophy *(133)*. This potential association was analyzed in detail among the Framingham Offspring cohort and found to be largely, although not entirely, confounded by age, gender, and resting BP *(125)*.

Snader and associates studied 594 adults who underwent exercise testing and coronary angiography within 90 d of one another at the Cleveland Clinic Foundation *(14)*; all increased systolic BP during exercise by at least 10 mmHg. Exercise hypertension was present in 196 patients (33%). Severe coronary disease was less common in patients with exercise hypertension (14 vs 25%, OR, 0.51; 95% CI, 0.32–0.81; $p = 0.004$). When resting and exercise types of hypertension were considered together, resting hypertension was associated with a greater likelihood of severe CAD, whereas exercise hypertension was independently associated with a lower likelihood. After adjusting for resting BP, age, gender, other coronary risk factors, and exercise capacity, exercise hypertension remained predictive of a lower likelihood of severe coronary disease (adjusted OR, 0.58; 95% CI, 0.34–0.97; $p = 0.04$).

Among 3445 adults evaluated for known or suspected CAD, exercise hypertension was associated with a lower likelihood of myocardial perfusion abnormalities, as assessed by thallium scanning, and was not associated with an increased mortality rate *(19)*. Exercise hypertension was defined as a peak systolic BP of at least 210 mmHg in men and at least 190 mmHg in women, and was present in 39% of the population. Patients with exercise-induced hypertension were less likely to have either fixed or reversible thallium perfusion defects (16 vs 25%; OR, 0.58; 95% CI, 0.49–0.69; $p < 0.001$) as well as reversible defects only (OR, 0.71; 95% CI, 0.57–0.90; $p < 0.001$). There was no association between exercise-induced hypertension and mortality during 6 yr of follow-up. These findings suggest that, among clinical populations, exercise hypertension is not an ominous finding and may even be a benign one.

CONCLUSION

There is a wealth of often-overlooked information contained in the exercise test. The focus of exercise test interpretation should turn away from the ST-segment and toward exercise capacity, HR, and other autonomic markers. Using these parameters, the exercise test can be an important tool for risk stratification and prevention. Future research is needed into how to use more expensive imaging tests more judiciously.

REFERENCES

1. Fletcher GF, Balady G, Froelicher VF, et al. Exercise standards. A statement for healthcare professionals from the American Heart Association. Writing Group. Circulation 1995;91:580–615.
2. Detrano R, Froelicher VF. Exercise testing: uses and limitations considering recent studies. Prog Cardiovasc Dis 1988;31:173–204.
3. Detrano R, Gianrossi R, Mulvihill D, et al. Exercise-induced ST segment depression in the diagnosis of multivessel coronary disease: a meta analysis. J Am Coll Cardiol 1989;14:1501–1508.
4. Detrano R, Gianrossi R, Froelicher V. The diagnostic accuracy of the exercise electrocardiogram: a meta-analysis of 22 years of research. Prog Cardiovasc Dis 1989;32:173–206.
5. Detrano R. Variability in the accuracy of the exercise ST-segment in predicting the coronary angiogram: how good can we be? J Electrocardiol 1992;24:54–61.
6. Gianrossi R, Detrano R, Mulvihill D, et al. Exercise-induced ST depression in the diagnosis of coronary artery disease. A meta-analysis. Circulation 1989;80:87–98.
7. Philbrick JT, Horwitz RI, Feinstein AR. Methodologic problems of exercise testing for coronary artery disease: groups, analysis and bias. Am J Cardiol 1980;46:807–812.
8. Philbrick JT, Horwitz RI, Feinstein AR, et al. The limited spectrum of patients studied in exercise test research. Analyzing the tip of the iceberg. JAMA 1982;248:2467–2470.
9. Choi BC. Sensitivity and specificity of a single diagnostic test in the presence of work-up bias [see comments]. J Clin Epidemiol 1992;45:581–586.

10. Diamond GA. Reverend Bayes' silent majority. An alternative factor affecting sensitivity and specificity of exercise electrocardiography. Am J Cardiol 1986;57:1175–1180.
11. Ransohoff DF, Feinstein AR. Problems of spectrum and bias in evaluating the efficacy of diagnostic tests. N Engl J Med 1978;299:926–930.
12. Froelicher VF, Lehmann KG, Thomas R, et al. The electrocardiographic exercise test in a population with reduced work-up bias: diagnostic performance, computerized interpretation, and multivariable freedom. Ann Intern Med 1998;128:965–974.
13. Christian TF, Miller TD, Bailey KR, Gibbons RJ. Exercise tomographic thallium-201 imaging in patients with severe coronary artery disease and normal electrocardiograms [see comments]. Ann Intern Med 1994;121:825–832.
14. Snader CE, Marwick TH, Pashkow FJ, et al. Importance of estimated functional capacity as a predictor of all-cause mortality among patients referred for exercise thallium single-photon emission computed tomography: report of 3,400 patients from a single center. J Am Coll Cardiol 1997;30:641–648.
15. Cole CR, Blackstone EH, Pashkow FJ, et al. Heart rate recovery immediately after exercise as a predictor of mortality. N Engl J Med 1999;341:1351–1357.
16. Lauer MS, Okin PM, Larson MG, et al. Impaired heart rate response to graded exercise. Prognostic implications of chronotropic incompetence in the Framingham Heart Study. Circulation 1996;93:1520–1526.
17. Lauer MS, Francis GS, Okin PM, et al. Impaired chronotropic response to exercise stress testing as a predictor of mortality. JAMA 1999;281:524–529.
18. Brener SJ, Pashkow FJ, Harvey SA, et al. Chronotropic response to exercise predicts angiographic severity in patients with suspected or stable coronary artery disease. Am J Cardiol 1995;76:1228–1232.
19. Campbell L, Marwick TH, Pashkow FJ, et al. Usefulness of an exaggerated systolic blood pressure response to exercise in predicting myocardial perfusion defects in known or suspected coronary artery disease. Am J Cardiol 1999;84:1304–1310.
20. Lauer MS, Pashkow FJ, Harvey SA, et al. Angiographic and prognostic implications of an exaggerated exercise systolic blood pressure response and rest systolic blood pressure in adults undergoing evaluation for suspected coronary artery disease. J Am Coll Cardiol 1995;26:1630–1636.
21. Schweikert RA, Pashkow FJ, Snader CE, et al. Association of exercise-induced ventricular ectopic activity with thallium myocardial perfusion and angiographic coronary artery disease in stable, low-risk populations. Am J Cardiol 1999;83:530–534.
22. Okin PM, Kligfield P. Heart rate adjustment of ST segment depression and performance of the exercise electrocardiogram: a critical evaluation. J Am Coll Cardiol 1995;25:1726–1735.
23. Peters RK, Cady LD Jr, Bischoff DP, et al. Physical fitness and subsequent myocardial infarction in healthy workers. JAMA 1983;249:3052–3056.
24. Paffenbarger RS Jr, Hyde RT, Wing AL, Hsieh CC. Physical activity, all-cause mortality, and longevity of college alumni. N Engl J Med 1986;314:605–613.
25. Leon AS, Connett J, Jacobs DR Jr, Rauramaa R. Leisure-time physical activity levels and risk of coronary heart disease and death. The Multiple Risk Factor Intervention Trial. JAMA 1987;258:2388–2395.
26. Ekelund LG, Haskell WL, Johnson JL, et al. Physical fitness as a predictor of cardiovascular mortality in asymptomatic North American men. The Lipid Research Clinics Mortality Follow-up Study. N Engl J Med 1988;319:1379–1384.
27. Blair SN, Kohl HWD, Paffenbarger RS Jr, et al. Physical fitness and all-cause mortality. A prospective study of healthy men and women. JAMA 1989;262:2395–2401.
28. van Saase JL, Noteboom WM, Vandenbroucke JP. Longevity of men capable of prolonged vigorous physical exercise: a 32 year follow up of 2259 participants in the Dutch eleven cities ice skating tour. Br Med J 1990;301:1409–1411.
29. Arraiz GA, Wigle DT, Mao Y. Risk assessment of physical activity and physical fitness in the Canada Health Survey mortality follow-up study. J Clin Epidemiol 1992;45:419–428.
30. Paffenbarger RS Jr, Hyde RT, Wing AL, et al. The association of changes in physical-activity level and other lifestyle characteristics with mortality among men. N Engl J Med 1993;328:538–545.
31. Lakka TA, Venalainen JM, Rauramaa R, et al. Relation of leisure-time physical activity and cardiorespiratory fitness to the risk of acute myocardial infarction. N Engl J Med 1994;330:1549–1554.
32. Lee IM, Hsieh CC, Paffenbarger RS Jr. Exercise intensity and longevity in men. The Harvard Alumni Health Study. JAMA 1995;273:1179–1184.
33. Blair SN, Kohl HW III, Barlow CE, et al. Changes in physical fitness and all-cause mortality. A prospective study of healthy and unhealthy men. JAMA 1995;273:1093–1098.

34. Lissner L, Bengtsson C, Bjorkelund C, Wedel H. Physical activity levels and changes in relation to longevity. A prospective study of Swedish women. Am J Epidemiol 1996;143:54–62.

35. Ellestad MH, Wan MK. Predictive implications of stress testing. Follow-up of 2700 subjects after maximum treadmill stress testing. Circulation 1975;51:363–369.

36. Bruce RA, DeRouen T, Peterson DR, et al. Noninvasive predictors of sudden cardiac death in men with coronary heart disease. Predictive value of maximal stress testing. Am J Cardiol 1977;39:833–840.

37. McNeer JF, Margolis JR, Lee KL, et al. The role of the exercise test in the evaluation of patients for ischemic heart disease. Circulation 1978;57:64–70.

38. Podrid PJ, Graboys TB, Lown B. Prognosis of medically treated patients with coronary-artery disease with profound ST-segment depression during exercise testing. N Engl J Med 1981;305:1111–1116.

39. Bruce RA, Hossack KF, DeRouen TA, Hofer V. Enhanced risk assessment for primary coronary heart disease events by maximal exercise testing: 10 years' experience of Seattle Heart Watch. J Am Coll Cardiol 1983;2:565–753.

40. McKirnan MD, Sullivan M, Jensen D, Froelicher VF. Treadmill performance and cardiac function in selected patients with coronary heart disease. J Am Coll Cardiol 1984;3:253–261.

41. Weiner DA, Ryan TJ, McCabe CH, et al. Prognostic importance of a clinical profile and exercise test in medically treated patients with coronary artery disease. J Am Coll Cardiol 1984;3:772–779.

42. Weiner DA, Ryan TJ, McCabe CH, et al. The role of exercise testing in identifying patients with improved survival after coronary artery bypass surgery. J Am Coll Cardiol 1986;8:741–748.

43. Weiner DA, Ryan TJ, McCabe CH, et al. Value of exercise testing in determining the risk classification and the response to coronary artery bypass grafting in three-vessel coronary artery disease: a report from the Coronary Artery Surgery Study (CASS) registry. Am J Cardiol 1987;60:262–266.

44. Weiner DA, Ryan TJ, Parsons L, et al. Long-term prognostic value of exercise testing in men and women from the Coronary Artery Surgery Study (CASS) registry. Am J Cardiol 1995;75:865–870.

45. Bogaty P, Dagenais GR, Cantin B, et al. Prognosis in patients with a strongly positive exercise electro-cardiogram. Am J Cardiol 1989;64:1284–1288.

46. Morris CK, Ueshima K, Kawaguchi T, et al. The prognostic value of exercise capacity: a review of the literature. Am Heart J 1991;122:1423–1431.

47. Mancini DM, Eisen H, Kussmaul W, et al. Value of peak exercise oxygen consumption for optimal timing of cardiac transplantation in ambulatory patients with heart failure. Circulation 1991;83:778–786.

48. Aaronson KD, Mancini DM. Is percentage of predicted maximal exercise oxygen consumption a better predictor of survival than peak exercise oxygen consumption for patients with severe heart failure? J Heart Lung Transplant 1995;14:981–989.

49. Mancini D, Katz S, Donchez L, Aaronson K. Coupling of hemodynamic measurements with oxygen consumption during exercise does not improve risk stratification in patients with heart failure. Circulation 1996;94:2492–2496.

50. Myers J, Gullestad L, Vagelos R, et al. Clinical, hemodynamic, and cardiopulmonary exercise test determinants of survival in patients referred for evaluation of heart failure. Ann Intern Med 1998;129:286–293.

51. Myers J, Buchanan N, Walsh D, et al. Comparison of the ramp versus standard exercise protocols. J Am Coll Cardiol 1991;17:1334–1342.

52. Weber KT, Janicki JS, McElroy PA. Determination of aerobic capacity and the severity of chronic cardiac and circulatory failure. Circulation 1987;76(Suppl VI):40–46.

53. Sawada SG, Ryan T, Conley MJ, et al. Prognostic value of a normal exercise echocardiogram. Am Heart J 1990;120:49–55.

54. Mark DB, Hlatky MA, Harrell FE Jr, et al. Exercise treadmill score for predicting prognosis in coronary artery disease. Ann Intern Med 1987;106:793–800.

55. Mark DB, Shaw L, Harrell FE Jr, et al. Prognostic value of a treadmill exercise score in outpatients with suspected coronary artery disease. N Engl J Med 1991;325:849–853.

56. Nallamothu N, Pancholy SB, Lee KR, et al. Impact on exercise single-photon emission computed tomographic thallium imaging on patient management and outcome. J Nucl Cardiol 1995;2:334–338.

57. Hayano J, Yamada A, Mukai S, et al. Severity of coronary atherosclerosis correlates with the respiratory component of heart rate variability. Am Heart J 1991;121:1070–1079.

58. Okin PM, Anderson KM, Levy D, Kligfield P. Heart rate adjustment of exercise-induced ST segment depression. Improved risk stratification in the Framingham Offspring Study. Circulation 1991;83:866–874.

59. Okin PM, Prineas RJ, Grandits G, et al. Heart rate adjustment of exercise-induced ST-segment depression identifies men who benefit from a risk factor reduction program. Circulation 1997;96:2899–2904.

60. Okin PM, Grandits G, Rautaharju PM, et al. Prognostic value of heart rate adjustment of exercise-induced ST segment depression in the multiple risk factor intervention trial. J Am Coll Cardiol 1996;27:1437–1443.

61. Cole CR, Pashkow FJ, Snader CE, et al. Computerized ST/HR index is a better predictor of mortality than standard ST or thallium [Abstract]. J Am Coll Cardiol 1999;33:542A.

62. Okin PM, Kligfield P. Identifying coronary artery disease in women by heart rate adjustment of ST-segment depression and improved performance of linear regression over simple averaging method with comparison to standard criteria. Am J Cardiol 1992;69:297–302.

63. Okin PM, Kligfield P. Effect of precision of ST-segment measurement on identification and quantification of coronary artery disease by the ST/HR index. J Electrocardiol 1992;24:62–67.

64. Ribisl PM, Liu J, Mousa I, et al. Comparison of computer ST criteria for diagnosis of severe coronary artery disease. Am J Cardiol 1993;71:546–551.

65. Lachterman B, Lehmann KG, Detrano R, et al. Comparison of ST segment/heart rate index to standard ST criteria for analysis of exercise electrocardiogram. Circulation 1990;82:44–50.

66. Herbert WG, Dubach P, Lehmann KG, Froelicher VF. Effect of beta-blockade on the interpretation of the exercise ECG: ST level versus delta ST/HR index. Am Heart J 1991;122:993–1000.

67. Cullen K, Stenhouse NS, Wearne KL, Cumpston GN. Electrocardiograms and 13 year cardiovascular mortality in Busselton study. Br Heart J 1982;47:209–212.

68. Miranda CP, Herbert WG, Dubach P, et al. Post-myocardial infarction exercise testing. Non-Q wave versus Q wave correlation with coronary angiography and long-term prognosis. Circulation 1991;84:2357–2365.

69. Stoletniy LN, Pai RG. Value of QT dispersion in the interpretation of exercise stress test in women. Circulation 1997;96:904–910.

70. Leroy F, Lablanche JM, Bauters C, et al. Prognostic value of changes in R-wave amplitude during exercise testing after a first acute myocardial infarction. Am J Cardiol 1992;70:152–155.

71. Bonoris PE, Greenberg PS, Christison GW, et al. Evaluation of R wave amplitude changes versus ST-segment depression in stress testing. Circulation 1978;57:904–910.

72. Bonoris PE, Greenberg PS, Castellanet MJ, Ellestad MH. Significance of changes in R wave amplitude during treadmill stress testing: angiographic correlation. Am J Cardiol 1978;41:846–851.

73. Battler A, Froelicher V, Slutsky R, Ashburn W. Relationship of QRS amplitude changes during exercise to left ventricular function and volumes and the diagnosis of coronary artery disease. Circulation 1979;60:1004–1013.

74. Cheng SL, Ellestad MH, Selvester RH. Significance of ST-segment depression with R-wave amplitude decrease on exercise testing. Am J Cardiol 1999;83:955–969.

75. Hollenberg M, Zoltick JM, Go M, et al. Comparison of a quantitative treadmill exercise score with standard electrocardiographic criteria in screening asymptomatic young men for coronary artery disease. N Engl J Med 1985;313:600–606.

76. Wagner S, Cohn K, Selzer A. Unreliability of exercise-induced R wave changes as indexes of coronary artery disease. Am J Cardiol 1979;44:1241–1246.

77. Lee JH, Crump R, Ellestad MH. Significance of precordial T-wave increase during treadmill stress testing. Am J Cardiol 1995;76:1297–1299.

78. Chikamori T, Doi YL, Furuno T, et al. Diagnostic significance of deep T-wave inversion induced by exercise testing in patients with suspected coronary artery disease. Am J Cardiol 1992;70:403–406.

79. Verrier RL, Stone PH. Exercise stress testing for T wave alternans to expose latent electrical instability [editorial]. J Cardiovasc Electrophysiol 1997;8:994–997.

80. Hohnloser SH, Klingenheben T, Zabel M, et al. T wave alternans during exercise and atrial pacing in humans. J Cardiovasc Electrophysiol 1997;8:987–993.

81. Schwartz PJ, Malliani A. Electrical alternation of the T-wave: clinical and experimental evidence of its relationship with the sympathetic nervous system and with the long Q-T syndrome. Am Heart J 1975;89:45–50.

82. Surawicz B, Fisch C. Cardiac alternans: diverse mechanisms and clinical manifestations. J Am Coll Cardiol 1992;20:483–499.

83. Zareba W, Moss AJ, le Cessie S, Hall WJ. T wave alternans in idiopathic long QT syndrome. J Am Coll Cardiol 1994;23:1541–1546.

84. Salerno JA, Previtali M, Panciroli C, et al. Ventricular arrhythmias during acute myocardial ischaemia in man. The role and significance of R-ST-T alternans and the prevention of ischaemic sudden death by medical treatment. Eur Heart J 1986;7:63–75.

85. Rosenbaum DS, Albrecht P, Cohen RJ. Predicting sudden cardiac death from T wave alternans of the surface electrocardiogram: promise and pitfalls. J Cardiovasc Electrophysiol 1996;7:1095–1111.

86. Gold MR, Bloomfield DM, Anderson KP, et al. T wave alternans predicts arrhythmia vulnerability in patients undergoing electrophysiology study [abstract]. Circulation 1998;98(Suppl):I647–I648.

87. Klingenheben T, Cohen RJ, Peetermans J, Hohnloser SH. Predictive value of T-wave alternans in patients with congestive heart failure. Circulation 1998;98(Suppl):I864.

88. Chikamori T, Kitaoka H, Matsumura Y, et al. Clinical and electrocardiographic profiles producing exercise-induced U-wave inversion in patients with severe narrowing of the left anterior descending coronary artery. Am J Cardiol 1997;80:628–632.

89. Choo MH, Gibson DG. U waves in ventricular hypertrophy: possible demonstration of mechano-electrical feedback. Br Heart J 1986;55:428–433.

90. Gerson MC, Phillips JF, Morris SN, McHenry PL. Exercise-induced U-wave inversion as a marker of stenosis of the left anterior descending coronary artery. Circulation 1979;60:1014–1020.

91. Gerson MC, McHenry PL. Resting U wave inversion as a marker of stenosis of the left anterior descending coronary artery. Am J Med 1980;69:545–550.

92. Salmasi AM, Salmasi SN, Nicolaides AN, et al. The value of exercise-induced U-wave inversion on ECG chest wall mapping in the identification of individual coronary arterial lesions. Eur Heart J 1985;6:437–443.

93. Grady TA, Chiu AC, Snader CE, et al. Prognostic significance of exercise-induced left bundle-branch block. JAMA 1998;279:153–156.

94. Berntsen RF, Gunnes P, Rasmussen K. Pattern of coronary artery disease in patients with ventricular tachycardia and fibrillation exposed by exercise-induced ischemia. Am Heart J 1995;129:733–738.

95. de Paola AA, Gomes JA, Terzian AB, et al. Ventricular tachycardia during exercise testing as a predictor of sudden death in patients with chronic chagasic cardiomyopathy and ventricular arrhythmias. Br Heart J 1995;74:293–295.

96. Casella G, Pavesi PC, Sangiorgio P, et al. Exercise-induced ventricular arrhythmias in patients with healed myocardial infarction. Int J Cardiol 1993;40:229–235.

97. Yang JC, Wesley RC Jr, Froelicher VF. Ventricular tachycardia during routine treadmill testing. Risk and prognosis. Arch Intern Med 1991;151:349–353.

98. Califf RM, McKinnis RA, McNeer JF, et al. Prognostic value of ventricular arrhythmias associated with treadmill exercise testing in patients studied with cardiac catheterization for suspected ischemic heart disease. J Am Coll Cardiol 1983;2:1060–1067.

99. Sami M, Chaitman B, Fisher L, et al. Significance of exercise-induced ventricular arrhythmia in stable coronary artery disease: a coronary artery surgery study project. Am J Cardiol 1984;54:1182–1188.

100. Busby MJ, Shefrin EA, Fleg JL. Prevalence and long-term significance of exercise-induced frequent or repetitive ventricular ectopic beats in apparently healthy volunteers. J Am Coll Cardiol 1989;14:1659–1665.

101. Ellestad MH. Chronotropic incompetence. The implications of heart rate response to exercise (compensatory parasympathetic hyperactivity?) [editorial]. Circulation 1996;93:1485–1487.

102. Hinkle LE Jr, Carver ST, Plakun A. Slow heart rates and increased risk of cardiac death in middle-aged men. Arch Intern Med 1972;129:732–748.

103. Hammond HK, Kelly TL, Froelicher V. Radionuclide imaging correlatives of heart rate impairment during maximal exercise testing. J Am Coll Cardiol 1983;2:826–833.

104. Heller GV, Ahmed I, Tilkemeier PL, et al. Influence of exercise intensity on the presence, distribution, and size of thallium-201 defects. Am Heart J 1992;123:909–916.

105. Beleslin BD, Ostojic M, Stepanovic J, et al. Stress echocardiography in the detection of myocardial ischemia. Head-to-head comparison of exercise, dobutamine, and dipyridamole tests. Circulation 1994;90:1168–1176.

106. Marwick TH, Nemec JJ, Pashkow FJ, et al. Accuracy and limitations of exercise echocardiography in a routine clinical setting. J Am Coll Cardiol 1992;19:74–81.

107. Hammond HK, Froelicher VF. Normal and abnormal heart rate responses to exercise. Prog Cardiovasc Dis 1985;27:271–296.

108. Dyer AR, Persky V, Stamler J, et al. Heart rate as a prognostic factor for coronary heart disease and mortality: findings in three Chicago epidemiologic studies. Am J Epidemiol 1980;112:736–749.

109. Paffenbarger RS, Hale WE. Work activity and coronary heart mortality. N Engl J Med 1975;292:545–550.

110. Willich SN, Lewis M, Lowel H, et al. Physical exertion as a trigger of acute myocardial infarction. Triggers and Mechanisms of Myocardial Infarction Study Group. N Engl J Med 1993;329:1684–1690.

111. Mittleman MA, Maclure M, Tofler GH, et al. Triggering of acute myocardial infarction by heavy physical exertion. Protection against triggering by regular exertion. Determinants of Myocardial Infarction Onset Study Investigators. N Engl J Med 1993;329:1677–1683.

112. Wilkoff BL, Miller RE. Exercise testing for chronotropic assessment. Cardiol Clin 1992;10:705–717.

113. Lauer MS, Pashkow FJ, Larson MG, Levy D. Association of cigarette smoking with chronotropic incompetence and prognosis in the Framingham Heart Study. Circulation 1997;96:897–903.

114. Okin PM, Lauer MS, Kligfield P. Chronotropic response to exercise. Improved performance of ST-segment depression criteria after adjustment for heart rate reserve. Circulation 1996;94:3226–3231.

115. Lauer MS, Mehta R, Pashkow FJ, et al. Association of chronotropic incompetence with echocardiographic ischemia and prognosis. J Am Coll Cardiol 1998;32:1280–1286.

116. Chin CF, Messenger JC, Greenberg PS, Ellestad MH. Chronotropic incompetence in exercise testing. Clin Cardiol 1979;2:12–18.

117. Mark AL. The Bezold-Jarisch reflex revisited: clinical implications of inhibitory reflexes originating in the heart. J Am Coll Cardiol 1983;1:90–102.

118. Francis GS, Goldsmith SR, Ziesche S, et al. Relative attenuation of sympathetic drive during exercise in patients with congestive heart failure. J Am Coll Cardiol 1985;5:832–839.

119. Colucci WS, Ribeiro JP, Rocco MB, et al. Impaired chronotropic response to exercise in patients with congestive heart failure. Role of postsynaptic beta-adrenergic desensitization. Circulation 1989;80: 314–323.

120. Cole C, Foody J, Blackstone E, Lauer M. Heart rate recovery after submaximal exercise testing as a predictor of mortality in a cardiovascularly healthy cohort. Ann Intern Med 2000;132:552–555.

121. Imai K, Sato H, Hori M, et al. Vagally mediated heart rate recovery after exercise is accelerated in athletes but blunted in patients with chronic heart failure. J Am Coll Cardiol 1994;24:1529–1535.

122. Schwartz PJ, La Rovere MT, Vanoli E. Autonomic nervous system and sudden cardiac death. Experimental basis and clinical observations for post-myocardial infarction risk stratification. Circulation 1992;85:I77–I91.

123. Dlin RA, Hanne N, Silverberg DS, Bar-Or O. Follow-up of normotensive men with exaggerated blood pressure response to exercise. Am Heart J 1983;106:316–320.

124. Wilson MF, Sung BH, Pincomb GA, Lovallo WR. Exaggerated pressure response to exercise in men at risk for systemic hypertension. Am J Cardiol 1990;66:731–736.

125. Lauer MS, Levy D, Anderson KM, Plehn JF. Is there a relationship between exercise systolic blood pressure response and left ventricular mass? The Framingham Heart Study. Ann Intern Med 1992;116:203–210.

126. Irving JB, Bruce RA, DeRouen TA. Variations in and significance of systolic pressure during maximal exercise (treadmill) testing. Am J Cardiol 1977;39:841–848.

127. Filipovsky J, Ducimetiere P, Safar ME. Prognostic significance of exercise blood pressure and heart rate in middle-aged men. Hypertension 1992;20:333–339.

128. Fagard RH, Pardaens K, Staessen JA, Thijs L. Prognostic value of invasive hemodynamic measurements at rest and during exercise in hypertensive men. Hypertension 1996;28:31–36.

129. Fagard R, Staessen J, Thijs L, Amery A. Relation of left ventricular mass and filling to exercise blood pressure and rest blood pressure. Am J Cardiol 1995;75:53–57.

130. Morrow K, Morris CK, Froelicher VF, et al. Prediction of cardiovascular death in men undergoing non-invasive evaluation for coronary artery disease. Ann Intern Med 1993;118:689–695.

131. Mundal R, Kjeldsen SE, Sandvik L, et al. Exercise blood pressure predicts cardiovascular mortality in middle-aged men. Hypertension 1994;24:56–62.

132. Mundal R, Kjeldsen SE, Sandvik L, et al. Exercise blood pressure predicts mortality from myocardial infarction. Hypertension 1996;27:324–329.

133. Gottdiener JS, Brown J, Zoltick J, Fletcher RD. Left ventricular hypertrophy in men with normal blood pressure: relation to exaggerated blood pressure response to exercise. Ann Intern Med 1990;112:161–166.

15

Aspirin and Antiplatelet Agents in the Prevention of Complications of Coronary Artery Disease

Andrew I. MacKinnon, MD, Scott A. Moore, MD, and Steven R. Steinhubl, MD

CONTENTS

INTRODUCTION

If not for the arterial thrombus, atherosclerosis—the principal cause of mortality in industrialized nations—might be an essentially benign disease. Although the relationship between atherosclerosis and thrombosis was recognized as early as 1852 by von Rokitansky *(1)*, not until the last several decades has its fundamental role been appreciated. The disruption of an atherosclerotic plaque with resultant intracoronary thrombus formation has been consistently demonstrated to be central to the pathophysiological process underlying unstable angina, acute myocardial infarction (MI), and sudden cardiac death *(2–5)*. There is also increasing evidence that asymptomatic plaque fissuring with associated nonocclusive thrombus is at least partially responsible for atherosclerotic plaque progression *(6–9)*. These findings suggest that antithrombotic therapy, and in particular antiplatelet therapy, is central to the prevention of intracoronary thrombosis and the prevention of the complications of coronary artery disease (CAD).

PATHOPHYSIOLOGY OF ARTERIAL THROMBUS FORMATION

The formation of a thrombus on injured arterial endothelium involves a complex interaction between platelets and a cascade of coagulation proteins that results in the

From: *Contemporary Cardiology: Preventive Cardiology:*
Insights Into the Prevention and Treatment of Cardiovascular Disease, Second Edition
Edited by: J. M. Foody © Humana Press Inc., Totowa, NJ

production of fibrin. First, the normally thrombosis-resistant endothelium is rendered prothrombotic by atherosclerosis. Disruption of the endothelial monolayer, as well as the high shear flow that is characteristic of stenosed coronary arteries initiate platelet adhesion. The initial binding of platelets to the vessel wall (adhesion) is strongly reliant on binding of specific platelet-membrane glycoprotein binding to adhesive proteins, such as von Willebrand factor and collagen *(10)*. Platelet activation can be initiated by any of more than 100 known agonists, including thromboxane A_2, thrombin, norepinephrine, collagen, and adenosine diphosphate (ADP). Activation leads to platelet degranulation and the release of serotonin, ADP, and thromboxane A_2 among others, which trigger the recruitment and activation of neighboring platelets *(11)*. These platelets ultimately become aggregated into a hemostatic plug via the binding of primarily fibrinogen and von Willebrand factor to glycoprotein IIb/IIIa integrins on adjacent platelets. The membrane surface of the activated platelets also serves to accelerate the conversion of prothrombin to thrombin, thereby promoting the development of an occlusive, stabilized thrombus containing platelets, thrombin, and fibrin.

ANTIPLATELET AGENTS

Many antiplatelet agents have been studied in the primary and secondary prevention of CAD to prevent adhesion, activation, aggregation, and thrombus formation. Because platelet function is multifaceted and antagonists function via different mechanisms, inhibition of platelet activation and function is therefore multifaceted. A number of antiplatelet agents are currently available or undergoing evaluation. This review presents the available data regarding the use of antiplatelet agents in the prevention of complications of CAD.

Aspirin

The benefits of willow bark as an antipyretic were first reported by Reverend Edmund Stone in 1763 *(12)*. The potential for aspirin to cause a bleeding tendency was recognized as early as 1891 *(13)*, but its inhibitory effect on platelets specifically was not discovered until the late 1960s *(14)*. Aspirin's first described use in CAD was in 1953, in a preventative role *(15)*. Although this nonrandomized observational study of daily aspirin use demonstrated 100% successful prevention of "coronary occlusion" among 1465 asymptomatic male patients, aspirin therapy has only recently become a cornerstone of therapy in CAD.

The mechanism by which aspirin induces a functional defect in platelets is through the inhibition of thromboxane A_2 production *(16,17)*. During platelet activation, the hydrolysis of membrane phospholipids yields arachidonic acid, which is converted to prostaglandin H_2 (PGH$_2$) by the catalytic activity of the cyclooxygenase enzyme, prostaglandin G/H synthase *(18)* (Fig. 1). PGH$_2$ is then converted via thromboxane synthase to thromboxane A_2. By the selective and irreversible acetylation of a single serine residue within prostaglandin G/H synthase, aspirin causes the permanent inactivation of cyclooxygenase activity. Because the nonnucleated platelets lack the biosynthetic capabilities necessary to synthesize new protein, the aspirin-induced defect cannot be repaired for the 8- to 10-d life-span of the platelet.

The ability of aspirin to inhibit cyclooxygenase activity also accounts for its variety of pharmacological effects in other tissues. This effect is of particular importance with respect to aspirin's use in the prevention of thrombosis, because aspirin inhibits the

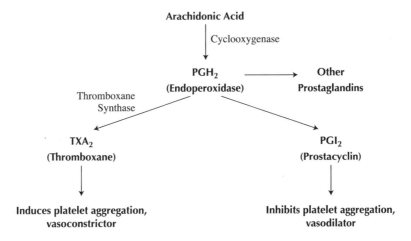

Fig. 1. Arachadonic acid metabolism in platelets and the vascular wall.

production of endothelial cell-produced prostacyclin; a vasodilator and inhibitor of platelet aggregation. This counter-balancing effect has raised the concern of a possible prothrombotic effect of aspirin therapy. Unlike platelets, endothelial cells possess the biosynthetic machinery necessary to produce new enzyme, and therefore recover their ability to synthesize prostacyclin within a few hours. Currently there is no direct evidence that prostacyclin inhibition of aspirin is clinically relevant.

Aspirin for Primary Prevention

The efficacy of aspirin to prevent a first ischemic event has now been evaluated in six large randomized trials involving more than 95,000 participants (19–23) (Table 1). The first of these, the British Doctors' Trial (21), enrolled 5139 male British Physicians between the ages of 50 and 78 yr. Two-thirds of the subjects were randomized to take 500 mg of aspirin daily and the remaining third were instructed to avoid aspirin and products containing aspirin. By the end of the 6-yr study, there was no significant difference between groups in the occurrence of MI, stroke, the combined endpoint of adverse vascular events, or total vascular mortality, but the 95% confidence intervals (CI) were very wide. A second trial, the US Physicians Health Study, was a double-blind, placebo-controlled trial that used a two-by-two factorial design to test simultaneously the effects of aspirin in reducing cardiovascular disease and β-carotene in the prevention of cancer. A total of 22,071 US male physicians, ranging in age from 40 to 84 yr, were randomized to receive 325 mg of aspirin or placebo every other day. The aspirin vs placebo component of the study was prematurely terminated owing to a marked reduction in the occurrence of MI (relative risk [RR], 0.56; 95% CI, 0.45–0.70; $p < 0.00001$) among those receiving aspirin. This reduction in risk was apparent only among those older than 50 yr of age. A trend toward an increased risk of any stroke (RR, 1.22; 95% CI, 0.93–1.60; $p = 0.15$) was observed, influenced primarily by the subgroup with hemorrhagic stroke (RR, 2.14; 95% CI, 0.96–4.77; $p = 0.06$). There was a significant decrease in the rate of fatal MI ($p = 0.004$) in the aspirin group, but this benefit was offset by an apparent increased risk for sudden death ($p = 0.09$), resulting in no reduction in total cardiovascular mortality (81 in the aspirin group vs 83 in the placebo group; $p = 0.87$).

Table 1
Relative Mean Percentage Decrease in Events with Aspirin Compared With Placebo
in Primary-Prevention Trials[a]

	US Physicians Health Study	British Doctors' Trial	Hypertension Optimal Treatment Trial	TPT	Primary Prevention Project	Women's Health Study
All MI	44%	3%	36%	20%	32%	NS
All stroke	(22%)	(17%)	2%	3%	17%	17%
Total vascular mortality	0%	6%	5%	(12.5%)	46%	5%

[a]Data are presented as mean percent reduction. Data in parenthesis represent a negative value (or increased percentage of events). MI, myocardial infarction; TPT, Thrombosis Prevention Trial.

When these two studies were evaluated together, a highly significant reduction (32%) in the risk of a nonfatal MI was demonstrated because of the much larger size of the US study *(24)*. Despite the trend toward an increased risk of stroke in the aspirin arm of both of these studies, the combined data still provided too few endpoints upon which any firm conclusions could be made. Before generalizing the findings of these trials to the entire male population, it is important to note that the participants in these studies represented a very health-conscious group of individuals. This likely explains the unusually low cardiovascular mortality rate among the participants—approx 15% of that expected for an age-matched group of white American men.

The Hypertension Optimal Treatment (HOT) study helped clarify aspirin's role in primary prevention in a more representative population *(23)*. The HOT study was the first large-scale, randomized trial to examine the role of aspirin for primary prevention in patients with hypertension, a population with a higher cardiovascular event rate than described in the earlier primary-prevention trials. More than 19,000 patients were randomized to one of three target blood pressure goals to determine whether there are additional benefits in lowering blood pressure of hypertensive patients to fully normotensive levels. Patients were also randomized to either low-dose aspirin (75 mg once daily) or placebo. After 3.8 yr of follow-up, major cardiovascular events (fatal and nonfatal MI, fatal and nonfatal stroke, all other cardiovascular deaths) were reduced by 15% in the aspirin group ($p = 0.03$). This benefit was largely caused by a 36% reduction in the rate of MI ($p = 0.002$). There was no significant difference in the rates of stroke, cardiovascular mortality, or total mortality. Importantly, aspirin did not increase the rates of fatal bleeding (including cerebral), but nonfatal major and minor bleeding, primarily gastrointestinal and nasal, were 1.8 times more frequent with aspirin ($p < 0.001$). In higher-risk patients, aspirin prevented 7.5 MIs per 1000 patients treated for 5 yr, without increasing the risk of hemorrhagic stroke. This is in contrast to the 4 events per 1000 patients treated for 5 yr in the Physicians' Health Study and British Doctors' Trial *(24)*.

The Thrombosis Prevention Trial (TPT) *(26)* confirmed the protective effect of aspirin and further evaluated the role of warfarin with or without aspirin in this population of men at risk for ischemic heart disease. These investigators found that, although the addition of low-dose warfarin (target international normalized ratio [INR], 1.5) to daily low-dose aspirin (75 mg) did demonstrate a trend toward decreased cardiac events, its use was associated with a significant increase in the risk of major hemorrhage. This was followed

by the Primary-Prevention Project *(25)*. This trial enrolled 4495 apparently healthy men (1912) and women (2583), aged from 50 to older than 80 yr, with one or more cardiac risk factors. They were randomized to take 100 mg/d of enteric-coated aspirin, 300 mg/d of vitamin E, both, or placebo. After a mean follow-up of 3.6 yr, the trial was prematurely stopped on ethical grounds because the results were consistent with the previous primary-prevention trials. Aspirin lowered the frequency of all the endpoints, with a significant reduction of cardiovascular death (RR, 0.56; 95% CI, 0.31–0.99) and total cardiovascular events (RR, 0.77; 95% CI, 0.62–0.95). Severe bleeding was more frequent in the aspirin group than the no-aspirin group (1.1 vs 0.3%; $p < 0.0008$). Vitamin E showed no effect on any prespecified endpoint.

When the data from these five studies is pooled and analyzed *(25)*, the role of aspirin in primary prevention is firmly established *(25)*. Among the 55,580 participants (11,466 women) aspirin was associated with a significant reduction (32%) in the risk of first MI and a significant reduction (15%) in the risk of all important vascular events, with only a modest increase in bleeding risk. Three of these trials included relatively small numbers of women, and similar reductions in events were seen in the female cohorts as were established for the male cohorts. Nonetheless, the majority of the population was male, leaving the role of aspirin for primary prevention of cardiovascular events in women up for debate. The Women's Health Study began in 1992 and randomized 39,876 women older than 45 yr of age to alternate-day 100 mg aspirin or placebo *(27)*. During follow-up, 477 major cardiovascular events were confirmed in the aspirin group, as compared with 522 in the placebo group. This represents a nonsignificant risk reduction (9%) in the aspirin group (RR, 0.91; 95% CI, 0.80–1.03; $p = 0.13$). Aspirin had no significant effect on the risk of fatal or nonfatal MI (RR, 1.02; 95% CI, 0.84–1.25; $p = 0.83$) or death from cardiovascular causes (RR, 0.95; 95% CI, 0.74–1.22; $p = 0.68$). Subgroup analyses did show that aspirin significantly reduced the risk of major cardiovascular events, ischemic stroke, and MI among women 65 yr of age or older. When compared with the previous primary-prevention trials of primarily male cohorts, this study raises several questions regarding the effects of aspirin in women compared with men. These questions require further investigation and are beyond the scope of this chapter.

Aspirin for Secondary Prevention

Patients with an established history of a cardiovascular event are at particular risk for subsequent cardiac events as well as cardiovascular death. A large number of randomized trials have been performed to determine whether aspirin therapy can modify the clinical course of these patients. An overview of 25 of the earliest antiplatelet trials involving approx 29,000 patients was reported in 1988 by the Antiplatelet Trialists' Collaboration *(28)*. They concluded that antiplatelet therapy decreased vascular mortality by 15% and nonfatal vascular events (stroke or MI) by 30%. This review has been revised twice during the past 10 yr. The latest revision, published in 2002, included an overview of 287 studies involving 135,000 patients in comparison of antiplatelet therapy vs control, and 77,000 patients in comparison of different antiplatelet regimens *(29)*. Overall, among these high-risk patients, allocation to antiplatelet therapy reduced the combined outcome of any serious vascular event by one-quarter; nonfatal MI by one-third, nonfatal stroke by one-quarter, and vascular mortality by one-sixth (with no apparent adverse effect on other deaths). In each of these high-risk categories, the absolute benefits substantially outweighed the absolute risks of major extracranial bleeding. Aspirin was the most

widely studied antiplatelet drug, with doses of 75 to 150 mg daily at least as effective as higher daily doses. The effects of doses lower than 75 mg daily were less certain. Overall, the results establish a one-third reduction in nonfatal vascular events, as well as a one-sixth decrease in vascular deaths in high-risk patients receiving antiplatelet therapy.

Stable Angina

Three prospective studies evaluated aspirin in patients with chronic stable angina. A subgroup analysis of the Physician's Health Study (20) evaluated 333 patients who at enrollment had stable angina (30). Although aspirin therapy did not influence the frequency or severity of angina episodes during 4 yr of study, it was associated with a 50% reduction in nonfatal first MI ($p < 0.019$). All fatal MIs occurred in the placebo group (0 vs 4), whereas, of the 13 strokes that occurred, 11 were among patients taking aspirin. A double-blind, randomized trial by Chesebro et al. involved 370 patients with stable CAD and evaluated the impact of combined aspirin and dipyridamole therapy vs placebo during a 5-yr period (31). There was a two-thirds reduction in the incidence of MI ($p = 0.007$) in treated patients and a trend for a reduction in new angiographic lesion formation (30% placebo vs 21% treated; $p = 0.06$). Finally, the largest trial evaluating aspirin therapy in patients with stable angina was a Swedish trial of 2035 patients (32). All patients received sotalol, aspirin, or aspirin placebo, and were followed for more than 4 yr. Patients receiving aspirin demonstrated a 34% reduction (95% CI, 24–49%; $p = 0.003$) in MI and sudden death. In aggregate, these studies suggest that aspirin therapy in 1000 patients with stable angina would prevent 51 important cardiovascular events during a 4-yr period—a benefit approx 10 times greater than that seen in primary-prevention trials.

Non-ST Elevation Acute Coronary Syndromes

The 1-yr mortality of patients with unstable angina ranges from 5 to 14%, with the majority of deaths occurring within several weeks of diagnosis (33). The benefit of aspirin therapy alone or in combination with heparin in the acute treatment of unstable angina has been proven in several randomized trials. In the landmark study, Heparin, Aspirin or Both to Treat Acute Unstable Angina, Theroux and colleagues (34) demonstrated a greater than 70% reduction in cardiac death or MI from 11.9% in the placebo group to 3.3% with aspirin alone and 1.6% with the combination of aspirin and heparin ($p = 0.0042$). The Research Group on Instability in Coronary Artery Disease in Southeast Sweden (35) demonstrated a 57% ($p = 0.033$) reduction in MI and death with aspirin compared with placebo, whereas intermittent intravenous heparin showed no significant influence on these endpoints. One-year follow-up of these patients continued to show an approx 50% reduction ($p < 0.0001$) in death and MI in aspirin-treated patients compared with placebo (36). The results of these studies and others (37,38) suggest that aspirin therapy can reduce the occurrence of death and MI by approx 50% in patients with non-ST elevation acute coronary syndromes (ACS).

ST Elevation MI and Post-MI

The ability of aspirin to reduce the risk of recurrent cardiovascular complications compared with placebo in patients who have survived a MI has been studied in eight trials involving nearly 16,000 patients (39). When considered collectively, these studies demonstrate a one-third reduction in the risk of nonfatal MI and a one-fourth decrease in the

occurrence of MI, stroke, or vascular death. In terms of absolute risk reduction, treatment of 1000 patients with a previous MI for 2 yr will prevent 36 major cardiovascular events.

The role of aspirin in the treatment of an evolving MI has been well-established. The Second International Study of Infarct Survival *(40)* randomized 17,187 patients to receive or not receive streptokinase with or without aspirin daily for 1 mo, beginning within 24 h of a suspected MI. Aspirin alone and streptokinase alone decreased 35-d vascular mortality similarly (23 and 25%, respectively), whereas the combination decreased mortality by 42% compared with placebo.

Adverse Effects

As with most medical therapies, but in particular with therapies designed to be preventive in nature, the physician must optimize the benefits and minimize the risks. Patients who regularly take nonsteroidal anti-inflammatory drugs have an increased risk of gastrointestinal bleeding or other events that result in hospitalization or death *(41)*. The gastrointestinal side-effects of aspirin are clearly dose related, but even doses as low as 75 mg/d cause peptic ulcer disease *(42)*. A dose-related risk of hemorrhagic stroke has also been suggested by several trials evaluating high- and low-dose aspirin *(43,44)*. Buffered aspirin preparations and enteric-coated aspirin are better tolerated than plain aspirin, but are still associated with similar rates of peptic ulcers *(45,46)*. Therefore, to minimize side-effects, the lowest effective dose should be used.

For aspirin therapy to be effective it must be prescribed to the patient. Despite the overwhelming evidence supporting its use, as well as its incomparably low cost and side-effect profile, studies have shown that up to one-third of elderly patients do not receive aspirin at the time of an acute MI *(47)*, and that a quarter do not receive it chronically after a MI *(48)*. With more than 1 million patients admitted to US hospitals each year with an acute MI, by increasing the use of aspirin to include essentially all patients, nearly 8000 premature deaths each year would be prevented *(49)*.

THIENOPYRIDINES

Ticlopidine was first introduced as an antiplatelet agent in the early 1980s, followed by clopidogrel in 1998. The active metabolite of these agents irreversibly binds to one of two platelet ADP receptors, $P2Y_{12}$, and prevents ADP-mediated platelet activation for the life of the platelet. One of multiple manifestations of the inhibition of the $P2Y_{12}$ receptor is the prevention of ADP-induced conformational changes in the glycoprotein IIb/IIIa receptor needed for high-affinity ligand binding *(50)*. Thienopyridines are inactive in vitro and require hepatic metabolism for the development of their antiplatelet activity *(51)*. Inhibition of platelet aggregation is both dose and time related, with onset of activity 24 to 48 h after oral administration, and near maximal activity at 3 to 5 d if no loading dose is used *(51)*. After a 300-mg loading dose of clopidogrel, in vitro data suggests near-maximal effects can be achieved within 3 to 6 h; however, clinical data suggest that up to 24 h may be required. More recently, a loading dose of 600 mg has been described as providing maximal platelet inhibition by 2 h *(52)*. Because their action is irreversible, similar to aspirin, the duration of effect persists for 7 to 10 d *(53)*.

Thienopyridines for Primary Prevention

Currently, there are no data available regarding the use of thienopyridines in a pure primary-prevention population. However, the ongoing Clopidogrel for High Athero-

thrombotic Risk and Ischemic Stabilization, Management, and Avoidance (CHARISMA) trial, in which more than 15,000 primary and secondary-prevention patients are being randomized to clopidogrel plus aspirin or aspirin alone will soon provide these data. As solitary therapy, the best data supporting the role of thienopyridines in a primary-prevention population comes from several large secondary-prevention trials for stroke and peripheral vascular disease, in which patients randomized to ticlopidine experienced a significant reduction in the incidence of MI. This suggests that, in patients at risk for CAD, particularly those with peripheral and cerebrovascular disease and those who are intolerant of aspirin, thienopyridines may have a role in the primary prevention of MI. In the Canadian American Ticlopidine Study (54), patients with a recent thromboembolic stroke were randomized to either ticlopidine or placebo. After 2 yr of follow-up, with ticlopidine there was a 30.2% RR reduction compared with placebo (95% CI, 7.5–48.3%; $p = 0.006$) in stroke, MI, or vascular death. A similar reduction in vascular events was demonstrated in the Swedish Ticlopidine Multicentre Study (55). In patients with a history of intermittent claudication treated with ticlopidine, there was a significant reduction in the rate of MI, stroke, or transient ischemic attacks (TIA) compared with placebo (13.8 vs 22.4%; $p = 0.017$). Other trials of secondary prevention in peripheral vascular disease have confirmed ticlopidine's efficacy, with 75% reductions in 6-mo vascular event rates compared with placebo (56,57). These data suggest that thienopyridines have a role in the primary prevention of complications of CAD and are acceptable alternatives for patients who cannot tolerate aspirin.

Thienopyridines for Secondary Prevention

The thienopyridines have been compared with aspirin in controlled trials for the secondary prevention of stroke, peripheral arterial occlusive disease, and MI (54,55,58–60). Each of these studies demonstrated a benefit with ticlopidine compared with aspirin. The Ticlopidine Aspirin Stroke Study (TASS) (58) was the first to suggest that, in the secondary prevention of stroke, ticlopidine may be more effective than aspirin. The 3-yr event rate for nonfatal stroke or death from any cause was 17% with ticlopidine and 19% for aspirin, a 12% risk reduction with ticlopidine ($p = 0.048$). In a second randomized trial, in patients admitted with unstable angina, treatment with ticlopidine compared with placebo lead to a significant reduction in subsequent cardiac events (61). The addition of ticlopidine to conventional treatment (β-blockers, calcium-channel blockers, and nitrates) in patients admitted with unstable angina resulted in a 46.3% reduction (7.3 vs 13.6%; $p = 0.009$) in the RR of nonfatal MI or vascular death at 6 mo follow-up. Of note, there was no aspirin arm in this study; therefore, the relative efficacy of ticlopidine compared with aspirin in secondary prevention after unstable angina cannot be assessed.

Ticlopidine has also been investigated in surgical revascularization. Platelets play an important role in early graft occlusion from thrombosis and may contribute to the process of intimal proliferation and late graft occlusion (62). A trial of 77 patients randomized to ticlopidine or placebo 3 d before coronary artery bypass graft (CABG) failed to show a benefit for ticlopidine over placebo at the 3-mo angiographic follow-up of saphenous vein graft patency (63). However, on-treatment analysis demonstrated a 67% reduction in the rate of occlusion (7.1 vs 21.8%; $p < 0.02$). In a subsequent study, ticlopidine's efficacy relative to placebo was demonstrated with statistically significant reductions in graft occlusion at 1-yr follow-up (15.9 vs 26.1%; $p < 0.01$) (64). Ticlopidine's efficacy in maintaining saphenous graft patency also applies to grafts used in peripheral arterial

revascularization with 2-yr graft patency of 82% compared with 51.2% for placebo (p = 0.002) (65).

The largest trial addressing the role of thienopyridines alone in secondary prevention is the Clopidogrel Vs Aspirin in Patients at Risk for further Ischemic Events (CAPRIE) trial (66). This was a prospective, randomized, blinded study involving more than 19,000 patients with atherosclerotic vascular disease. Patients with a recent ischemic stroke, MI, or symptomatic peripheral vascular disease were randomized to either daily aspirin or clopidogrel therapy. After a mean follow-up of approx 2 yr, those patients receiving clopidogrel had an annual risk of ischemic stroke, MI, or vascular death of 5.3% compared with 5.8% for those receiving aspirin (p = 0.043). These results suggest that for every 1000 patients with manifestations of atherosclerotic vascular disease receiving antiplatelet therapy for secondary prevention, clopidogrel would be expected to prevent five more major clinical events per year than aspirin, with a decreased incidence of side-effects. There are also several retrospective analyses of high-risk subgroups that suggest a more pronounced benefit of clopidogrel over aspirin in secondary prevention (67–69). These findings are subjects for future evaluation in prospective, randomized trials.

Thienopyridine Side-Effects

Ticlopidine and clopidogrel share similar long-term antiplatelet efficacy (70). However, the side-effect profiles are what separate the medications in terms of clinical application. The main side-effects reported with both medications include bleeding, gastrointestinal complaints, and rash. The incidence of these side-effects is relatively low for both medications, with clopidogrel being the better tolerated of the two overall.

The most frequently reported complaints for both agents are gastrointestinal—more commonly with ticlopidine than clopidogrel. Diarrhea is reported by as many as 20% of patients treated with ticlopidine, and nausea, dyspepsia, and anorexia are also frequent (71). In CAPRIE, diarrhea occurred in 4.5% of clopidogrel patients vs 3.36% of patients treated with aspirin (p < 0.05), and indigestion/nausea/vomiting developing in 15% of patients treated with clopidogrel and 17.6% of patients treated with aspirin (p < 0.05) (66). Rash is reported in 3 to 11% of patients treated with ticlopidine (72,73) and in up to 6% of clopidogrel patients (66). Risk of hemorrhage for both agents is low, and similar to aspirin (72).

Unique to ticlopidine is the occurrence of potentially life-threatening hematological complications. A review of an estimated 10 million patient-years of ticlopidine treatment identified 645 cases of agranulocytosis, pancytopenia, aplastic anemia, and bone marrow suppression, with an associated mortality of 16% (74). The most frequently recognized hematological complication associated with ticlopidine is neutropenia, which occurs in 2 to 3% of patients and is severe in 0.85% of patients. This typically occurs within the first 3 mo of treatment and seems to be reversible when the drug is discontinued (75). Close monitoring of the white blood cell count is therefore mandatory during the first 3 mo of therapy. Clopidogrel does not seem to share ticlopidine's marrow-suppressive effects. In CAPRIE (66), the rate of neutropenia (0.1%) was not significantly different from that observed with aspirin (0.17%).

A less common, but potentially more devastating complication associated with ticlopidine is thrombotic thrombocytopenic purpura (TTP). Ticlopidine's association with TTP was first described in 1991 in a report of four patients (76). A summary of 60 cases suggested the incidence might be higher than previously believed (77). Two groups

have evaluated the incidence of TTP in patients receiving short-term ticlopidine after stenting *(78,79)*. These results suggest an incidence of 1 in 1500 to 1 in 4500 patients treated. The clinical presentation of ticlopidine-associated TTP is similar to that of TTP in general, and there is a comparable mortality rate of 21 to 33%. Early recognition and management with plasmapheresis have consistently been shown to be the most important determinants of survival *(77,78)*. There have been several case reports of clopidogrel-induced TTP. However, the incidence of TTP from clopidogrel seems to be much lower, and is currently estimated at four cases per million patients treated *(80)*.

The side-effect profiles of ticlopidine and clopidogrel were directly compared in the Clopidogrel Aspirin Stent International Cooperative Study (CLASSICS). After successful stent placement, 1020 patients were randomized to a 28-d regimen of either:

1. 300-mg clopidogrel (loading dose) and 325 mg aspirin on day 1, followed by 75 mg/d clopidogrel and 325 mg/d aspirin.
2. 75 mg/d clopidogrel plus 325 mg/d aspirin.
3. 250 mg ticlopidine twice daily and 325 mg/d aspirin *(81)*.

The primary endpoint consisted of major peripheral or bleeding complications, neutropenia, thrombocytopenia, or early discontinuation of study drug. The primary endpoint occurred in 9.1% of patients in the ticlopidine group and 4.6% of patients in the combined clopidogrel group (RR, 0.50; 95% CI, 0.31–0.81; $p = 0.005$). Overall rates of major adverse cardiac events (cardiac death, MI, and target lesion revascularization) were low, and were comparable between treatment groups (0.9% with ticlopidine, 1.5% with 75 mg/d clopidogrel, and 1.2% with the clopidogrel loading dose). The authors concluded the safety/tolerability of clopidogrel (plus aspirin) is superior to that of ticlopidine (plus aspirin) ($p = 0.005$). Given the improved safety profile and the favorable pharmacokinetic properties (shorter time to onset of platelet inhibition with a loading dose), clopidogrel has emerged as the preferred thienopyridine for use in secondary prevention.

Combination Therapy With Aspirin and Thienopyridines

The recurrence of ischemic events despite aspirin therapy in some patients suggests the need for more complete inhibition of the platelet. A clear rationale exists for combination antiplatelet therapy because there are multiple pathways of platelet activation that are independent of aspirin's target, cyclooxygenase. Experimentally, it has been shown in healthy volunteers that the combination of ticlopidine and aspirin is more effective than either alone in inhibiting collagen-induced platelet aggregation *(82)*. This synergistic effect is a consequence of the combination of the different antiplatelet activities of these agents. In patients with a history of stroke or TIA, aspirin alone markedly inhibited platelet aggregation induced by arachidonic acid, but not by ADP or platelet-activating factor (PAF) *(83)*. Ticlopidine inhibited ADP-induced and PAF-induced platelet aggregation, but not arachidonic acid. The combination, by virtue of the complimentary mechanisms of action, markedly inhibited platelet aggregation in response to all three agonists. Similar results have been demonstrated in patients who have been treated with coronary stents, with significantly greater degrees of platelet inhibition with combination therapy than with monotherapy using either agent *(84)*.

The effect of combination therapy has been clearly demonstrated in several landmark trials (Table 2). Combination antiplatelet therapy compared with aggressive anticoagulant therapy plus aspirin has dramatically reduced the risk of subacute thrombosis after

Table 2
Studies of Combination Aspirin and Thienopyridine Therapy

	ISAR	STARS	CURE	CREDO	CLARITY	COMMIT
Patients	527	1,965	12,562	2,116	3,491	45,852
Aspirin alone	NA	325 qd	75–325 qd	81–325 qd	150–325 qd	NA
Aspirin combined	100 bid	325 qd	75–325 qd	81–325 qd	75–162 qd	162 qd
Thienopyridine	Ticlopidine 250 bid	Ticlopidine 250 bid	Clopidogrel 75 qd	Clopidogrel 75 qd	Clopidogrel 75 qd	Clopidogrel 75 qd
Loading dose	None	None	300 mg	300 mg	300 mg	300 mg
Duration	30 d	30 d	365 d	365 d	30 d	16 d (mean)
Fibrinolytic	NA	NA	NA	NA	99.7% of patients enrolled	49% of patients enrolled
Goal INR	3.5–4.5	2.0–2.5	NA	NA	NA	NA
RR/OR (combination)	RR, 0.25; $p < 0.001$	RR, 0.15; $p < 0.001$	RR, 0.8; $p < 0.001$	RR, 0.73; $p = 0.02$	OR, 0.64; $p < 0.001$	RR, 0.91; $p = 0.002$
Bleeding (combination)						
Major	NA	5.5%; $p < 0.001$	3.7%; $p = 0.001$	8.8%; $p = 0.07$	NS	NS
Minor	NA	NA	5.1%; $p < 0.001$	3.1%; $p = 0.23$	NS	NS
Bleeding (warfarin)	6.5%; $p < 0.001$	6.2%; $p < 0.001$	NA	NA	NA	NA

ISAR, Intracoronary Stenting and Antithrombotic Regimen; STARS, Stent Anticoagulation Regimen Study; CURE, Clopidogrel in Addition to Aspirin in Patients with ACS Without ST-segment Elevation; CREDO, Early and Sustained Dual Oral Antiplatelet Therapy After PCI; CLARITY, Addition of Clopidogel to Aspirin and Fibrinolytic Therapy for MI with ST-Elevation; COMMIT, Clopidogrel and Metoprolol in Myocardial Infarction Trial; qd, once daily; NA, not applicable; bid, twice daily; OR, odds ratio; NS, not significant; INR, international normalized ratio; RR, relative risk.

coronary stent implantation. The Intracoronary Stenting and Antithrombotic Regimen trial was the first randomized trial of antiplatelet vs anticoagulant therapy after coronary stenting (85). At 30 d, treatment with ticlopidine and aspirin was associated with a 1.6% rate of cardiac death, MI, CABG, or repeat percutaneous revascularization in contrast to the 6.2% rate with warfarin and aspirin (RR, 0.25; 95% CI, 0.06–0.77; $p = 0.01$). There were no major bleeding complications with the antiplatelet regimen, whereas 6.5% of patients in the warfarin arm experienced a major hemorrhagic event ($p < 0.001$). These results were confirmed in the Stent Anticoagulation Regimen Study (86), the first large, multicenter trial comparing combined antiplatelet therapy and anticoagulant therapy. The combination of ticlopidine and aspirin was shown to be more effective than aspirin alone (0.5 vs 3.6% event rate) or aspirin and warfarin (2.7%, $p = 0.001$ for the comparison of all three groups). These trials firmly established the efficacy of combined antiplatelet therapy in the prevention of subacute thrombosis.

This success with ticlopidine spurred further investigation regarding combination therapy of aspirin with clopidogrel. The Clopidogrel in Unstable Angina to Prevent Recurrent Ischemic Events (CURE) (87) trial randomized 12,562 patients with unstable angina or non-Q MI to aspirin alone or a loading dose (300 mg) of clopidogrel followed

by 75 mg/d plus aspirin (75–300 mg). The composite endpoint of cardiovascular death, nonfatal MI, or stroke occurred in 9.3% of the clopidogrel group compared with 11.4% in controls (RR, 0.8; 95% CI, 0.72–0.90; $p < 0.001$). Clopidogrel also significantly reduced the incidence of recurrent ischemia, in-hospital refractory or severe ischemia, heart failure, and revascularization procedures. The rate of major bleeding was significantly higher in the clopidogrel group (RR 1.38; $p = 0.01$), but there was no significant increase in the rates of life-threatening bleeding or hemorrhagic strokes. This landmark trial firmly established the role of combination aspirin and clopidogrel therapy in ACS.

The Clopidogrel for the Reduction of Events During Extended Observation (CREDO) *(88)* trial studied the effect of combination therapy with clopidogrel in a more stable interventional population. CREDO enrolled 2116 patients undergoing, or at high likelihood for, a planned coronary intervention who were randomized to either pretreatment with 300 mg clopidogrel or aspirin alone. At the time of the intervention, all patients received 75 mg clopidogrel and 325 mg of aspirin, which were continued daily for 28 d. Patients randomized to clopidogrel pretreatment were maintained on this regimen for 1 yr, whereas the other group continued daily aspirin alone. At 12 mo, long-term therapy with clopidogrel was associated with a reduction in the combined risk of death, MI, or stroke (RR, 0.73; 95% CI, 0.56–0.96; $p = 0.02$). There was a nonsignificant trend in reduction of combined risk of death, MI, or urgent target-vessel revascularization (RR, 0.82; 95% CI, 0.58–1.1; $p = 0.23$). However, subgroup analysis showed a nearly significant reduction in the secondary endpoint in those patients receiving clopidogrel at least 6 h before their intervention (RR, 0.61; 95% CI, 0.37–1.02; $p = 0.051$). There was no significant increase of major bleeding at 1 yr in the dual antiplatelet regimen ($p = 0.07$).

Two recent studies evaluated the efficacy of adding clopidrogrel to aspirin in patients with ST-elevation MI receiving thrombolytic therapy. The Addition of Clopidogrel to Aspirin and Fibrinolytic Therapy for MI with ST-Segment Elevation trial *(89)* enrolled 3491 patients presenting within 12 h after the onset of ST-elevation MI. They were randomized to receive clopidogrel (300 mg loading dose, then 75 mg/d) or placebo. All patients were then to receive a fibrinolytic agent, aspirin, and heparin (when appropriate), and were scheduled to undergo angiography at 48 to 192 h after enrollment. The primary endpoint was a composite of an occluded infarct-related artery on angiography, or death or recurrent MI before angiography. At 30 d, clopidogrel therapy provided a 20% RR reduction in the primary endpoint (11.6 vs 14.1%; $p = 0.03$). As with the other combination therapy trials, no significantly increased rate of major bleeding was seen. This was followed by the larger Clopidogrel and Metoprolol in Myocardial Infarction Trial (COMMIT) trial, which was presented at the 2005 meeting of the American College of Cardiology Scientific Sessions. The COMMIT trial *(90)* enrolled 45,852 patients who were within 24 h of developing ST-elevation MI (ST change or new left bundle-branch block). These patients were randomized to clopidogrel (75 mg once daily, no loading dose) vs placebo. All patients received 162 mg of aspirin, and 49% of patients received thrombolytics. The primary endpoint was a composite of death, reinfarction, or stroke at hospital discharge. The data from this trial has yet to be published. However, the presentation of the American College of Cardiology showed that, at a mean of 16 d, the addition of clopidogrel to this patient population provided a 9% RR reduction of the primary endpoint (9.3 vs 10.1%; $p = 0.002$). Mortality alone was also significantly reduced (7.7 vs 8.1%; $p = 0.03$), as was reinfarction (2.1 vs 2.4%; $p = 0.02$). These trials confirm the benefit of a multifaceted approach to antiplatelet therapy across a wide spectrum of cardiovascular events.

OPTIMAL DOSING OF ASPIRIN IN COMBINATION THERAPY

As noted in these trials, the benefit of combination therapy with aspirin and the thienopyridines is not without risk. The CLASSICS trial showed a 1.5% risk of major bleeding with combination of 325 mg aspirin and 75 mg of clopidogrel. CURE showed a significant (1%) increase in major bleeding with combination therapy, and an insignificant (0.4%) increase in life-threatening bleeding. CREDO also showed a 2.1% increase in major bleeding with combination therapy, though this increase did not reach statistical significance. The bleeding risk is offset by the benefit derived from dual antiplatelet therapy. However, it raises the questions of the optimal dose and duration of these medications needed to provide benefit, yet limit the risk of bleeding.

The question of dose was addressed in a substudy of the CURE trial *(91)*. The 12,562 patients enrolled in the CURE study were divided into three groups based on the dose of aspirin used:

1. ≤100 mg aspirin.
2. 101–199 mg aspirin.
3. ≥200 mg aspirin.

The combined rate of cardiovascular death, MI, or stroke was reduced with combination therapy, regardless of the aspirin dose used. However, as the dose of aspirin increased, the risk of major bleeding increased in both the aspirin plus placebo group (1.9, 2.8, and 3.7%, respectively; $p = 0.001$) and in the combination therapy group (3.0, 3.4, and 4.9%, respectively; $p = 0.0009$). The investigators concluded that adding clopidogrel to aspirin is beneficial regardless of the aspirin dose used. Further, the optimal daily dose of aspirin, with or without clopidogrel, seems to be between 75 mg and 100 mg. The question of duration of combination therapy remains to be clearly determined. CREDO showed a significant benefit from continuing combination therapy for 1 yr after percutaneous intervention. However, the optimal duration of therapy has yet to be firmly established. Further trials, such as CHARISMA, will be important in helping to determine the optimal duration of combination therapy.

Combination Therapy for Primary Prevention

Whereas combination therapy with aspirin and clopidogrel has proven benefits in secondary prevention of cardiovascular events, the benefit of combination therapy has not been studied in primary prevention to this point. The CHARISMA trial was designed to better answer this question *(92)*. This study was designed to evaluate the efficacy and safety of combination therapy in patients with established coronary, cerebral, or peripheral artery disease, and in those patients without a history of vascular events but who are at heightened risk. CHARISMA randomized more than 15,000 patients to clopidogrel plus aspirin vs placebo plus aspirin. The primary endpoint is a composite of vascular death, MI, or stroke. Rates of bleeding will also be compared between the two arms. This study should help us further understand the benefits and safety of long-term combination therapy for cardiovascular disease.

PLATELET GLYCOPROTEIN IIB/IIIA RECEPTOR INHIBITORS

The final common pathway of aggregation, irrespective of how it is initiated, involves the binding of the IIb/IIIa receptors of adjacent platelets. By blocking these platelet receptors, aggregation can be essentially eliminated. Coller and colleagues were the first

to demonstrate that a murine monoclonal antibody (7E3), directed against the IIb/IIIa receptor, could inhibit binding of fibrinogen to platelets, thereby inhibiting platelet aggregation *(93)*. This monoclonal antibody was later redesigned as a half-murine, half-human chimeric Fab fragment (c7E3 Fab, abciximab) using recombinant techniques. Subsequently, a number of other parenteral glycoprotein IIb/IIIa receptor antagonists have been developed and clinically evaluated, including the peptide inhibitor, eptifibatide, and the nonpeptide inhibitors, tirofiban and lamifiban *(94)*. More than 10 large-scale, placebo-controlled, randomized trials involving more than 35,000 patients have been performed to evaluate the short-term, intravenous use of these agents in the setting of percutaneous coronary interventions (PCIs) or ACS. In the setting of a PCI, randomization to a GPIIb/IIIa antagonist is associated with a greater than 50% RR reduction in the incidence of death and MI at 30 d, whereas, in the ACS population, their overall relative benefit in the same endpoint is approx 10%.

In the realm of secondary prevention, a need clearly exists for longer-term inhibition of this receptor complex, because the favorable short-term benefits of parenteral IIb/IIIa inhibitors, particularly target vessel revascularization, have not been maintained with longer follow-up in some trials *(95–97)*. With ACS, activation of the hemostatic system persists for months after the acute event *(98)*, supporting a potential role for oral GPIIb/IIIa agonists in long-term secondary prevention. To this end, a number of oral GPIIb/IIIa antagonists have been evaluated, but surprisingly not only was long-term treatment with an oral GPIIb/IIIa antagonist found not to be beneficial, they actually significantly increased mortality. Further study to better explain the mechanism behind this is critical.

Dipyridamole

Dipyridamole, a primidopyrimidine derivative with vasodilator properties, was introduced for the treatment of angina in 1961. Its antithrombotic properties were first reported in 1965 *(99)*. The basis for any antiplatelet and antithrombotic properties is not clear, but may be related to:

1. Inhibition of platelet phosphodiesterase, resulting in an increase in intraplatelet cyclic adenosine monophosphate (cAMP).
2. Stimulation of endogenous prostaglandin release from the endothelium.
3. Inhibition of adenosine uptake, with subsequent degradation by the vasculature.

Dipyridamole alone is a weak inhibitor of platelet aggregation in vitro. The potential antithrombotic effect of dipyridamole has been assessed in a large number of studies, but typically in combination with aspirin rather than compared directly with a placebo. Doses from 75 to 400 mg daily in divided doses have been investigated. In early clinical trials of stroke and CAD in which aspirin alone has been compared with the combination of aspirin and dipyridamole, dipyridamole contributed no benefit *(100)*. However, a recent trial evaluating a long-acting formulation of dipyridamole in stroke patients demonstrated a significant benefit in the reduction of recurrent strokes but not MIs or cardiovascular death with dipyridamole alone compared with placebo, and an even greater benefit when dipyridamole was used in combination with aspirin *(101)*. Based on the results of this trial, a combination formulation of aspirin and a long-acting preparation of dipyridamole (Aggrenox) is currently approved for the prevention of recurrent strokes.

Cilostazol

Cilostazol is approved for the treatment of intermittent claudication, related to its vasodilator properties *(102)*. Cilostazol, similar to dipyridamole, selectively inhibits platelet phosphodiesterase type III, thereby increasing intracellular concentrations of cAMP and inhibiting platelet aggregation *(103)*. Antiplatelet activity is detected within 6 h of oral ingestion and persists for 48 h after drug withdrawal *(104)*. In a cAMP-dependent mechanism, it also acts as an arterial vasodilator *(105)*. Cilostazol is well-tolerated, with the most commonly reported side-effects being headache, diarrhea, and dizziness *(106)*.

In the setting of peripheral vascular disease, cilostazol has been shown to significantly improve symptoms of intermittent claudication with up to 40% increases in maximal walking distance *(107)*. This benefit is assumed to be primarily caused by its vasodilatory effects, but may also be related to its antiplatelet properties. Based on animal models of carotid artery balloon injury demonstrating significantly decreased rates of neointimal proliferation *(108)*, the role of cilostazol in PCI has also been investigated. In a preliminary study of 36 patients undergoing Palmaz-Schatz coronary stent implantation, randomization to cilostazol was associated with a significantly greater minimal luminal diameter at 6 mo compared with aspirin *(109)*. In a larger study of 211 patients undergoing percutaneous transluminal coronary angioplasty (PTCA), angiographic follow-up was performed 3 mo after randomization to either cilostazol or aspirin *(110)*. Angiographic restenosis was significantly less frequent with cilostazol compared with aspirin (17.9 vs 39.5%; $p < 0.001$) and target lesion revascularization was also less frequent with cilostazol (11.4 vs 28.7%; $p < 0.001$). When compared with ticlopidine, in aspirin-treated patients after coronary stent implantation, cilostazol has similar efficacy in preventing subacute thrombosis and may confer an advantage in reducing 6-mo angiographic restenosis, with a decreased side-effect profile *(111–116)*.

The most recent trial investigating cilostazol is the Cilostazol for RESTenosis (CREST; *117*) trial. The preliminary results of this trial were reported at the American Heart Association Scientific Sessions in 2003. This trial evaluated 705 patients undergoing elective PCI with bare-metal stenting. The patients were randomized to cilostazol (100 mg twice daily for 6 mo) vs placebo. All patients received aspirin and clopidogrel for the duration of the study, with 6-mo clinical and angiographic follow-up. The primary endpoint was in-segment minimum luminal diameter. The addition of cilostazol conferred a 39.5% RR reduction of in-segment restenosis. Notably, there was also less restenosis in diabetic patients (17 vs 37%; $p = 0.01$) and in small (<3 mm) vessels (22 vs 34%; $p = 0.01$). This study has yet to be published, but suggests a benefit of adding cilostazol in the setting of PCI, particularly in those patients at risk for restenosis.

Cilostazol is thought to decrease neointimal proliferation after balloon angioplasty via its antiplatelet actions and subsequent decreases in platelet-derived growth factors *(118)*. By a mechanism that is not yet understood, cilostazol is also thought to be capable of direct inhibition of smooth muscle cell proliferation *(119)*. This may be the primary mechanism of reduction of late lumen loss after PTCA with cilostazol. However, not all interventional trials have demonstrated a benefit with cilostazol. In fact, two recently published trials have shown increased rates of in-stent thrombosis with cilostazol when compared with ticlopidine *(120,121)*. For this reason, further investigation of cilostazol in the setting of coronary intervention is needed.

Combination Therapy With Anticoagulant and Antiplatelet Agents

Because both platelets and the coagulation cascade are integral in the pathophysiology of intracoronary thrombosis, therapy using a combination of antiplatelet and anticoagulant agents may offer an additive benefit. This hypothesis is supported by studies among patients with prosthetic heart valves that have demonstrated a decreased risk of thromboembolic complications with combination therapy *(122)*. The TPT was initiated to evaluate primary prevention with either low-dose aspirin (75 mg daily), low-dose warfarin (INR target of 1.5), both, or neither in 5493 men at "greater than average risk" for ischemic heart disease *(22)*. Overall, warfarin use, either alone or in combination with aspirin, was associated with a 21% reduction ($p = 0.003$) in all events (coronary death and fatal and nonfatal MI), with the benefit largely caused by a 39% reduction in fatal events. Aspirin therapy, either alone or in combination with warfarin, was associated with a 20% reduction in events ($p = 0.004$), with most of the benefit caused by a 32% reduction in nonfatal events. Combination therapy with warfarin and aspirin was associated with a 15% relative reduction in the event rate compared with aspirin alone. This small effect must be considered in light of the increased rates of hemorrhagic (0.9%) and fatal (1.5%) stroke with the warfarin and aspirin combination, as well as significantly higher rates of intermediate (6.2%) and minor bleeding (48%). These results suggest a small potential benefit for combining warfarin and aspirin for primary prevention. Whether the increased risk of adverse events and the requirement for close monitoring of the INR outweigh these benefits is left up to the individual provider.

The role of combined antiplatelet and anticoagulant therapy in secondary prevention has been addressed in several trials. The Coumadin Aspirin Reinfarction Study (CARS) compared the efficacy of fixed, low-dose warfarin and aspirin with aspirin alone for secondary prevention in patients with clinically stable CAD *(123)*. The trial was prematurely terminated because of a lack of efficacy in the combination arms vs aspirin alone. The combination arms of this study used rather low, set doses (1 or 3 mg) of warfarin, which may have limited efficacy. The Antithrombotic Therapy in Acute Coronary Syndromes Research Group studied the combination of aspirin and anticoagulant therapy (heparin followed by warfarin) vs aspirin alone in 214 nonprevious aspirin users with either unstable angina or non-ST-elevation MI *(124)*. Those randomized to receive warfarin had a target INR of 2 to 3, and active treatment was maintained for 12 wk. Although combination therapy significantly reduced the incidence of primary ischemic events within the first 14 d (27% aspirin alone; 10% combination therapy; $p = 0.004$), by 12 wk, there was only a trend favoring combination therapy (28% aspirin alone; 19% combination therapy; $p = 0.09$). These results are consistent with the benefit demonstrated by some studies of the acute treatment of unstable angina with a combination of aspirin and heparin *(34,125)*, but they do not offer strong support for prolonged oral anticoagulant therapy for these patients.

The Organization to Assess Strategies for Ischemic Syndromes (OASIS) pilot study also addressed the role of combination therapy after unstable angina or non-ST-elevation MI *(126)*. Phase 1 of this study randomized 309 patients to either fixed, low-dose warfarin (3 mg/d) or standard therapy, with 87% of patients receiving aspirin in each group. This portion of OASIS confirmed the findings of the CARS trial—there was no significant reduction in events at 6 mo of follow-up with the combination of fixed, low-dose warfarin plus aspirin. In phase 2, 197 patients were randomized to either adjusted-dose warfarin with a target INR of 2 to 2.5 or standard therapy, with 85% of patients in each group

Table 3
Trials of Combined Antiplatelet and Antithrombotic Therapy

	CHAMP	WARIS-2	ASPECT-2
No. of patients	5059	3630	999
Aspirin dose (alone)	162	160	100
Aspirin dose (combination)	81	75	100
Warfarin dose or target INR	1.5–2.5	2.0–2.5	2.0–2.5
Follow-up	2.7 yr	4 yr	2 yr
Hazard ratio (combination)	NS	0.71 ($p = 0.001$)	0.50 ($p = 0.03$)
Bleeding risk (combination)			
Major	1.56 ($p < 0.001$)	1.25 ($p < 0.001$)	1.03 ($p = $ NS)
Minor	NA	NA	3.13 ($p < 0.0001$)

CHAMP, Combination Hemotherapy and Mortality Prevention; WARIS, Warfarin Re-infarction Study; ASPECT, Anticoagulants in the Secondary Prevention of Events in Coronary Thrombosis; NS, not significant; NA, not applicable.

receiving aspirin. At 3 mo, there was a trend favoring combination therapy, with a 58% relative reduction in the risk of the primary endpoint of cardiovascular death, new MI, and refractory angina (5.8 vs 12.1%; RR, 0.42; 95% CI, 0.15–1.15; $p = 0.08$). The substantially higher event rate in the aspirin arm compared with the event rate of the phase 1 study suggests a higher-risk population and a potential bias favoring combination therapy. The event rates for major bleeding were too small for statistical comparison, but again, minor bleeding was significantly more frequent with combination therapy. These data suggest that adjusted-dose warfarin, unlike fixed, low-dose warfarin, in combination with aspirin, may have a role in secondary prevention.

With consistently higher rates of bleeding and without a clearly demonstrated benefit in smaller populations, combination therapy with aspirin and warfarin was subsequently studied in several larger randomized trials (Table 3). The Warfarin, Aspirin, or Both After Myocardial Infarction (WARIS-II) trial studied the effects of combining aspirin with warfarin in patients after acute MI (127). This trial enrolled 3630 post-MI patients to receive warfarin with a goal INR of 2.8 to 4.2 (1216 patients), 160 mg of aspirin (1206 patients), or 75 mg aspirin plus warfarin with a goal INR of 2.0 to 2.5 (1208 patients). The patients were followed for a mean of 4 yr for the composite endpoint of death, nonfatal MI, or thromboembolic cerebral stroke. The endpoint occurred in 241 (20%) in the aspirin group, 203 (16.7%) in the warfarin group, and 181 (15%) in the combination group (RR, 0.71 when compared with aspirin alone; 95% CI, 0.6–0.83; $p = 0.001$). The difference between the two warfarin groups did not reach statistical significance. Major, nonfatal bleeding complications were seen in 62% of patients in the warfarin groups, as opposed to 17% in the aspirin group ($p < 0.001$).

The Aspirin and Coumadin After Acute Coronary Syndromes (ASPECT-2) study compared aspirin with warfarin or combination therapy in patients with ACS (128). This trial randomized 999 patients after ACS to 100 mg aspirin (336 patients), warfarin with a goal INR of 3.0 to 4.0 (330 patients), or 100 mg aspirin plus warfarin with goal INR of 2.0 to 2.5 (333 patients). The patients were followed for 2 yr for the combined endpoint of MI, stroke, and death. This endpoint occurred in 31 (9%) patients in the aspirin group, 17 (5%) patients in the warfarin group, and 16 (5%) patients in the combination group.

Compared with aspirin therapy, the hazard ratio was 0.55 ($p = 0.0479$) for warfarin alone, and 0.50 ($p = 0.03$) for warfarin plus aspirin. Again, however, this benefit was offset by a significant increase in bleeding complications. Major bleeding occurred in 2% in the combination group as opposed to 1% in the aspirin or warfarin arms ($p = 0.2$). Minor bleeding was 15% in the combination group vs 5 and 8% in the single-therapy arms ($p < 0.0001$).

The Clinical Trial Comparing Combined Warfarin and Aspirin with Aspirin Alone in Survivors of Acute Myocardial Infarction (CHAMP) study also compared aspirin with combination therapy (129). This trial randomized 5059 patients to 81 mg aspirin (2537 patients) or 81 mg aspirin plus warfarin (2522 patients), with a goal INR of 1.5 to 2.5. The patients were followed for a mean of 2.7 yr for the primary endpoint of death and combined secondary endpoint of MI, stroke, and major hemorrhage. This trial failed to show a significant reduction in death or stroke between the two groups. However, as with the other trials, it did observe a significant increase in the rates of bleeding with 1.28 vs 0.72 events per 100 person-years of follow-up, respectively ($p < 0.001$).

Together, these trials suggest a benefit from combination aspirin and warfarin therapy in patients after ACS. However, this benefit is offset by a significant increase in bleeding complications. Given the benefits of aspirin plus clopidogrel in these patients, with the relatively low added risk of bleeding, the role of combination therapy with warfarin has yet to be firmly established.

Combination anticoagulant and antiplatelet therapy has also been investigated in surgical revascularization. The Post Coronary Artery Bypass Graft Trial Investigators addressed the role of low-dose warfarin and aspirin for the prevention of the progression of saphenous vein graft disease (130). In this study, 1351 patients who had undergone bypass surgery 1 to 11 yr before were randomized using a two-by-two factorial design to either aggressive or moderate cholesterol-lowering therapy, plus either warfarin or placebo. All patients were encouraged to take 81 mg of aspirin daily. The warfarin dose was regulated to maintain the INR less than 2 (mean INR, 1.4). After a mean follow-up of 4.3 yr, those randomized to warfarin showed no significant difference in angiographic outcomes or the combined clinical endpoint of death, nonfatal MI, stroke, CABG, or PTCA compared with placebo. Although these results cannot exclude a benefit of more aggressive long-term anticoagulation, they do not support low-dose combination therapy over aspirin alone.

CONCLUSION

Antithrombotic therapy, as it is currently used, prevents heart attacks and saves lives. For every 1000 individuals free of diagnosed atherosclerotic disease treated with aspirin during a 5-yr period, up to 7 important cardiac events will be prevented. More importantly, by targeting preventative therapy to those at higher risk, a 10-fold greater benefit can be achieved. In fact, when aspirin is used in patients after MI or with unstable angina, an almost one-fourth reduction in mortality can be realized. Although aspirin is extremely inexpensive, generally well-tolerated, and at least as effective as all other currently studied antithrombotic preventative regimens, there are those individuals in whom it is not a viable therapeutic option. For these patients, data supports the use of the thienopyridine derivatives as an effective aspirin alternative. Further, more aggressive long-term antiplatelet protection, in the form of the combination of a thienopyridine and aspirin, has shown incremental benefit in secondary prevention of cardiovascular events.

However, as discussed in this chapter, the value of each of these therapies must be weighed against the potential harm implicit to regimens including combinations of antiplatelet and anticoagulant medications. Other potential pitfalls in our treatment strategies include the concepts of aspirin and thienopyridine resistance, and differing effects of antiplatelet agents between sexes. These topics are neither clearly defined nor completely understood, and remain subjects for further investigation. Ultimately, as our understanding of the pathophysiology of all aspects of cardiovascular disease continues to grow, further innovations in antithrombotic therapy will undoubtedly lead to even more dramatic results in the prevention of ischemic heart disease while limiting potential complications to our patients.

REFERENCES

1. von Rokitansky C. A Manual of Pathologic Anatomy. The Sydenham Society, London, 1852, pp. 265–275.
2. Falk E, Unstable angina with fatal outcome: Dynamic coronary thrombosis leading to infarction and/or sudden death. Autopsy evidence of recurrent mural thrombosis with peripheral embolization culminating in total vascular occlusion. Circulation 1989;71:699–708.
3. DeWood MA, et al. Prevalence of total coronary occlusion during the early hours of transmural myocardial infarction. N Engl J Med 1980;303:897–902.
4. Davies MJ, Thomas AC. Plaque fissuring—the cause of acute myocardial infarction, sudden ischaemic death, and crescendo angina. Br Heart J 1985;53:363–373.
5. Buja LM, Willerson JT. Clinicopathologic correlates of acute ischemic heart disease syndromes. Am J Cardiol 1981;47:343–356.
6. Bini A, et al. Identification and distribution of fibrinogen, fibrin and fibrin(ogen) degradation products in atherosclerosis. Arteriosclerosis 1989;9:109–121.
7. MacIsaac AI, Thomas JD, Topol EJ. Toward the quiescent plaque. J Am Coll Cardiol 1993;22:1228–1241.
8. Fuster V, et al. The pathogenesis of coronary artery disease and the acute coronary syndromes. N Engl J Med 1992;326:242–250, 310–318.
9. Davies MJ, et al. Factors influencing the presence or absence of acute coronary thrombi in sudden ischemic death. Eur Heart J 1989;10:203–208.
10. Kaplan AV, et al. Roles of thrombin and platelet membrane glycoprotein IIb/IIIa in platelet-subendothelial deposition after angioplasty in an ex vivo whole artery model. Circulation 1991;84:1279–1288.
11. Holmsen H, Weiss HJ. Secretable storage pools in platelets. Ann Rev Med 1979;30:119–134.
12. Stone E. An account of the success of the bark of the willow in the cure of agues. Philos Trans R Soc Lond [Biol] 1763;53:195–200.
13. Binz C. Vorlesungen Ueber Pharmakologie. 2nd ed. Berlin, 1891.
14. Weiss HJ, Aledort LM. Impaired platelet-connective-tissue reaction in man after aspirin ingestion. Lancet 1967;2:495–497.
15. Craven LL. Experiences with aspirin (acetylsalicylic acid) in the nonspecific prophylaxis of coronary thrombosis. Mississippi Valley Medical Journal 1953;75:38–44.
16. Vane JR. Inhibition of prostaglandin synthesis as a mechanism of action for aspirin-like drugs. Nature 1971;231:231–235.
17. Smith JB, Willis AL. Aspirin selectively inhibits prostaglandin production in human platelets. Nature 1971;231:235–237.
18. Patrono C. Aspirin as an antiplatelet drug. N Engl J Med 1994;330(18):1287–1294.
19. Steering Committee of the Physicians' Health Study Research Group. Preliminary report: Findings from the aspirin component of the ongoing physicians' health study. N Engl J Med 1988;318(4):262–264.
20. Steering Committee of the Physicians' Health Study Research Group. Final report on the aspirin component of the ongoing physicians' health study. N Engl J Med 1989;321(3):129–135.
21. Peto R, et al. Randomised trial of prophylactic aspirin in British male doctors. Br Med J 1988;296:313–316.
22. The Medical Research Council's General Practice Research Framework. Thrombosis prevention trial: randomised trial of low-intensity oral anticoagulation with warfarin and low-dose aspirin in the primary prevention of ischaemc heart disease in men at increased risk. Lancet 1998;351:323–341.
23. Hansson L, Zanchetti A, Carruthers S. Effects of intensive blood pressure lowering and low-dose aspirin in patients with hypertension: results of the Hypertension Optimal Treatment (HOT) randomised trial. Lancet 1998;351:1755–1762.

24. Hennekens CH, et al. An overview of the British and American aspirin studies. N Engl J Med 1988;318:923–924.
25. Eidelman RS, et al. An update on aspirin in the primary prevention of cardiovascular disease. Arch Intern Med 2003;163(17):2006–2010.
26. Collaborative Group of the Primary Prevention Project. Low-dose aspirin and vitamin E in people at cardiovascular risk: a randomized trial in general practice. Lancet 2001;357:89–95.
27. Ridker PM, et al. for the Women's Health Study Research Group. A randomized trial of low-dose aspirin in the primary prevention of cardiovascular disease in women. N Engl J Med 2005;352:1293–1304.
28. Collaborative overview of randomised trials of antiplatelet therapy—III: Reduction in venous thrombosis and pulmonary embolism by antiplatelet prophylaxis among surgical and medical patients. Antiplatelet Trialists' Collaboration. BMJ 1994;308(6923):235–46.
29. Collaborative meta-analysis of randomised trials of antiplatelet therapy for prevention of death, myocardial infarction, and stroke in high risk patients. BMJ 2002;324(7329):71–86.
30. Ridker PM, et al. Low-dose aspirin therapy for chronic stable angina. A randomised, placebo-controlled clinical trial. Ann Intern Med 1991;114:835–839.
31. Chesebro JH, et al. Antithrombotic therapy and progression of coronary artery disease. Antiplatelet versus antithrombins. Circulation 1992;86(Suppl III):III-100–III-111.
32. Juul-Moller S, et al. Double-blind trial of aspirin in primary prevention of myocardial infarction in patients with stable chronic angina pectoris. Lancet 1992;340:1421–1425.
33. Rahimtoola SH. Coronary bypass surgery for unstable angina. Circulation 1984;69:842–848.
34. Theroux P, et al. Aspirin, heparin or both to treat acute unstable angina. N Engl J Med 1988;319:1105–1111.
35. The RISC Group. Risk of myocardial infarction and death during treatment with low dose aspirin and intravenous heparin in men with unstable coronary artery disease. Lancet 1990;336:827–830.
36. Wallentin LC, and the RISC Group. Aspirin (75mg/day) after an episode of unstable coronary artery disease: long-term effects on the risk of myocardial infarction, occurrence of severe angina and the need for revascularization. J Am Coll Cardiol 1991;18:1587–1593.
37. Lewis HD Jr, et al. Protective effects of aspirin against acute myocardial infarction and death in men with unstable angina: Results of a Veterans Administration Cooperative Study. N Eng J Med 1983;309:396–403.
38. Holdright D, et al. Comparison of the effect of heparin and aspirin versus aspirin alone on transient myocardial ischemia and in-hospital prognosis in patients with unstable angina. J Am Coll Cardiol 1994;24:39–45.
39. Antiplatelet Trialists' Collaboration. Collaborative overview of randomised trials of antiplatelet therapy—II: Maintenance of vascular graft or arterial patency by antiplatelet therapy. BMJ 1994;308:159–168.
40. ISIS-2 Collaborative Group. Randomised trial of intravenous streptokinase, oral aspirin, both, or neither among 17,187 cases of suspected acute myocardial infarction: ISIS-2. Lancet 1988;2:349–360.
41. Gabriel SE, Jaakkimainen L, Bombardier C. Risk of serious gastrointestinal complications related to nonsteroidal anti-inflammatory drugs: a meta-analysis. Ann Intern Med 1991;115:787–796.
42. Weil J, et al. Prophylactic aspirin and risk of peptic ulcer bleeding. Br Med J 1995;310:827–830.
43. The Dutch TIA Study Group. A comparison of two doses of aspirin (30 mg vs. 283 mg a day) in patients after transient ischemic attack or minor ischemic stroke. N Engl J Med 1991;325:1261–1266.
44. Farrell B, et al. The United Kingdom transient ischemic attack (UK-TIA) aspirin trial: final results. J Neurol Neurosurg Psychiatry 1991;54:1044–1054.
45. Hofteizer JW, et al. Comparison of the effects of regular and enteric coated aspirin on gastroduodenal mucosa of man. Lancet 1980;2:609–612.
46. Leonards JR, Levy G. Effect of pharmaceutical formulation on gastrointestinal bleeding from aspirin tablets. Arch Intern Med 1972;129:457–460.
47. Krumholz HM, et al. Aspirin in the treatment of acute myocardial in elderly medicare beneficiaries. Patterns of use and outcomes. Circulation 1995;92:2841–2847.
48. Krumholz HM, et al. Aspirin for secondary prevention after acute myocardial infarction in the elderly: prescribed use and outcomes. Ann Intern Med 1996;124:292–298.
49. Hennekens CH, Jonas MA, Buring JE. The benefits of aspirin in acute myocardial infarction: Still a well kept secret in the U.S. Arch Intern Med 1994;154:37–39.
50. Hardisty R, Powling M, Nokes T. The action of ticlopidine on human platelets: studies on aggregation, secretion, calcium mobilization and membrane glycoproteins. Thromb Haemost 1990;64:150–155.
51. Defreyn G, et al. Pharmacology of ticlopidine: a review. Semin Thromb Hemost 1989;15:159–166.

52. Muller I, Seyforth M, Rudiger S, et al. Effect of a high loading dose of clopidogrel on platelet function in patients undergoing coronary stent placement. Heart 2001;85:92–93.
53. McTavish D, Faulds D, Goa K. Ticlopidine: an updated review of its pharmacology and therapeutic use in platelet-dependent disorders. Drugs 1990;40:238–259.
54. Gents M, Blakely J, Easton J. The Canadian American Ticlopidine Study (CATS) in thromboembolic stroke. Lancet 1989;1(1215–1120).
55. Janzon L, et al. Prevention of myocardial infarction and stroke in patients with intermittent claudication; effects of ticlopidine. Results from STIMS, the Swedish Ticlopidine Multicentre Study. J Intern Med 1990;227:301–308.
56. Arcan J, Blanchard J, Boissel J. Multi-center double-blind study of ticlopidine in the treatment of intermittent claudication and prevention of its complications. Angiology 1988;39:802–811.
57. Blanchard J, Carreras L, Kindermans M. Results of EMATAP: a double-blind palcebo-controlled multicentre trial of ticlopidine in patients with peripheral arterial disease. Nouv Rev Fr Hematol 1993;35:523–528.
58. Hass W, Easton J, Adams JH, et al. A randomized trial comparing ticlopidine hydrochloride with aspirin for the prevention of stroke in high risk patients. N Engl J Med 1989;321:501–507.
59. Knudsen JB, et al. The efect of ticlopidine on platelet functions in acute myocardial infarction. A double blind controlled trial. Thromb Haemost 1985;53(3):332–336.
60. Sadowski Z, et al. Comparison of ticlopidine and aspirin in unstable angina[abstract]. Eur Heart J 1995;16(Suppl.):259.
61. Balsano F, et al. Antiplatelet treatment with ticlopidine in unstable angina. A controlled multicenter clinical trial. Circulation 1990;82:17–26.
62. Fuster V, Chesebro JH. Role of platelets and platelet inhibitors in aorto-coronary vein graft disease. Circulation 1986;73:227–232.
63. Chevigne M, David J, Rigo P. Effect of ticlopidine on saphenous vein patency rates: a double-blind study. Ann Thorac Surg 1984;37:371–378.
64. Limet R, David J, Rigo P. Prevention of aorta-coronary bypass graft occlusion. Beneficial effect of ticlopidine on early and late patency rates of venous coronary bypass grafts: a double-blind study. J Thorac Cardiovasc Surg 1987;94:773–783.
65. Becquemin J. Effect of ticlopidine on the long-term patency of saphenous-vein bypass grafts in the legs. N Engl J Med 1997;337:1726–1731.
66. CAPRIE, a randomised, blinded, trial of clopidogrel versus aspirin in patients at risk of ischaemic events. Lancet 1996;348:1329–1339.
67. Ringleb PA, Bhatt DL, Hirsch AT, et al. Benefit of clopidogrel over aspirin is amplified in patients with a history of ischemic events. Stroke 2004;35:528–532.
68. Bhatt DL, Chew DP, Hirsch AT, Ringleb PA, Hacke W, Topol EJ. Superiority of clopidogrel versus aspirin in patients with prior cardiac surgery. Circulation 2001;103:363–368.
69. Bhatt DL, Marso SP, Hirsch AT, Ringleb PA, Hacke W, Topol EJ. Amplified benefit of clopidrogel versus aspirin in patients with diabetes mellitus. Am J Med 2004;90:625–628.
70. Megumi T, Kurz HI, Lasala JM. Randomized comparison of ticlopidine and clopidogrel after intracoronary stent implantation in a broad patient population. Circulation 2001;104:539–543.
71. Sharis P, Cannon C, Loscalzo J. The antiplatelet effects of ticlopidine and clopidogrel. Ann Intern Med 1998;129:394–405.
72. Bellavance A. Efficacy of ticlopidine and aspirin for prevention of reversible cerebrovascular ischemic events: the ticlopidine and aspirin stroke study. Stroke 1993;24:1452–1457.
73. Bertrand M, Legrand V, Boland J. Randomized multicenter comparison of conventional anticoagulation versus antiplatelet therapy in unplanned and elective coronary stenting: the Full Anticoagulation Versus Aspirin and Ticlopidine (FANTASTIC) study. Circulation 1998;98:1597–1603.
74. Wysowksi DK, Bacsanyi J. Blood dyscrasias and hematologic reactions in ticlopidine users. JAMA 1996;276(12):952.
75. Schror K. Antiplatelet drugs: a comparative review. Drugs 1995;50:7–28.
76. Page Y, et al. Thrombotic thrombocytopenic purpura related to ticlopidine. Lancet 1991;337:774–776.
77. Bennet CL, et al. Thrombotic thrombocytopenic purpura associated with ticlopidine. A review of 60 cases. Ann Intern Med 1998;128:541–544.
78. Steinhubl SR, Tan WA, Foody JM. Incidence and clinical cause of TTP due to ticlopidine following coronary stenting. JAMA 1999;281:806–810.
79. Bennett C, et al. Thrombotic thrombocytopenic purpura after stenting and ticlopidine. Lancet 1998;352:1036–1037.

80. Zakarija A, Bandarenko N, Pandy DK, et al. Clopidogrel-associated TTP: an update of pharmacovigilance efforts conducted by independent researchers, pharmaceutical suppliers, and the Food and Drug Administration. Stroke 2004;35(2):533–537.

81. Bertrand ME, Rupprecht HJ, Urban P, Gershlick AH, Investigators FT. Double-blind study of the safety of clopidogrel with and without a loading dose in combination with aspirin compared with ticlopidine in combination with aspirin after coronary stenting. Circulation 2000;102:624–629.

82. Splawinska B, et al. The efficacy of and potency of antiplatelet activity of ticlopidine is increased by aspirin. Int J Clin Pharmacol Ther 1996;34:352–356.

83. Uchiyama S, et al. Combination theray with low-dose aspirin and ticlopidine in cerebral ischemia. Stroke 1989;20:1643–1647.

84. Rupprecht H-J, et al. Comparison of antiplatelet effects of aspirin, ticlopidine, or their combination after stent implantation. Circulation 1998;97:1046–1052.

85. Schomig A, et al. A randomized comparison of antiplatelet and anticoagulant therapy after placement of coronary-artery stents. N Engl J Med 1996;334:1084–1089.

86. Leon MB, et al. A clinical trial comparing three anti-thrombotic regimens following coronary artery stenting. N Eng J Med 1998;339:1665–1671.

87. Yusuf S, Zhao F, Mehta SR, Chrolavicius S, Tognoni G, Fox KK; Clopidogrel in Unstable Angina to Prevent Recurrent Events Trial Investigators. Effects of clopidogrel in addition to aspirin in patients with acute coronary syndromes without ST-segment elevation. N Engl J Med 2001;345(7):494–502.

88. Steinhubl SR, Berger PB, Man JT 3rd, et al. for the CREDO investigators. Early and sustained dual oral antiplatelet therapy following percutaneous coronary intervention. JAMA 2002;288(19):2411–2420.

89. Sabatine MS, Cannon CP, Gibson CM, et al. Addition of clopidogrel to aspirin and fibrinolytic therapy for myocardial infarction with ST-segment elevation. N Engl J Med 2005;352.

90. COMMIT investigators. Clopidogrel and Metoprolol in Myocardial Infarction Trial. Initial results of ACC investigator meeting. March 9, 2005.

91. Peters. Effects of aspirin dose when used alone or in combination with clopidogrel in patients with acute coronary syndromes. Circulation 2003;108:1682–1687.

92. Bhatt DL, Topol EJ. Clopidogrel added to aspirin versus aspirin alone in secondary prevention and high-risk primary prevention: rationale and design of the Clopidogrel for High Atherothrombotic Risk and Ischemic Stabilization, Management, and Avoidance (CHARISMA) trial. Am Heart J 2004;148(2):263–268.

93. Coller B, Peerschke E, Scudder L. A murine monoclonal antibody that completely blocks the binding of fibrinogen to platelets produces a thrombasthenic-like state in normal platelets and binds to glycoproteins IIb and/or IIIa. J Clin Invest 1983;72:325–338.

94. Lefkovits J, Plow E, Topol E. Platelet glycoprotein IIb/IIIa receptors in cardiovascular medicine. N Engl J Med 1995;332:1553–1559.

95. The Platelet Receptor Inhibition in Ischemic Syndrome Management (PRISM) study investigators, A comparison of aspirin plus tirofiban with aspirin plus heparin for unstable angina. N Engl J Med 1998;338:1498–1505.

96. The EPILOG Investigators. Platelet glycoprotein IIb/IIIa receptor blockade and low-dose heparin during percutaneous coronary revascularization. N Engl J Med 1997;336:1689–1696.

97. The RESTORE investigators. Effects of platelet glycoprotein IIb/IIIa blockade with tirofiban on advers cardiac events in patients with unstable angina or acute myocardial infarction undergoing coronary angioplasty. Circulation 1997;1997:1445–1453.

98. Merlini PA, et al. Persistant activation of the coagulation system in unstable angina and myocardial infarction. Circulation 1994;90:61–68.

99. Emmons PR, et al. Effect of dipyridamole on human platelet behaviour. Lancet 1965;2:603–606.

100. FitzGerald GA. Dipyridamole. N Engl J Med 1987;316(20):1247–1257.

101. Diener H, et al. European Stroke Prevention Study 2. Dipyridamole and acetylsalicylic acid in the secondary prevention of stroke. J Neurol Sci 1996;143:1–13.

102. Anonymous. Cilostazol. Med Letter Drugs Ther 1999;7:44.

103. Kimura Y, et al. Effect of cilostazol on platelet agregation and experimental thrombosis. Arzneimittelforschung/Drug Res 1985;35:1144–1149.

104. Yasunaga K, Mase K. Antiaggregatory effect of oral cilostazol and recovery of platelet aggregability in patients with cerebrovascular disease. Arzneimittelforschung/Drug Res 1985;35:1189–1192.

105. Tanaka T, et al. Effect of cilostazol, a selective cAMP phosphodiesterase inhibitor on the contraction of vascular smooth muscle. Pharmacology 1988;36:313–320.

106. Sarkin E, Markham A. Cilostazol. Drugs Aging 1999;14:63–71.

107. Dawson D, Cutler B, Strandness D. Cilostazol has beneficial effects in treatment of intermitent claudication: results from a multicenter, randomized, prospective, double-blinded trial. Circulation 1998;98:678–686.
108. Ishizaka N, et al. Effects of a single local administration of cliostazol on neointima formation in balloon injured rat carotid arteries. Atherosclerosis 1999;142:41–46.
109. Yamasaki M, et al. Effect of cilostazol on late lumen loss after Palmaz-Schatz stent implantation. Cath and Cardiovasc Diag 1998;44:387–391.
110. Tsuchikane E, et al. Impact of cilostazol on restenosis after percutaneous balloon angioplasty. Circulation 1999;100:21–26.
111. Yoon Y, et al. Comparison of cilostazol and ticlopidine after coronary artery stenting: immediate and long-term results. J Am Coll Cardiol 1999;33 (Supp A):40A.
112. El-Beyrouty. Cilostazol for prevention of thrombosis and restenosis after intracoronary stenting. Ann Pharmacother 2001;35(9):1108–1113.
113. Yoon Y, Shim WH, Lee DH, et al. Usefulness of cilostazol versus ticlopidine in coronary artery stenting. Am J Cardiol 1999;84(12):1375–1380.
114. Park SW, Lee CW, Kim HS, et al. Comparison of cilostazol versus ticlopidine therapy after stent implantation. Am J Cardiol 1999;84(5):511–514.
115. Kamishirado H, Inoue T, Mizoguchi K, et al. Randomized comparison of cilostazol versus ticlopidine hydrochloride for antiplatelet therapy after coronary stent implantation for prevention of late restenosis. Am Heart J 2002;144(2):303–308.
116. Tanabe Y, Ito E, Nakagawa I, Suzuki K. Effect of cilostazol on restenosis after coronary angioplasty and stenting in comparison to conventional coronary artery stenting with ticlopidine. Int J Cardiol 2001;78(3):285–291.
117. Douglas JS, Weintraub WS, Holmes D. CREST. Not yet published, 2003.
118. Matsumoto Y, et al. Effects of cilostazol, an antiplatelet drug, on smooth muscle cell proliferation after endothelial cell denudation in rats. Jpn J Pharmacol 1992;58:284.
119. Takahashi S, et al. Effect of cilostazol, a cyclic AMP phosphodiesterase inhibitor, on the proliferation of rat aortic smooth muscle cells in culture. J Cardiovasc Pharmacol 1992;20:900–906.
120. Sekiguchi M, Hoshizaki H, Adachi H, et al. Effects of antiplatelet agents on subacute thrombosis and restenosis after successful coronary stenting. Circ J 2004;68:610–614.
121. Kawata M, Kuramoto E, Kataoka T, et al. Comparative inhibitory effects of cilostazol and ticlopidine on subacute stent thrombosis and platelet function in acute myocardial infarction patients with percutaneous coronary intervention. Int Heart J 2005;46(1):13–22.
122. Chesebro JH, et al. Trial of combined warfarin and dipyridamole or aspirin therapy in prosthetic heart valve replacement: Danger of aspirin compared with dipyridamole. Am J Cardiol 1983;51:1537–1541.
123. Coumadin Aspirin Reinfarction Study (CARS) Investigators. Randomised double-blind trial of fixed low-dose warfarin with aspirin after myocardial infarction. Lancet 1997;350:389–396.
124. Cohen M, et al. Combination antithrombotic therapy in unstable rest angina and non-Q-wave infarction in nonprior aspirin useers. Primary end points analysis from the ATACS trial. Circulation 1994;89:81–88.
125. Oler A, et al. Adding heparin to aspirin reduces the incidence of myocardial infarction and death in patients with unstable angina. JAMA 1996;276:811–815.
126. Anand S, et al. Long-term oral anticoagulant therapy in patients with unstable angina or suspected non-Q-wave myocardial infarction: organization to assess strategies for ischemic syndromes (OASIS) pilot study results. Circulation 1998;98:1064–1070.
127. Hurlen. Warfarin, aspirin, or both after myocardial infarction. N Engl J Med 2002;347(13):969–974.
128. van Es RF, Jonkor JJ, Verheugt FW, et al. Aspirin and coumadin after acute coronary syndromes (the ASPECT-2 study): a randomised controlled trial. Lancet 2002;360:109–113.
129. Fiore LD, Ezekowitz MD, Brophy MT, et al. Department of veterans affairs cooperative studies program clinical trial comparing combined warfarin and aspirin with aspirin alone in survivors of acute myocardial infarction. Circulation 2002;105:555–563.
130. The Post Coronary Artery Bypass Graft Trial Investigators. The effect of aggressive lowering of low-density lipoprotein cholesterol levels and low-dose anticoagulation on obstructive changes in saphenous vein coronary artery bypass grafts. N Engl J Med 1997;336:153–162.

16 Pharmacoeconomics of Cardiovascular Medicine

Melanie Oates, PhD, MBA, RN,
William F. McGhan, PharmD, PhD,
and Ron Corey, PhD, MBA, RPH

CONTENTS

INTRODUCTION

The growth of managed care in the 1980s and 1990s and the resulting emphasis on cost containment have impacted the practice of cardiovascular medicine in the 21st century. In this age of limited economic resources, it is no longer appropriate to embrace all advancements, however minor, in health care technology. Instead, today's physician often must choose treatments with a careful consideration of the expected improvement in patient outcomes compared with the added costs to both patients and third-party payers. This frame of reference does not imply a reduction in quality of care. Instead, it implies an awareness of the quality of health care offered per dollar spent.

From: *Contemporary Cardiology: Preventive Cardiology:*
Insights Into the Prevention and Treatment of Cardiovascular Disease, Second Edition
Edited by: J. M. Foody © Humana Press Inc., Totowa, NJ

CARDIOVASCULAR DISEASE

Cardiovascular disease (CVD) is the leading cause of death in this country. Coronary heart disease (CHD) accounts for nearly 500,000 of those deaths *(1)*. The American Heart Association (AHA) estimated that in 1996, 58.8 million Americans suffered from some form of CVD. According to the National Center for Health Statistics, nearly 633 yr of potential life were lost to heart disease for every 100,000 persons younger than 65 yr of age *(2)*. The economic burden of heart disease is also high, with 1999 direct plus indirect costs for CVD plus stroke in the United States estimated to exceed $286 billion *(3–5)*.

HEALTH ECONOMIC ANALYSIS

Health economic analysis uses tools for comprehensively examining the economic impact of alternative drug therapies and other medical interventions. Health economics identifies, measures, and compares the costs and consequences of medical products and services. The health care system is facing a multitude of economic challenges. The realizations of limited resources and the impact of cost containment is causing administrators and policy makers in the managed care field, and throughout the health system, to vigilantly apply health economic principles in examining the costs and benefits of both proposed and existing drugs and services. With health care reform, all health service sectors will experience increasing pressure and demands that all patient care interventions be evaluated in terms of clinical and social outcomes related to costs incurred.

All of the following groups may have differing agendas, and it is important in health economic evaluations to consider these various perspectives. It must be kept in mind, in considering all these perspectives, that the most important perspective to include in all health economic evaluations is that of society as a whole. Some of the various health economic perspectives include:

1. Individual patients.
2. Employers.
3. Health Maintenance Organizations (HMOs).
4. Hospitals.
5. Insurance companies.
6. Medicaid and Medicare (government).

In considering the foregoing points of view, it is important to consider who pays the cost of the intervention and who gets the benefits. For example, an employer may be very interested in a new therapy (e.g., for treating migraine or asthma) that decreases the loss of work days, but the HMO may be concerned about an increase in the pharmacy drug budget. Because Medicare's diagnosis-related groups do not include quality-of-life or outcome adjustments, some people have expressed concern that the federal government is allowing budgetary considerations to override the individual patient's desire for improved quality of life and long-term health outcomes.

QUANTITATIVE TOOLS

Health economics brings to the health arena sophistication in the types of quantitative tools that are available to assist health care managers and providers in making decisions for their patients, including:

1. Cost of illness.
2. Cost minimization.

Table 1
Comparison of Evaluation Techniques Regarding Inputs and Outputs

Technique	Inputs	Outputs
Cost of illness	Dollars	N/A
Cost–effectiveness analysis	Dollars	Natural units
Cost–benefit analysis	Dollars	Dollars
Cost–utility analysis	Dollars	Utilities/preferences
Cost–minimization analysis	Dollars	Assumed equal

N/A, not applicable.

3. Cost benefit.
4. Cost-effectiveness.
5. Cost utility *(6)*.

All health economic principles can be framed in the traditional paradigm of comparing inputs vs outputs. The inputs are the resources consumed (i.e., the cost of therapy, health care program, and so on) and the health improvements. The outputs are often effectiveness measures, such as changes in blood pressure (BP) or cholesterol, and utility scales, which are comparisons between healthy states and patient assessments of care. The most difficult step is translating all of this activity into dollars, as is required in cost benefit analysis. Table 1 compares the evaluation techniques and the different sets of inputs and outputs.

Assigning a dollar value to each step in care of a patient can be complicated. There are obvious costs, such as the drug costs, hospital costs, and clinic costs. But what about the costs of patient's waiting time, travel time, or even cholesterol changes? The answer to these questions depends on the health economic methodology chosen.

1. *Cost-of-illness studies* are important because they help policy makers and planners to identify what diseases and health problems should be targeted. These studies are basically cost identification studies that can take place at national or local levels. Cost studies have been performed on most diseases, including asthma, arthritis, depression, CVD, and migraine.
2. *Cost-minimization analysis* compares costs for comparable treatments with the same clinical effectiveness, such as me-too situations. When competing choices have equal effectiveness, the cost-minimization objective is finding the least expensive way to reach an identical endpoint in therapy. Table 2 describes a "me-too" angiotensin-converting enzyme (ACE) analysis in which effectiveness is presumed equal.
3. *Cost–benefit analysis* measures costs and consequences only in dollars. This can be a complex analysis because all outcomes, such as BP changes, must be assigned a dollar value. Table 3 compares different formulas for cost–benefit calculations, and Table 4 provides an example of a cost–benefit analysis.
4. *Cost-effectiveness analysis* measures costs in relation to therapeutic objectives. For example, the benefits of a hypertension medication may be the percentage reduction in diastolic BP. Table 5 illustrates how cost-effectiveness ratios can be used to rank therapies.
5. *Cost–utility analysis* measures costs and therapeutic objects against intervention preferences by the patient. Thus, the total costs of cancer chemotherapeutic agents would be adjusted by the number of years-of-life gained (YLG) and the patient's preference for various health states. Table 6 provides an example of a cost–utility analysis.

Table 2
Cost-Minimization Analysis: Example Applied to Drug Therapy

| | | Cost of therapies ($) | |
		Drug A	Drug B
Costs			
Acquisition cost		250	350
Administration		75	0
Monitoring		75	25
Adverse effects		100	25
	Subtotal	500	400
Outcomes			
Drug effectiveness		90%	90%
	Result = cost of drug A > cost of drug B		

In cost minimization, both interventions (drugs) are considered to be equally effective; and in this example, the cost minimization question is answered by stating that drug B is $100 less than drug A.

Table 3
Sample Comparison Using Three Different Cost–Benefit Equations

	Costs (t1)	Benefits (t1)	1 Cost benefit ratio (B/C)	2 Net present value (B - C)	3 Internal rate of return (B - C) C
A	$10,000	$15,000	1.5:1	$5,000	50%
B	$100,000	$180,000	1.8:1	$80,000	80%

Another limitation is the economic confusion that can surround the terms "direct costs" and "indirect costs." Direct costs are costs that can usually be related to writing a check or monitored by standard health care billing procedures. Direct costs can include hospital or clinic expenses, health professional fees, product costs, and administration overhead. These costs are usually the ones targeted for reductions in health care costs.

Indirect costs are the more intangible factors, such as the days that the patient is too sick to work, an early death that reduces lifelong wage earnings, or even time spent waiting for the doctor. These expenses are usually not measured from hospital bills, yet they can account for as much as 60% of the total costs of an illness. Morbidity, the days lost from work, generally accounts for approx 22%. Premature mortality, which is permanent loss from the work force, is approx 38% (7). These numbers significantly affect total health care costs, yet are not often considered fully in health care debates. In the context of total health expenditures in the United States, we are already spending more than $1 trillion for health care. This nationally reported statistic only represents direct costs. Therefore, if we estimate that this is half of the total cost of illness in the United States, illness in this country would include another $1 trillion in indirect costs from lost productivity and early death, for a total cost of illness of $2 trillion. Health economic

Table 4
Cost–Benefit Analysis: Example Applied to Drug Therapy

		Cost of therapies ($)	
		Drug A	Drug B
Costs			
Acquisition cost		300	400
Administration		50	0
Monitoring		50	0
Adverse effects		100	0
	Subtotal	500	400
Benefits			
Days at work ($)		1000	1000
Extra months of life ($)		2000	3000
	Subtotal ($)	3000	4000
Benefit–cost ratio:		3000/500	4000/400
		= 6:1	= 10:1

Table 5
Cost–Effectiveness Analysis: Example Applied to Drug Therapy

		Cost of therapies ($)	
		Drug A	Drug B
Costs			
Acquisition cost		300	400
Administration		50	0
Monitoring		50	0
Adverse effects		100	0
	Subtotal	500	400
Outputs			
Extra years of life		1.5	1.6
Cost–effectiveness ratio:		500/1.5	400/1.6
		= $333	= $250
		per extra year of life	

analysis allows us to evaluate the impact of new health interventions, as illustrated in Figure 1. The point illustrated in this circle is that we want to develop health interventions that decrease the total costs of illness, even if the direct expenditures may have to increase. For example, we could certainly reduce the direct costs of care if we denied paying for polio vaccine, but we certainly would risk dramatic increases in indirect and, thus, total, costs of illness.

HEALTH ECONOMICS AND OUTCOME MANAGEMENT

Health economics is a central component of the outcomes model. As in continuous quality improvement, the health economic outcomes model is a continuous process with six recursive steps:

Table 6
Cost-Utility Analysis: Example Applied to Drug Therapy

		Cost of therapies ($)	
		Drug A	Drug B
Costs			
Acquisition cost		300	400
Administration		50	0
Monitoring		50	0
Adverse effects		100	0
	Subtotal	500	400
Utilities			
Extra years of life		1.5	1.6
Quality of life		.33	.25
QALYs[a]		0.50	0.40
Cost-utility ratio:		500/0.5	400/0.4
		= $1000	= $1000
		per extra quality of life year	

[a]QALYs, quality-adjusted life years.

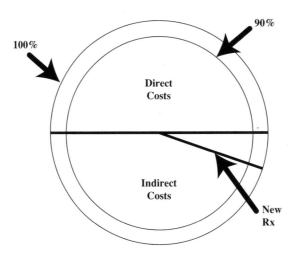

Fig. 1. Direct and indirect costs of illness; consideration of new therapy costs. An increase in direct costs with new therapy (Rx) may decrease indirect costs and total costs.

1. Setting outcome goals, with treatment protocols and standards.
2. Designing clinical and economics evaluations that are implemented through randomized control trials, postmarketing epidemiology, or individual patient monitoring.
3. Implementing the interventions.
4 Measuring (collecting data on) the patients' clinical and economic outcomes.
5. Analyzing the outcomes data.
6. The final continuous, recursive step is translating these analyses and feedback into improved procedures, protocols, and guidelines.

In a health economic outcomes program, the inputs and outcomes are illustrated as follows:

1. Specific input parameters.
    a. Acquisition costs.
    b. Efficacy.
    c. Side effects.
    d. Compliance.
    e. Administration costs.
    f. Acquisition costs.
    g. Monitoring costs.
2. Outcome parameters: impact on total system.
    a. Changes in cost of illness.
    b. Potential increases in productivity.
    c. Improved quality of life.
    d. Other outcomes.

GENERAL STEPS IN A HEALTH ECONOMIC STUDY

In evaluating or planning a health economic study, there are several steps that should be addressed in the specific health economic methodology (e.g., cost-effectiveness vs cost benefit).

To illustrate this, the steps associated with cost-effectiveness analysis are listed as follows:

Step 1. Before incorporating health economic evaluations into any research project, the investigator must first establish the *perspective* from which to evaluate the various costs, benefits, and outcomes. That is, will the costs and consequences be those of society, specific patients, a third-party payer, HMO, or hospital? Depending on whose perspective is taken, the results may vary greatly.

Step 2. Describe/specify the *treatment alternatives*. The alternatives included in a health economic evaluation should be those acceptable to the patient and practitioners. The competing alternatives should be dosed at comparable levels.

Step 3. For each treatment alternative, specify the *possible outcomes* (i.e., patient pathways) and their probabilities. This can be retrospective, using information from clinical studies, medical literature, and/or expert panels. It can also be a product of a current clinical trial. The pathways can often be clearly presented in the form of decision trees or similar diagrams.

Step 4. Specify and monitor the *health care resources* that are consumed in each pathway. Resources include: drugs, physician services, hospital "hotel," and ancillary services, lab tests, and so on. This can be performed retrospectively or concurrently with a clinical trial. If this is performed retrospectively, each patient pathway is described in terms of the health care resources that are likely to be consumed. If concurrent with a clinical trial, the "artificial" use of services—required by the trial's protocol—must be considered. The perspective of the study (e.g., insurer, hospital, society) affects the resources that are included in a study. For instance, a diagnosis-related group-paid hospital is not concerned with the increased intensity of nursing home care that may be associated with shorter hospital stays.

Step 5. Assign *dollar values* to the resources consumed. Dollar values are assigned to each resource. In drug studies, hospital services require special attention because of their

relative magnitude. Also, drug prices need to be selected carefully because of their availability.

Step 6. Specify and monitor *non-health care resources* consumed in each pathway. Generally, this is not a concern in drug studies. Often these resources, such as the economic impact a patient's treatment has on the family, are difficult to measure. The resources should be estimated, or at least noted and brought into discussion as a caveat when reporting the results of the study. The qualitative endpoints can support the quantitative analysis.

Step 7 Specify the unit of *effectiveness*. The appropriate unit depends on the disease/ condition and the results of treatment. Some possibilities are patient lives saved, YLG, or reduction in morbidity attributed to the disease (these data are derived from the clinical portion of the trial).

Step 8. Specify other *noneconomic attributes* of the alternatives (e.g., pain or side effects). These may be difficult to quantify and may lead to using quality-of-life determination and cost–utility analysis.

Step 9. Analyze the data using the appropriate health economic *methodology* (e.g., cost-effectiveness analysis, cost-minimization analysis). The appropriate analysis will be determined by how the study was set up, the perspective, and the type and quality of the data gathered.

Step 10. Conduct a *sensitivity analysis*. Ratios are recalculated, using different values for those items not known with certainty. Sensitivity analysis essentially defines a range of confidence for the results of the study.

CHALLENGES AND OPPORTUNITIES

There are many challenges that we must face in the future, including:

1. Dealing with health care reform.
2. Supporting research on new drugs and paying for appropriate use of new or unapproved uses of current drugs.
3. Including individual patient variation and patient preferences into drug protocols.

The standard tools for health economic analyses make it possible to ask basic questions such as "how much does illness cost in my organization" and "what is the most cost-beneficial way to treat the illness?" Final, conclusive answers, however, can be difficult to find because there is a need for continuing data collection on the cost of treating many illnesses, especially when new drugs or procedures affect older therapies. We need further economic research on how to account for factors such as stress on the family, home health care intervention, life extension based on quality-of-life years, and so on.

This section of the chapter provided a general overview of health economic analyses in health care. In the following sections, we review the economic factors in the treatment or prevention of selected cardiovascular conditions.

ECONOMIC CONSIDERATIONS IN COMMON CARDIOVASCULAR CONDITIONS

Economic evaluations of cardiovascular treatment programs have used the variety of analytic methods discussed in the preceding section. Comparison of the costs and effectiveness of one treatment relative to another can help decision makers determine the appropriate allocation of scarce resources. Numerous pharmacoeconomic evaluations of

cardiovascular treatments have been conducted during the past 20 yr. Some of the more recent and relevant examples are summarized next. Although this is not an exhaustive review, it provides the reader with insight into the previous research conducted.

MYOCARDIAL INFARCTION: THROMBOLYTIC THERAPY

Myocardial infarction (MI) occurs in more than 1 million persons per year in the United States, with approximately one-third of the victims dying. More than 250,000 of these deaths occur before the patient reaches the hospital, within 1 h of the onset of symptoms *(4,5)*. An estimated 4 million people across the globe die each year from MI *(8)*.

MI imposes a substantial economic burden on the US health care system. The costs (in 1993 dollars) of treating an acute MI range from $14,470 to $31,397 for a patient who dies soon after the event, according to a 1995 report issued by the Office of Technology Assessment. The figure escalates to $74,217 (at a 5% discount rate) for a patient who survives for 5 yr *(9,10)*.

The high death rate from acute MI plus the substantial treatment costs incurred even among patients who expire leads to consideration of the acceptable costs to prevent death in some of these patients. In theory, no cost is too great to save a life, but, in practice, finite resources dictate that limits must be set. The decision to use or to not use a new or expensive treatment regimen is often made by comparing the costs per YLG or the costs per quality-adjusted YLG (QALY) for the new treatment to that of currently accepted standards of treatment. An arbitrary upper limit of acceptable expenditure may be set based on community standards. There is no absolute standard for acceptable treatment costs, because ability and willingness to pay will vary depending on wealth as well as cultural factors. Expert opinion is that health care interventions that cost less than $20,000/QALY are acceptable, whereas interventions with costs that exceed $100,000/QALY are inappropriate *(8)*. It is in this context of acceptable costs per YLG that economic analyses of treatments for acute MI must be viewed.

Treatment of acute MI includes reperfusion techniques, such as percutaneous transluminal coronary angioplasty, coronary artery bypass graft, and intravenous thrombolytic therapy, with agents such as streptokinase, alteplase (recombinant tissue plasminogen activator [rt-PA]), anistreplase, reteplase, and saruplase. Thrombolysis has become the treatment of choice for eligible patients *(8)*. Clinical trials have demonstrated the survival benefit of thrombolysis, which has been shown to result in an 18% proportional reduction in mortality if the thrombolytic agent is administered within 24 h of the infarct *(11)*. The least expensive of the thrombolytic drugs is streptokinase, which was the first thrombolytic agent to be widely used in MI.

Pharmacoeconomic studies have shown thrombolytic therapy with streptokinase to be cost-effective for the treatment of acute MI in a number of circumstances. Early computer models of thrombolytic cost-effectiveness suggested that the routine administration of either streptokinase or rt-PA was likely to increase the volume of coronary angioplasty and coronary artery bypass surgeries performed in the United States *(12)*.

However, subsequent studies did not find this to be an economic disincentive to thrombolysis. Simoons et al. *(13)* studied 533 patients from the Netherlands Interuniversity Trial of Streptokinase and concluded that thrombolysis improved survival after MI without substantially increasing the need for other costly revascularization procedures, such as coronary artery bypass graft or percutaneous transluminal coronary angioplasty. A

lack of consensus among cardiologists regarding the benefits of streptokinase for older patients prompted a 1992 investigation by Krumholz et al. *(14)*. Pooled clinical data from trials in elderly patients indicated that administration of streptokinase within 6 h of symptom onset would reduce mortality by 13%. Using a decision analytic model, the authors estimated that the cost of streptokinase treatment for an 80-yr-old patient would be $21,200 per year-of-life saved (YLS), whereas the cost of treating a 70-yr-old would be $21,600 per YLS. Both figures are less than an arbitrary cost-effectiveness cutoff point of $55,000 per YLS *(14)*.

The value of streptokinase therapy may depend on the site of the infarct. Midgette et al. *(15)* investigated the effects of infarct location on the cost-effectiveness of streptokinase for acute MI. The authors combined a meta-analysis of short-term survival data from clinical trials of streptokinase with a simple decision-tree model. They determined that the marginal cost-effectiveness (dollars per life saved) of thrombolytic therapy varies depending on the infarct site. For definitively diagnosed acute MI, the cost per life saved was calculated to be $9900, $56,600, and $28,400, respectively, for anterior, inferior, and other infarcts. The marginal costs increased as the diagnosis of acute MI became less certain, approaching $132,000 per life saved when the probability of an inferior infarct was 50%. Nevertheless, the authors concluded that given a societal willingness to pay of $250,000 per life saved, streptokinase therapy should be administered in most cases of suspected acute MI *(15)*.

The cost-effectiveness of thrombolysis with rt-PA was evaluated by Levin and Jonsson *(16)*, who analyzed data from 314 patients in the Anglo-Scandinavian Study of Early Thrombolysis trial. Although the direct plus indirect cost for the rt-PA patient group was 8% higher (5700 Swedish kroner) than that of the placebo group, the 12-mo survival rate for the rt-PA patients was 7.1% higher. The authors concluded that the cost-effectiveness of thrombolysis treatment is high compared with other treatments for CHD, because of the benefit of increased survival *(16)*.

The use of rt-PA rather than streptokinase increases the cost of thrombolytic therapy, because the acquisition cost of rt-PA may be 5 to 15 times greater than that of streptokinase *(8)*. An important recent evaluation of the comparative cost-effectiveness of streptokinase and rt-PA was conducted by Mark et al. *(17)*, using data from the Global Utilization of Streptokinase and Tissue Plasminogen Activator for Occluded Coronary Arteries (GUSTO) study. The 41,021-patient GUSTO study found a statistically significant relative decrease of 15% and an absolute decrease of 1% in 30-d mortality among patients treated with an accelerated rt-PA regimen (administration of the drug during a period of 1.5 h rather than the conventional 3-h administration) compared with patients treated with streptokinase. The investigators concluded that the $32,678 extra cost per YLS by the use of rt-PA was in line with the costs of other routine therapies, including coronary bypass surgery. The use of rt-PA rather than streptokinase was shown to produce 1 extra disabling stroke per 1000 patients treated. When the increased risk of stroke was considered, the cost per YLS increased from $32,538 to $42,400, depending on assumptions for the level of poststroke care. These figures were still below the investigators' $50,000 per YLS benchmark for cost-effectiveness. Although the routine substitution of rt-PA for streptokinase would cost the US health care system almost $500 million per year, the authors calculated that this substitution would also offer an additional 3.5 million yr of life for MI patients *(17)*.

In reviewing the GUSTO cost-effectiveness study, Gillis and Goa *(8)* noted that the added costs of rt-PA may be a decision factor for some hospital formularies. Furthermore, Stanek et al. *(18)* determined that rt-PA was preferred by potential patients when there was a zero-cost assumption, but that potential patients' preference shifted toward streptokinase when they were asked to pay for the drug themselves *(18)*.

PRIMARY AND SECONDARY PREVENTION: CHOLESTEROL AND LIPID REDUCTION

Pooled data from studies of secondary prevention of ischemic heart disease and CHD suggest that each 1% reduction in serum cholesterol levels results in a 1.9% reduction in recurrent CHD events. Early studies of the cost-effectiveness of cholesterol-lowering agents focused on the drugs cholestyramine and colestipol. In general, the studies reported that these cholesterol-lowering drugs were less cost-effective than other common treatment regimens. For example, a 1988 study by Kinosian and Eisenberg reported that cholestyramine and colestipol cost more than $60,000, per YLS except when used by smokers, for whom costs were only $51,500 per YLS *(19)*. However, the newer statin drugs (hydroxymethylglutaryl (HMG)–coenzyme A (CoA) reductase inhibitors) have been shown to be much more cost-effective. A review of treatment costs in the British National Health Service demonstrated that annual costs per 10% drop in cholesterol levels were more than three times lower for simvastatin or pravastatin compared with cholestyramine *(20)*.

Several large-scale, placebo-controlled trials have demonstrated the survival benefit of the statins. These studies demonstrated the need for further research on morbidity and mortality outcomes, not just clinical endpoints such as low-density lipoprotein reduction. The Scandinavian Simvastatin Survival Study, conducted in 1987, was designed to test whether lipid-lowering therapy could decrease mortality in coronary artery disease. This landmark study demonstrated the true outcome associated with this therapy was not just lowering the amount of cholesterol in the blood but also impacted mortality and morbidity *(21)*.

The West of Scotland Coronary Prevention Study was conducted using pravastatin to investigate the effectiveness of the drug in preventing coronary events in men with moderate hypercholesterolemia and no history of MI. Results of this trial among 6595 subjects showed that pravastatin reduced the risk of fatal and nonfatal coronary events by approx 30% compared with placebo. In addition, the need for coronary angiography and revascularization procedures was significantly lower among men who received pravastatin. There were no excess deaths from noncardiovascular causes among the pravastatin patients *(22)*.

Goldman et al. evaluated the cost-effectiveness of HMG-CoA reductase inhibitors in the primary and secondary prevention of CHD. Using a computer simulation called The Coronary Heart Disease Policy Model, the authors estimated the risk-specific incidence of heart disease and the risk of recurrent coronary events in persons with preexisting coronary disease. The Coronary Heart Disease Policy Model takes the perspective of society as a whole, rather than that of the individual patient. The model was used to estimate the costs and effectiveness of the HMG-CoA reductase inhibitor, lovastatin, among specific subsets of the population. Lovastatin at a 20 mg per day dose was demonstrated to be cost-effective for secondary prevention of CHD among patients with

moderate or severe hypercholesterolemia, with costs (1989 dollars) below $20,000 per YLS for men and women of all ages. Increasing the dosage to 40 mg per day added costs ranging from $8600 to $38,000 for men, and $29,000 to $49,000 for women. Increasing the dosage to 80 mg per day added incremental costs of more than $70,000 per YLS. For men with cholesterol levels below 250 mg/dL, the costs for 20 mg lovastatin were calculated to range from $16,000 to $38,000 per YLS. The secondary prevention costs for women with the same pretreatment cholesterol levels ranged from $23,000 per YLS for women 75 to 84 yr of age, to $210,000 per YLS for women 35 to 44 yr of age. The use of lovastatin for primary prevention was cost-effective only for selected groups, such as men aged 35–44 who also had hypertension, smoked, and were more than 13% above ideal weight. In general, the lovastatin study indicated that cost-effectiveness of drug therapy was higher for men, older patients, and patients with higher risk of CHD. Additional morbidity/mortality studies have been conducted or are in progress with other statins (fluvastatin, simvastatin, atorvastatin, and rosuvastatin). All economic analyses of the statins have shown that appropriate use translates to economic savings *(23)*.

HYPERTENSION

Hypertension is the most common cardiovascular condition in the United States, afflicting an estimated 50 million persons *(1–5)*. The AHA estimates that the total direct costs plus indirect costs for the treatment of hypertension in the United States exceeds $33 billion per year *(1–5)*. Hypertension medication accounts for up to 81% of direct costs by the third year of treatment *(24)*. Hypertension is a notable risk factor for the development of a number of diseases. A 15-yr follow-up of the nearly 350,000 men in the Multiple Risk Factor Intervention Trial demonstrated that the relative risk of stroke mortality among men with stage 4 hypertension is more than 18 times the risk of men with optimal BP *(25)*. Hypertension also contributes to the development of CHD, with relative risks of CHD mortality 6.9 times higher for men with stage 4 hypertension than for men with optimal BP. The major cause of the development of congestive heart failure (CHF) is hypertension, according to the Framingham Heart Study *(26)*. Meta-analysis of hypertension treatment trials demonstrated that treatment of hypertension reduces the incidence of CHF by 52% *(27)*. Meta-analysis also demonstrated a positive impact on stroke mortality, with the risk of fatal stroke reduced by 45% with the treatment of hypertension *(28)*. Epidemiological studies show that a 35 to 40% decline in stroke risk was associated with lowering diastolic BP by 5 to 6 mmHg. The risk of CHD fell by 20 to 25% for the same decrease in BP *(29)*.

Modern economic analysis of hypertension treatment began with Weinstein and Stason's 1976 study *(30)*, which evaluated the costs of treatment per QALY. The model developed by Weinstein and Stason indicated that hypertension treatment is more cost-effective with increasing age and with higher pretreatment BP levels. Although some of the assumptions used by Weinstein and Stason have been shown to be in error, the analysis is still considered to be among the best in the field *(31)*. Edelson and colleagues *(32)* estimated that one-third of the US population has hypertension. The authors evaluated the cost-effectiveness of hypertension treatment using the Coronary Heart Disease Policy Model, which is a computer simulation of overall mortality, morbidity, and cost of CHD in the US population. Estimated antihypertensive and anticholesterol effects of various antihypertensive regimens were derived from a meta-analysis of 153 reports in a literature search for studies that met prospectively determined criteria. Cost of medi-

cation was estimated from average wholesale price (plus 10% markup and $2 pharmacy fee/100 units) in the 1987 *Redbook (33)*. A 5% yearly discount rate was used. For 20 yr of simulated therapy from 1990 through 2010, the cost per YLS was projected to be $10,900 for propranolol HCL, $16,400 for hydrochlorothiazide, $31,600 for nifedipine, $61,900 for prazocin HCL, and $72,100 for captopril. Propranolol was the preferred initial option under most assumptions in this study *(32)*.

Several recent studies have investigated the cost-effectiveness of drug treatment for hypertension. The cost-effectiveness of hypertension treatment seems to be highly sensitive to the price of the medications *(34)*. In general, the older, less-expensive drugs, such as diuretics and β-blockers were found to be more cost-effective. As in the study by Edelson *(32)*, ACE inhibitors and other newer drug products are more costly and, therefore, were usually found to be less cost-effective. For example, Pearce and associates *(35)* calculated the cost-effectiveness of antihypertensives in the prevention of MI, stroke, or death. Drug acquisition costs to prevent one major adverse event in middle-aged patients ranged from $4730 for the diuretic, hydrochlorothiazide, to $346,236 for nifedipine gastrointestinal therapeutic system, a calcium-channel blocker. Enalapril, an ACE inhibitor, cost $156,520 for prevention of one major adverse event *(35)*. Hoerger et al. *(34)* found that a combination of hydrochlorothiazide and bisoprolol, a β-blocker, was more cost-effective than amlodipine, a calcium-channel blocker, or enalapril. It was estimated that the acquisition cost *(33)* of enalapril would have to decrease by 57.9%, and that of amlodipine by 50.9%, to equal the cost-effectiveness of the hydrochlorothiazide/ bisoprolol combination. Similarly, Griebenow et al. *(36)* found a 50% difference in cost per mmHg BP reduction for a combination of reserpine and clopamide vs enalapril. Cost-effectiveness of antihypertensive medication is also influenced by patient age. For example, in the Pearce *(35)* study, the cost of preventing one adverse event in the elderly was only $1595 with hydrochlorothiazide and $52,780 with enalapril. Johannesson *(37)*, in a review of 19 hypertension cost-effectiveness trials, demonstrated by regression analysis that the average cost per YLG for men with a diastolic BP of 95 decreased from $83,333 at age 40 to $5000 at 70 yr of age. Costs for women were slightly higher, declining from $85,000 at age 40 to $8333 at 70 yr of age. Schueler *(38)* reviewed the cost-effectiveness literature for hypertension and concluded that a treatment approach characterized by therapeutic restraint is warranted. Therapeutic restraint implies the use of less expensive medications, initiated at older ages and only after high diastolic BPs are measured. Under the assumptions of therapeutic restraint, the use of diuretics alone or with β-blockers is recommended as initial therapy for hypertension. It must be noted, however, that the conditions of daily practice may not match the ideal conditions of a clinical trial. A medication that the patient does not take will not be cost-effective, no matter how inexpensive the drug. Compliance with therapeutic recommendations is an issue in the treatment of hypertension, which is usually an asymptomatic disorder. A medication or treatment regimen that is not tolerable to the patient, perhaps because of side effects or inconvenience, may be discontinued or used suboptimally, leading to reduced effectiveness. Rizzo and colleagues performed multivariate analysis of compliance with ACE inhibitors, calcium antagonists, β-blockers, and diuretics.

They found that higher rates of compliance were associated with ACE inhibitors and calcium antagonists. Poor compliance was associated with higher health care costs *(39)*. Clinicians' choice of antihypertensive therapy must be guided, therefore, not only by drug acquisition cost but also by patient preferences and individual needs.

CONGESTIVE HEART FAILURE

CHF is the leading diagnosis among older adults who are hospitalized in the United States, afflicting almost 5 million Americans *(40)*. Approximately 400,000 patients are diagnosed with CHF each year *(41)*, and more than 46,000 annual deaths may be attributed to the disorder *(40)*. Annual costs for the treatment of CHF in the United States exceed $10 billion *(42)*. Mortality from CHF averages 50% during 5 yr, with an annual death rate of 10% *(42)*. Despite progress in treatment, the mortality of CHF remains high, although recent analyses suggest that the yearly age-adjusted death rates are dropping among patients 65 yr of age and older. Although the age-adjusted death rates for CHF increased throughout most of the 1980s, the period from 1988 to 1995 showed a 1.1% average annual decline in deaths caused by CHF among Americans older than 65 yr of age *(40)*. Experts at the Centers for Disease Control and Prevention suggest that this improvement may be caused by new treatment strategies and earlier detection of heart disease or its precursors, such as hypertension. However, the incidence and prevalence of heart failure is likely to grow as the population ages. Aging of the cardiovascular system, hypertension, coronary artery disease, and valvular heart disease are more prevalent among adults older than 65 yr of age, leading to an increased incidence of heart failure in this age group *(43)*. Moreover, a 1982 follow-up of the Framingham Study showed that the incidence of heart failure more than doubled every 10 yr for persons between the ages of 45 and 75 yr *(44)*. As a result of growth in the population of older Americans, the total death toll from CHF is expected to continue to increase *(40)*.

CHF is most often a consequence of the several conditions discussed in the previous sections of this chapter including hypertension, MI, and dyslipidemia. Hypertension is the leading cause of CHF in the United States *(27)*. Treatment of hypertension reduces the incidence of heart failure by 52% *(28)*. MI is the second major cause of CHF *(45)*. The economics of therapies for the prevention of CHF are, therefore, identical to the economics of therapies for the prevention and control of the major risk factors for CHF, hypertension, and MI. Although drug therapy is the mainstay of CHF treatment, nondrug interventions, including surgical options, nursing interventions, and implantable cardiac devices, are also used. Heart transplantation is indicated for adults with life-threatening CHF that has not responded adequately to more conservative treatment. The AHA reported that approx 40,000 Americans age 65 yr or younger could benefit from a heart transplant in a given year, but that only 2290 of these procedures were actually performed in 1997. Aravot and associates *(46)* investigated the impact of heart transplantation on patients 60 yr of age or older. Quality of life was evaluated using the Nottingham Health Profile, a validated, generic quality-of-life instrument. At 1 yr after transplantation, 84% of the patients (21 of 25 patients) were still alive, and quality of life among the survivors was improved compared with pretransplant levels *(46)*. A 1986 study by Evans calculated the cost-effectiveness for heart transplantation as $23,500 per YLS, a figure that compares favorably with other major medical–surgical interventions *(47)*.

CONCLUSION

The impact of CVD can be measured in economic and noneconomic terms. The direct and indirect costs associated with CVD are very high. Physicians need to balance these costs when making treatment decisions. The efficacy of these treatment alternatives may need to be balanced by the economic outcomes. This chapter discussed the various economic approaches used to measure the health economic impact of treatment choices.

Cost-effectiveness is the most widely used method to balance the inputs (costs) and outputs (outcomes) of these choices. Applying these techniques can assist the clinician in making more efficient use of the limited health care resources.

The second part of this chapter presented a review of the economic analyses of several CVDs. The objective is to introduce the previous research as the beginning of the quest for more efficient clinical decisions. As the population ages and the cost of health care increases, the clinician in all practice settings needs to understand the balance between effectiveness and cost-effectiveness to make the difficult treatment decisions required in this environment.

REFERENCES

1. American Heart Association. Cardiovascular Disease Statistics. In: Science and Professional Statistics. http:\\www.americanheart.org., 1999.
2. National Center for Health Statistics. Highlights of a new report from the National Center for Health Statistics (NCHS). Monitoring Health Care in America. Quarterly Report, March 1996.
3. American Heart Association. Cardiovascular Diseases. http:\\www.americanheart.org., 1999.
4. American Heart Association. Economic Cost of Cardiovascular Diseases. http:\\www.american heart.org., 1999.
5. American Heart Association. Heart Transplants and Statistics. http:\\www.americanheart.org., 1999.
6. Bootman JL, Townsend RJ, McGhan WF. Principles of Pharmacoeconomics, 2nd ed. Harvey Whitney Books, Cincinnati, OH, 1996.
7. Rice DP. Cost of illness studies: fact or fiction. Lancet 1994;344;1519–1520.
8. Gillis JC, Goa KL. Streptokinase: a pharmacoeconomic appraisal of its use in the management of acute myocardial infarction. Pharmacoeconomics 1996;10(3):281–310.
9. US Congress, Office of Technology Assessment, Effectiveness and Costs of Osteoporosis Screening and Hormone Replacement Therapy, Volume I: Cost Effectiveness Analysis, OTA-BP-H-160, US Government Printing Office, Washington, DC, August, 1995.
10. US Congress, Office of Technology Assessment, Effectiveness and Costs of Osteoporosis Screening and Hormone Replacement Therapy, Volume II: Evidence on Benefits, Risks, and Costs, OTA-BP-H-144, US Government Printing Office, Washington, DC, August 1995.
11. Fibrinolytic Therapy Trialists (FTT) Collaborative Group. Indications for fibrinolytic therapy in suspected acute myocardial infarction: collaborative review of early mortality and major morbidity from all randomized trials of more than 1000 patients. Lancet 1994;343:311–322.
12. Steinberg EP, Topol EJ, Sakin JW, et al. Cost and procedure implications for thrombolytic therapy for acute myocardial infarction. J Am Coll Cardiol 1988;12(6):58A–68A.
13. Simoons ML, Vos J, Martens LL. Cost–utility analysis of thrombolytic therapy. Eur Heart J 1991;12: 694–699.
14. Krumholz HM, Pasternak RC, Weinstein MC, et al. Cost effectiveness of thrombolytic therapy with streptokinase in elderly patients with suspected acute myocardial infarction. N Engl J Med 1992;327(1):7–13.
15. Midgette AS, Wong JB, Beshansky JR, et al. Cost-effectiveness of streptokinase for acute myocardial infarction: a combined meta-analysis and decision analysis of the effects of infarct location and of likelihood of infarction. Medical Decision Making 1994;14(2):108–117.
16. Levin LA, Jonsson B. Cost-effectiveness of thrombolysis—a randomized study of intravenous rt-PA in suspected myocardial infarction. Eur Heart J 1992;13:2–8.
17. Mark DB, Hlatky MA, Califf RM, et al. Cost effectiveness of thrombolytic therapy with tissue plasminogen activator as compared with streptokinase for acute myocardial infarction. N Engl J Med 1995;332(21):1418–1424.
18. Stanek EJ, Cheng JW, Peeples PJ, et al. Patient preferences for thrombolytic therapy in acute myocardial infarction. Medical Decision Making 1997;17(4):464–471.
19. Kinosian BP, Eisenberg JM. Cutting into cholesterol: cost-effective alternatives for treating hypercholesterolemia. JAMA 1988;259:2249–2254.
20. Reckless JPD. Cost-effectiveness of hypolidaemic drugs. Postgrad Med J 1993;69(Suppl 1):S30–S33.
21. Pederson TR. Coronary artery disease: The Scandinavian Simvastatin Survival Study experience. Am J Cardiol 1998;82(10B):55T–56T.

22. Shepherd J, Cobbe SM, Ford I, et al. Prevention of coronary heart disease with pravastatin in men with hypercholesterolemia. N Engl J Med 1995;333:1301–1307.
23. Hay JW, Yu WM, Ashraf T. Pharmacoeconomics of lipid-lowering agents for primary and secondary prevention of coronary artery disease. Pharmacoeconomics 1999;15(1):47–74.
24. Odell TW, Gregory MC. Cost of hypertension treatment. J Gen Intern Med 1995;10(12):686–688.
25. Stamler J. The INTERSALT study: background, methods, findings and implications. Am J Clin Nutr 1997;65(2 Suppl):626S–642S.
26. Kannel WB, Castelli WP, McNamara PM, et al. Role of blood pressure in the development of congestive heart failure: the Framingham Study. N Engl J Med 1972;287(16):781–787.
27. Moser M, Herbert PR. Prevention of disease progression, left ventricular hypertrophy and congestive heart failure in hypertension treatment trials. J Am Coll Cardiol 1996;27(5):1214–1218.
28. Collins R, Peto R, MacMahon S, et al. Blood pressure, stroke, and coronary heart disease. Part 2. Short term reductions in blood pressure: overview of randomised drug trials in their epidemiological context. Lancet 1990;335(8693):827–838.
29. MacMahon S, Peto R, Cutler J, et al. Blood pressure, stroke, and coronary heart disease. Part 1. Prolonged differences in blood pressure: prospective observational studies corrected for the regression dilution bias. Lancet 1990;335(8692):765–774.
30. Weinstein MC, Stason WB. Hypertension: A Policy Perspective. Harvard University Press, Cambridge, MA, 1976.
31. Johannesson M, Jonsson B. A review of cost-effectiveness analyses of hypertension treatment. Pharmacoeconomics 1992;1(4):250–264.
32. Edelson JT, Weinstein MC, Tosteson ANA, et al. Long-term cost-effectiveness of various initial monotherapies for mild to moderate hypertension. JAMA 1990;263(3):407–413.
33. Redbook, vol. 6. Montvale, NJ, Medical Economics Company, 1987.
34. Hoerger TJ, Bala MV, Eggleston JL, et al. A comparative cost-effectiveness study of three drugs for the treatment of mild-to-moderate hypertension. P&T 1998;23(5):245–267.
35. Pearce KA, Furberg CD, Psaty BM, Kirk J. Cost-minimization and the number needed to treat in uncomplicated hypertension. Am J Hypertens 1998;11(5):618–629.
36. Griebenow R, Pittrow DB, Weidinger G, et al. Low-dose reserpine/thiazide combination in first-line treatment of hypertension: efficacy and safety compared to an ACE inhibitor. Blood Pressure 1997;6(5):299–306.
37. Johannesson M. The impact of age on the cost-effectiveness of hypertension treatment: an analysis of randomized drug trials. Medical Decision Making 1994;14(3):236–244.
38. Schueler K. Cost-effectiveness issues in hypertension control. Can J Public Health 1994;85(Suppl 2):S54–S56.
39. Rizzo JA, Simons WR. Variations in compliance among hypertensive patients by drug class: implications for health care costs. Clin Ther 1997;19(6):1446–1457.
40. Centers for Disease Control and Prevention. Changes in mortality from heart failure—United States, 1980–1995. MMWR 1998;47:633–637.
41. Patterson JH, Adams KF. Pathophysiology of heart failure. Pharmacotherapy 1993;13:73S–81S.
42. Konstam MA, Dracup K, Baker DW, et al. Heart failure: evaluation and care of patients with left-ventricular systolic dysfunction. Clinical Practice Guideline No. 11. AHCPR Publication No. 94-0612. Rockville, MD: Agency for Health Care Policy and Research, Public Health Service, US Department of Health and Human Services, June 1994.
43. Rich MW. Epidemiology, pathophysiology, and etiology of congestive heart failure in older adults. J Am Geriatr Soc 1997;45(8):968–974.
44. Kannel WB, Savage D, Castelli WP. Cardiac failure in the Framingham Study: twenty-year follow up. In: Braunwald E, Mock MB, Watson JT, eds. Congestive Heart Failure: Current Research and Clinical Applications. Grune & Stratton, New York, 1982, pp. 15–30.
45. Vasan RS, Levy D. The role of hypertension in the pathogenesis of heart failure. A clinical mechanistic overview. Arch Intern Med 1996;156(16):1789–1796.
46. Aravot DJ, Banner NR, Khaghani A, et al. Cardiac transplantation in the seventh decade of life. Am J Cardiol 1989;63(1):90–93.
47. Evans RW. Cost-effectiveness analysis of transplantation. Surg Clin North Am 1986;66:503–517.

17 Innovative Models for the Delivery of Preventive Cardiovascular Care

Joseph P. Frolkis, MD, PhD, FACP

CONTENTS

INTRODUCTION
BACKGROUND
RATIONALE
CONCLUSION
REFERENCES

INTRODUCTION

Our increasingly sophisticated understanding regarding the epidemiology, pathophysiology, and treatment of cardiovascular disease (CVD) has only served to underscore the continuing need for primary and secondary prevention efforts. Many of these insights have been incorporated into updated practice guidelines. At the same time, however, there is little evidence that the "treatment gap"—the troubling disparity between such endorsed guidelines and actual clinical practice—has narrowed. This is particularly true in ambulatory settings, and in clinical encounters in which a solo physician is the source of preventive services. The resulting need to translate research into practice for more effective CVD prevention is undiminished, as is the opportunity to develop innovative models for such care.

BACKGROUND

CVD Epidemiology

Approximately 1 million deaths yearly are attributable to CVD, making it the leading cause of mortality in the United States *(1,2)*. Coronary heart disease (CHD) causes more than half of all CVD deaths, making it alone the overall national leader in mortality *(1,3)*. Although only 13% of women identify this fact correctly, CVD (and CHD specifically) is also the leading cause of death in women, and more women have succumbed to CVD than men since 1984. *(4)*. Similarly, CVD generally, and CHD specifically, is the primary killer of people older than 65 yr; most new CHD events and 85% of CHD deaths occur

From: *Contemporary Cardiology: Preventive Cardiology:*
Insights Into the Prevention and Treatment of Cardiovascular Disease, Second Edition
Edited by: J. M. Foody © Humana Press Inc., Totowa, NJ

in this cohort *(1,5)*. Because the proportion of the US population older than 65 yr is expected to grow from 12% currently to 20% by 2030, the public health implications are obvious and sobering.

In addition to mortality, of course, CVD imposes a terrible of burden of suffering on those who survive, including the loss of normal ventricular function in half of those with a history of myocardial infarction (MI) *(6)*, and significant functional impairment in many of the 4 million survivors of stroke *(7)*. This sobering human cost is accompanied by a staggering financial one, with current estimates of combined direct and indirect annual CVD expenses approaching $400 billion *(1,8)*.

Recent epidemiological trends in CVD have important implications for the future of preventive cardiology. There has been a marked decrease in age-adjusted mortality rates for both CHD and stroke in the United States during the last 30 yr *(3)*, probably as a result of decreased levels of serum cholesterol *(9)*, blood pressure *(10)*, and cigarette smoking *(11)*. Improved survival rates for initial MI and more-effective secondary prevention in those who have experienced an initial event also contribute to this trend *(12)*. These improved survival rates, however, combined with the increasing prevalence of CVD with age and the concurrent rise in the percentage of the population that is elderly, have produced a paradoxical *increase* in the overall prevalence of CVD, which is projected to continue into the next century *(13)*. Thus, the population at risk for both initial and recurrent CVD events, and therefore likely to benefit from aggressive risk factor control, will increase in the future.

These population trends have been accompanied by a growing understanding of the epidemiological behavior of the risk factors for CVD. It is now appreciated, for instance, that CVD is unlikely to occur when a patient has only a single risk factor. Much more commonly, two or more such factors co-occur in a given patient *(2,14,15)*. The presence of multiple CVD risk factors significantly increases the relative and absolute risks of CVD and CHD in both men and women *(16)*, and it has become apparent that risk factors are at least additive, and probably synergistic, in their effects *(17,18)*. Such findings clarify the multifactorial nature of CVD, and underscore the importance of simultaneously assessing all risk factors in a given patient in the process of estimating future risk *(16,19)*. Moreover, the clinical relevance of the specific clustering of CVD risk factors into the metabolic syndrome, affecting approx 25% of the adult US population, and 40% of those 60 yr and older, has recently been appreciated *(20–25)*. Reflecting the unprecedented epidemic of physical inactivity and obesity *(26)*, diabetes, and CVD, the metabolic syndrome confers a relative risk for CHD *mortality* of almost 4 *(27)*. The need to directly address all components of the metabolic syndrome has now been incorporated into the National Cholesterol Education Program (NCEP) Adult Treatment Panel (ATP) III recommendations *(28)*. Finally, although there has been some debate regarding the percentage of patients with documented CHD who do not exhibit abnormalities of traditional risk factors *(29,30)*, epidemiological reports that are more recent indicate that 80 to 90% of CHD patients, in fact, have abnormalities of one or more of these risk factors *(31)*.

Effectiveness of Risk Factor Control

In addition to the scientific data on the potent and interactive nature of CVD risk factors and the increasing population burden of CVD, there is consistent and encouraging evidence regarding the reduction of CVD incidence that can be produced through control of the modifiable risk factors for the disease. Although a complete review of the supporting

literature is beyond the scope of this chapter, it may be helpful to present a brief summary of the current consensus on several of the major traditional CVD risk factors that are amenable to modification in the preventive cardiology setting.

The sizeable evidence base of randomized clinical trials of lipid lowering with the hydroxymethylglutaryl–coenzyme A (HMG-CoA) reductase inhibitors (the statin trials) for both primary and secondary prevention have demonstrated striking reductions in relative risks for morbid and mortal CVD events for men and women across a wide range of ages and lipid levels *(32–41)*. Each of these trials also documented a statistically significant decrease in the need for revascularization procedures. In addition, at least five of the secondary prevention trials *(33,35,36,38,39)* found a significant decrease in cerebrovascular events in patients treated with statins, an effect supported by studies documenting regression of carotid atherosclerosis as a result of aggressive lipid lowering *(42,43)*, and by a recent meta-analysis showing that cholesterol lowering with the statins reduces the risk of stroke *(44)*. The cumulative impact of these results led the ATP III panel to release an update of their 2001 guidelines in 2004 *(45)*, in which a new low-density lipoprotein (LDL)-cholesterol goal of less than 70 mg/dL was introduced for very high-risk patients.

The reduction in risk for CVD events that accompanies cigarette cessation *(46,47)*, control of elevated blood pressure *(48–52)*, and the use of antithrombotic agents *(53,54)* is similarly well-documented and unequivocal. Each of these risk factors confers a twofold to threefold increase in risk for CVD when present and untreated.

Dietary therapy remains a cornerstone of treatment for those at risk for CVD and for patients with documented disease, as proposed in the guidelines of the NCEP *(28,55)*. The potential impact of altered patterns of nutrient intake was confirmed in a follow-up report of a trial involving a so-called "Mediterranean" diet. Patients randomized to such treatment enjoyed 50 to 70% reductions in risk for morbid and mortal CVD events when compared with patients who ate a prudent Western diet *(56)*. More recently, a similar diet was shown to decrease high-sensitivity (hs)-C-reactive protein (CRP), and improve insulin resistance and endothelial function *(57)*.

It has long been recognized that diabetes is a potent risk factor for CHD, stroke, and peripheral arterial disease, which occur twice as often in diabetic men and up to four times as often in diabetic women as in their nondiabetic counterparts *(2,58)*. CVD is the leading cause of mortality in diabetes, causing 80% of all deaths; CHD is responsible for 75% of all CVD-related mortality in diabetics *(59)*. It is now recognized that even diabetics without documented CHD have a risk for MI comparable to nondiabetics who have already suffered an MI *(60)*. Such evidence has led both the American Diabetes Association *(61)* and the NCEP–ATP III Panel *(28)* to recommend that LDL levels in diabetics be lowered to less than 100 mg/dL, just as in patients with diagnosed CHD. Moreover, diabetic patients with documented CVD are now included in the very high-risk category, with suggested LDL targets of less than 70 mg/dL *(45)*. In fact, there is agreement that strict control of all the traditional risk factors is critical in modifying CVD occurrence in diabetics. One recent study showed that although the prevalence of CVD was constant across increasing quartiles of glycohemoglobin in a diabetic population, it was strongly associated with age, hypertension, cigarette use, and the ratio of total cholesterol to high-density lipoprotein (HDL) cholesterol *(62)*.

Physical inactivity doubles risk for both CVD mortality and CHD morbidity *(63)*. Increased physical activity, in turn, decreases all-cause mortality, CVD mortality, and CVD morbidity *(64–67)*. The beneficial effects of exercise have been documented in both

genders, the elderly, and smokers, even when performed at moderate levels *(64,67,68)*. In addition to enhancing fibrinolytic activity, improving carbohydrate metabolism, and lowering weight, blood pressure, and serum triglyceride levels *(53)*, exercise has been shown to be an independent predictor of decreased angiographic progression of CHD *(69)*. Poor fitness levels in young adults are associated with increased future rates of diabetes, hypertension, and the metabolic syndrome *(70)*. Conversely, even moderate-intensity aerobic exercise improves endothelial function *(71)*. Exercise and weight reduction can ameliorate components of the metabolic syndrome *(72)* and reduce the incidence of developing diabetes in high-risk groups *(73)*. Physical inactivity, similar to obesity is now recognized as an independent "life habit" risk factor by the NCEP–ATP III panel.

Obesity increases CVD risk both directly and indirectly. It has been known for some time that obesity is indirectly causal via its effect on hypertension, diabetes, elevated triglycerides, and low levels of HDL cholesterol, and its association with physical inactivity and diets high in cholesterol and saturated fats *(74–76)*. More recently, it has been noted that much of the excess CVD risk associated with obesity is accounted for by the pattern of central adiposity, probably through the mechanism of insulin resistance *(75,76)*. Although most patients cannot maintain successful weight loss *(77,78)*, it is now recognized that CVD risk factors such as hypertension, hypercholesterolemia, and glucose intolerance can be favorably altered by even modest reductions in excess weight *(74–78)*. Further, adipose tissue has now been recognized as an important site of cytokine activity, and associated with hs-CRP *(79)*. Weight loss can reduce elevated hs-CRP levels, providing another potential pathway for its impact on CVD risk.

There is an extensive literature demonstrating a causal linkage between various psychosocial factors and CVD. Hostility *(80)*, depression *(81–83)*, hopelessness *(84)*, worry *(85)*, and social isolation *(86,87)* have all been shown to be associated with total and CVD mortality and with nonfatal and total CHD incidence. Depression in older women was associated with increased risk of CVD death and all-cause mortality *(88)*. Psychosocial factors are thought to affect CVD risk both directly and indirectly. Direct effects are hypothesized to be mediated by the process of cardiovascular reactivity, whereby exaggerated responses to stress by the sympathetic and pituitary–adrenal axis produce ischemic and arrhythmogenic events *(89)*. A recent study found that depressive mood was associated with increased levels of CRP, interleukin-6, and intercellular adhesion molecule-1 *(90)*. Indirect effects include facilitating poor lifestyle choices concerning cigarette use, physical inactivity, and obesity *(91)*. Psychosocial factors have an impact on CVD risk comparable to other major risk factors, increasing incidence from twofold to fourfold *(89,91)*. Although major clinical trials are lacking in this area, behavior modification and stress management interventions have demonstrated favorable effects in secondary prevention studies *(82,92)*. Because psychological issues can negatively affect compliance with efforts to modify other CVD risk factors, systems to assess and address these issues must be built into preventive cardiological care.

The Limits of Intervention

Several lines of scientific inquiry have shed new light on the pathophysiology of CVD, with important implications for preventive cardiology. It is now known that most acute coronary events are caused by the rupture of "vulnerable" atherosclerotic plaques with subsequent superimposed thrombosis *(93)*. Such plaques are characterized by a large

lipid core, a thinned fibrous cap heavily infiltrated by matrix-degrading macrophages, evidence of increased inflammation, and a paucity of smooth muscle cells *(94)*. Perhaps most strikingly, it seems that the majority of the lesions responsible for such events are not the severely stenotic targets of interventional procedures, such as coronary artery bypass grafting and balloon angioplasty, but lesions of mild-to-moderate severity producing stenosis of 70% or less *(95)*. Because it has been estimated that there are numerous such lesions in the coronary arterial tree, the failure of targeted interventional therapies to convincingly reduce overall cardiovascular mortality should not be surprising, and further supports the logic of a preventive approach. Further, results of the so-called "regression trials" *(96)*, including two recent studies which drove LDL levels below the then-recommended NCEP–ATP III targets *(40,41)*, and the growing recognition of the role of endothelial dysfunction *(97,98)* and plaque stabilization *(99)* have helped explain the marked reductions in clinical events that accompany aggressive lipid lowering even in the absence of dramatic angiographic change. Combined with the striking relative risk reductions for morbid and mortal CVD events demonstrated in the statin trials described earlier, these recent insights have validated the critical role of preventive practices and even fueled calls for comparative trials of lipid lowering vs revascularization *(100)*.

RATIONALE

The Treatment Gap

It has been demonstrated previously that CVD is prevalent and costly, that it is associated with risk factors that are easily measured and amenable to modification, and that such modification is both effective and based on plausible pathophysiological hypotheses. Moreover, with the changing demographics of our society and the concerning prevalence of inactivity, obesity, diabetes, and the metabolic syndrome, the need for both primary and secondary prevention has never been greater *(101,102)*. These facts alone would provide substantial justification for coordinated preventive cardiology programs that focus on simultaneous control of all risk factors. Current patterns of clinical practice, however, offer additional proof of the need for such programs.

Based on scientific data such as those presented earlier, major professional organizations and expert panels have issued guidelines for the assessment and treatment of CVD risk factors *(55,103–106)*. Unfortunately, there is consistent data demonstrating that patients are not deriving the benefit of these clinical guidelines *(107,108)*. For hypercholesterolemia, it has been shown that fewer than one-third of those who need treatment are receiving it, even if one includes rudimentary dietary advice *(109)*. Even in patients documented to be at high risk, physicians are not inquiring about the presence of risk factors *(110–113)* or initiating appropriate therapy when they are found to be present *(111,113,114)*. This is true for patients on the coronary care unit (CCU) *(113)*, awaiting bypass *(110)*, before discharge from a CHD-related hospitalization *(108)*, or treated in the community *(115,116)*. When hyperlipidemia is treated, even in patients with known CHD, NCEP targets for LDL cholesterol are being met less than 20% of the time *(117–119)*. Similar data exist for the other risk factors *(116)*. It is estimated, for instance, that fewer than 30% of smokers receive documented counseling regarding cigarette cessation before leaving the hospital after MI *(120)*, whereas one study *(113)* found that fewer than 5% of smokers admitted to a CCU had been counseled. The rates of use of β-blockers (45%), angiotensin-converting enzyme (ACE) inhibitors (59%), and aspirin (77%) after

MI are similarly disappointing *(120)*. National data from National Health and Nutrition Examination Survey suggest that, from 1991 to 1994, substantial decreases occurred in awareness (from 73 to 68%), rates of treatment (from 55 to 54%), and control (from 29 to 27%) of blood pressure. Although the rate of control had risen slightly (to 34%) by the time of the publication of the Joint National Committee on the Detection, Evaluation, and Treatment of High Blood Pressure Seventh report in 2003, this is a problematic "success" story *(105)*. A study of the ambulatory treatment of hypertension found that only 25% of patients were adequately controlled, even using older cut points of 140/90 mmHg *(121)*. Similar poor rates of blood pressure control were recently observed in a community-based cohort study of older adults, and were particularly low in the oldest women *(122)*.

Awareness of and concern regarding this treatment gap between treatment guidelines and actual practice is growing *(123,124)*. There is, in addition, increasing recognition that the results of carefully controlled clinical trials are not always applicable to the reality of everyday patient care. In response, efforts have been initiated to analyze barriers to the implementation of risk-factor management *(124)*. Such barriers include the structural and reimbursement realities of attempting to provide preventive services in the setting of a busy practice or acute care facility. Physicians—the traditional source of preventive services—have limited time, little confidence in their knowledge concerning prevention, and no financial incentive to provide such services. Physicians also overestimate their own compliance with screening guidelines. Although physicians can be quite knowledgeable regarding the content of specific guidelines and believe generally in the importance of prevention, they comply with recommendations only 20 to 60% of the time *(125–128)*. There is also concern that the increasing complexity of guidelines will lead to even lower physician compliance with treatment recommendations, and some evidence that physicians may have negative attitudes regarding guidelines that themselves constitute barriers to their use *(129)*. A growing body of literature has examined the impact of electronic medical records, chart prompts, "academic detailing," clinical "report cards," and "pay for performance" plans in affecting behavior change in providers *(130–133)*. Although some studies have shown encouraging results, there is as yet no consistency to the outcomes. At least until such mechanisms are mandated, the weight of the evidence suggests that making physicians the sole focus of improved risk factor management may be problematic.

Nontraditional Models of Care

One model that has emerged as an effective solution to the inadequate implementation of aggressive risk factor control is the multidisciplinary team in which the nurse acts as the case manager, with physician supervision *(134)*. Although the structure of such teams varies across institutions and practice settings, they often include dietitians, pharmacists, and psychologists *(135–139)*. Such programs have had success in the management of hypertension *(140,141)*, diabetes *(142)*, smoking cessation *(143–145)*, chronic heart failure *(146)*, and hyperlipidemia *(135–139,147–150)*. Simultaneous modification of all risk factors present in a given patient has also proven effective *(137,150)*.

In addition to this documented clinical effectiveness, nurse-managed programs have shown promise in terms of cost effectiveness *(124,139,151–153)*, probably because of a combination of lower salaries for nonphysician professionals, the use of standardized clinical algorithms, and improved patient compliance. These characteristics make such programs potentially attractive to managed care providers, although, to date, preventive

services remain undervalued and poorly reimbursed for both physicians and nurses. Because clinical trial results have demonstrated that risk-factor modification reduces future CVD events and the need for costly, interventional, hospital-based care, it may be that preventive services can gain more acceptance when viewed as a cost-saving component of an overall health care system.

Other models have used the effect of a community pharmacist intervention on cholesterol risk management. In the Study of Cardiovascular Risk Intervention by Pharmacists, a randomized controlled trial was conducted in 54 community pharmacies from 1998 to 2000 *(154)*. This intervention targeted patients at high risk for cardiovascular events based on the presence of atherosclerotic disease or diabetes mellitus with another risk factor. Of the 675 patients enrolled, approx 40% were women, and the average age was 64 yr. Patients randomized to the pharmacist intervention received education and a brochure on risk factors, point-of-care cholesterol measurement, referral to their physician, and regular follow-up for 16 wk. Pharmacists faxed a simple form to the primary care physician identifying risk factors and any suggestions based on evidence-based guidelines. Usual-care patients received the same brochure and general advice only, with minimal follow-up. The primary endpoint of the study was a composite of proportion of patients receiving a fasting cholesterol panel or addition or increase in dose of cholesterol-lowering medication. Despite its small size, the external monitoring committee recommended early study termination because of the significant benefit of the pharmacist intervention. Patients in the intervention arm were significantly more likely than those in the control arm to receive appropriate lipid testing and intervention (57 vs 31%, respectively; odds ratio, 3.0; 95% confidence interval, 2.2–4.1; $p < 0.001$). Based on the results of this study, a community-based intervention program improved the process of cholesterol management in high-risk patients. This program demonstrates the value of community pharmacists working in collaboration with patients and physicians and serves as a unique model for addressing low rates of guideline adherence with respect to lipid lowering.

Other models have developed a multidisciplinary model to address cardiovascular risk factors and the fact that life-saving therapies are underused in patients receiving conventional care. One such program, the Cardiac Hospitalization Atherosclerosis Management Program (CHAMP) was designed and implemented at the University of California Los Angeles (UCLA) Medical Center starting in 1994 *(155)*. CHAMP focused on initiation of aspirin, cholesterol-lowering medication (HMG-CoA reductase inhibitor titrated to achieve LDL cholesterol <100 mg/dL), β-blocker, and ACE-inhibitor therapy, in conjunction with diet and exercise counseling before hospital discharge in patients with established coronary artery disease. This treatment program was based on the hypothesis that initiation of therapy in the hospital setting would result in higher use rates both at the time of discharge and during longer-term follow-up. Implementation of this program involved the use of a focused treatment guideline, standardized admission orders, educational lectures by local thought leaders, and tracking/reporting of treatment rates. To assess the impact of the program, treatment rates and clinical outcome were compared in patients discharged in the 2-yr periods before and after CHAMP was implemented. In the pre- and post-CHAMP patient groups, aspirin use at discharge improved from 68 to 92% ($p < 0.01$), β-blocker use improved from 12 to 62% ($p < 0.01$), ACE inhibitor use increased from 6 to 58% ($p < 0.01$), and statin use increased from 6 to 86% ($p < 0.01$). This increased use of treatment persisted during subsequent follow-up. There was also a significant

increase in patients achieving a LDL cholesterol level of at most 100 mg/dL (6 vs 58%; $p < 0.001$) and a reduction in recurrent MI and 1-yr mortality. Compared with conventional guidelines and care, CHAMP was associated with a significant increase in use of medications that have been previously demonstrated to reduce mortality; more patients achieved an LDL cholesterol of at most 100 mg/dL, and there were improved clinical outcomes in patients after hospitalization for acute MI. Hospital-based treatment protocols such as CHAMP have the potential to significantly increase treatment use of therapies previously demonstrated to improve survival and thus substantially improve the outcome of the 2 million patients diagnosed and hospitalized each year with coronary artery disease.

CONCLUSION

CVD remains the leading cause of death in the United States. The prevalence of CVD is likely to increase into the next century, with a larger and older population requiring secondary preventive services. CVD is usually associated with *multiple* risk factors, which interact to increase the likelihood of an initial or recurrent event, and modification of CVD risk factors has been proven to decrease the incidence of CVD for both primary and secondary prevention. Moreover, the changing demographics of the population, with increasingly normative obesity and sedentariness, unfortunately present an ample opportunity to address CVD risk factors that are ideally controlled through often labor-intensive lifestyle alteration. Despite the large body of evidence supporting the use of therapies to improve outcomes in patients with or at risk for CVD, these interventions are underused. Nationally, even patients at high risk for CVD are inadequately screened and insufficiently treated for traditional CVD risk factors.

In view of these findings and facts, new models must be developed so that society may realize the full potential of preventive interventions. Given the growing fiscal and logistic pressures associated particularly with ambulatory practice, we recognize that physicians may not be the best—and certainly should not be the sole—providers of preventive cardiological care. A preventive cardiology program using a multidisciplinary team for the simultaneous and aggressive management of CVD risk factors may be most effective in decreasing risk factor burden and attaining recommended treatment targets. Although important barriers remain before the potential impact of preventive cardiology can be fully realized, new models must be developed to address the epidemic of CVD.

REFERENCES

1. American Heart Association. Heart Disease and Stroke Statistics. Dallas, TX, 2005.
2. Levy D. Atherosclerotic cardiovascular disease: An epidemiologic perspective. In: Topol EJ, ed. Textbook of Cardiovascular Medicine, 1998, Lippincott-Raven, Philadelphia, PA, p. 12–30.
3. National Center for Health Statistics: Vital Statistics of the United States. 1993, Washington, DC: US Government Printing Office, Public Health Service.
4. Mosca L, Ferris A, Fabunmi R, Robertson RM; American Heart Association. Tracking women's awareness of heart disease: an American Heart Association national study. Circulation 2004;109(5):573–579.
5. Kannel WB, Vokonas PS. Demographics of the prevalence, incidence, and management of coronary heart disease in the elderly and in women. Ann Epidemiol 1992;2(1–2):5–14.
6. Castelli WP. Lipids, risk factors and ischaemic heart disease. Atherosclerosis 1996;124(Suppl):S1–9.
7. Wolf P. Cerebrovascular risk. In: Izzo H, ed. Hypertension Primer: The Essentials of High Blood Pressure, 3rd ed. Lippincott Williams & Wilkins, Baltimore, MD, 2003, pp. 239–243.
8. American Heart Association. Statistical Update, American Heart Association. 1999.

9. Johnson CL, Rifkind BM, Sempos CT, et al. Declining serum total cholesterol levels among US adults. The National Health and Nutrition Examination Surveys. JAMA 1993;269(23):3002–3008.

10. Thom TJ, Roccella EJ. Trends in blood pressure control and mortality. In: Izzo H, ed. Hypertension Primer: The Essentials of High Blood Pressure, 3rd ed. Lippincott Williams & Wilkins, Baltimore, MD, 2003, pp. 299–301.

11. Goldman L, Cook EF. The decline in ischemic heart disease mortality rates. An analysis of the comparative effects of medical interventions and changes in lifestyle. Ann Intern Med 1984;101(6):825–836.

12. Rosamond WD, Chambless LE, Folsom AR, et al. Trends in the incidence of myocardial infarction and in mortality due to coronary heart disease, 1987 to 1994. N Engl J Med 1998;339(13):861–867.

13. Kelly DT. Paul Dudley White International Lecture. Our future society. A global challenge. Circulation 1997;95(11):2459–2464.

14. Kannel WB. The Framingham Experience. In: Marmot M, Elliott P, eds. Coronary Heart Disease Epidemiology: From Aetiology to Public Health. 1992, Oxford University Press, New York, pp. 67–82.

15. Kannel WB. Cardiovascular risk factors and hypertension. In: Izzo H, ed. Hypertension Primer: The Essentials of High Blood Pressure, 3rd ed. Lippincott Williams & Wilkins, Baltimore, MD, 2003.

16. Lowe LP, Greenland P, Ruth KJ, Dyer AR, Stamler R, Stamler J. Impact of major cardiovascular disease risk factors, particularly in combination, on 22-year mortality in women and men. Arch Intern Med 1998;158(18):2007–2014.

17. Califf RM, Armstrong PW, Carver JR, D'Agostino RB, Strauss WE. 27th Bethesda Conference: matching the intensity of risk factor management with the hazard for coronary disease events. Task Force 5. Stratification of patients into high, medium and low risk subgroups for purposes of risk factor management. J Am Coll Cardiol 1996;27(5):1007–1019.

18. Kannel WB, Wilson PW. An update on coronary risk factors. Med Clin North Am 1995;79(5):951–971.

19. Ballantyne CM. Current thinking in lipid lowering. Am J Med 1998;104(6A):33S–41S.

20. Grundy SM, Brewer HB Jr, Cleeman JI, et al. Definition of metabolic syndrome: Report of the National Heart, Lung, and Blood Institute/American Heart Association conference on scientific issues related to definition. Circulation 2004;109(3):433–438.

21. Deedwania PC. Metabolic syndrome and vascular disease: is nature or nurture leading the new epidemic of cardiovascular disease? Circulation 2004;109(1):2–4.

22. Hu G, Qiao Q, Tuomilehto, J, et al. Prevalence of the metabolic syndrome and its relation to all-cause and cardiovascular mortality in nondiabetic European men and women. Arch Intern Med 2004;164(10):1066–1076.

23. Lteif AA, Han K, Mather KJ. Obesity, insulin resistance, and the metabolic syndrome: determinants of endothelial dysfunction in whites and blacks. Circulation 2005;112(1):32–38.

24. Kereiakes DJ, Willerson JT. Metabolic syndrome epidemic. Circulation 2003;108(13):1552–1553.

25. Malik S, Wong ND, Franklin SS, et al. Impact of the metabolic syndrome on mortality from coronary heart disease, cardiovascular disease, and all causes in United States adults. Circulation 2004;110(10):1245–1250.

26. Manson JE, Skerrett PJ, Greenland P, Van Itallie TB. The escalating pandemics of obesity and sedentary lifestyle. A call to action for clinicians. Arch Intern Med 2004;164(3):249–258.

27. Lakka HM, Laaksonen DE, Lakka TA, et al. The metabolic syndrome and total and cardiovascular disease mortality in middle-aged men. JAMA 2002;288(21):2709–2716.

28. Detection, Evaluation, and Treatment of High Blood Cholesterol in Adults (Adult Treatment Panel III) Final Report. 2002, National Cholesterol Education Program. National Institute of Health.

29. Canto JG, Iskandrian AE. Major risk factors for cardiovascular disease: debunking the "only 50%" myth. JAMA 2003;290(7):947–949.

30. Magnus P, Beaglehole R. The real contribution of the major risk factors to the coronary epidemics: time to end the "only-50%" myth. Arch Intern Med 2001;161(22):2657–2660.

31. Greenland P, Knoll MD, Stamler J, et al. Major risk factors as antecedents of fatal and nonfatal coronary heart disease events. JAMA 2003;290(7):891–897.

32. Downs JR, Clearfield M, Weis S, et al. Primary prevention of acute coronary events with lovastatin in men and women with average cholesterol levels: results of AFCAPS/TexCAPS. Air Force/Texas Coronary Atherosclerosis Prevention Study. JAMA 1998;279(20):1615–1622.

33. Sacks FM, Pfeiffer MA, Moye LA, et al. The effect of pravastatin on coronary events after myocardial infarction in patients with average cholesterol levels. Cholesterol and Recurrent Events Trial investigators. N Engl J Med 1996;335(14):1001–1009.

34. Shepherd J, Cobbe SM, Ford I, et al. Prevention of coronary heart disease with pravastatin in men with hypercholesterolemia. West of Scotland Coronary Prevention Study Group. N Engl J Med 1995;333(20): 1301–1307.

35. Prevention of cardiovascular events and death with pravastatin in patients with coronary heart disease and a broad range of initial cholesterol levels. The Long-Term Intervention with Pravastatin in Ischaemic Disease (LIPID) Study Group. N Engl J Med 1998;339(19):1349–1357.

36. Randomised trial of cholesterol lowering in 4444 patients with coronary heart disease: the Scandinavian Simvastatin Survival Study (4S). Lancet 1994;344(8934):1383–1389.

37. Shepherd J, Blauw GJ, Murphy MB, et al. Pravastatin in elderly individuals at risk of vascular disease (PROSPER): a randomized controlled trial. Lancet 2002;360:1623–1630.

38. Heart Protection Study Collaborative Group. MRC/BHF Heart Protection Study of cholesterol lowering with simvastatin in 20,536 high-risk individuals: a randomized placebo-controlled trial. Lancet 2002;360:7–22.

39. Sever PS, Dahlof B, Poulter NR, et al. Prevention of coronary and stroke events with atorvastatin in hypertensive patients who have average or lower-than-average cholesterol concentrations, in the Anglo-Scandinavian Cardiac Outcomes Trial–Lipid Lowering Arm (ASCOT–LLA): a multicentre randomized controlled trial. Lancet 2003;361:1149–1158.

40. Nissen SE, Tuzcu EM, Schoenhagen P, et al. Statin therapy, LDL cholesterol, C-reactive protein, and coronary artery disease. N Engl J Med 2005;352:29–38.

41. Cannon CP, Braunwald E, McCabe CH, et al. Intensive versus moderate lipid lowering with statins after acute coronary syndromes. N Engl J Med 2004;350:1495–1504.

42. Furberg CD, Adams HP Jr, Applegate WB, et al. Effect of lovastatin on early carotid atherosclerosis and cardiovascular events. Asymptomatic Carotid Artery Progression Study (ACAPS) Research Group. Circulation 1994;90(4):1679–1687.

43. Furberg CD, Byington RP, Crouse JR, Espeland MA. Pravastatin, lipids, and major coronary events. Am J Cardiol 1994;73(15):1133–1134.

44. Hebert PR, Gaziano JM, Chan KS, Hennekens CH. Cholesterol lowering with statin drugs, risk of stroke, and total mortality. An overview of randomized trials. JAMA 1997;278(4):313–321.

45. Grundy SM, Cleeman JI, Merz CN, et al. Implications of recent clinical trials for the National Cholesterol Education Program Adult Treatment Panel III guidelines. Circulation 2004;110(2):227–239.

46. The Health Benefits of Smoking Cessation: A Report of the Surgeon General. Department of Health and Human Services, Rockville, MD, 1990.

47. The Health Consequences of Smoking: Cardiovascular Disease. A Report of the Surgeon General. Department of Health and Human Services: Rockville, MD, 1983.

48. Prevention of stroke by antihypertensive drug treatment in older persons with isolated systolic hypertension. Final results of the Systolic Hypertension in the Elderly Program (SHEP). SHEP Cooperative Research Group. JAMA 1991;265(24):3255–3264.

49. Collins R, Peto R, MacMahon S, et al. Blood pressure, stroke, and coronary heart disease. Part 2, Short-term reductions in blood pressure: overview of randomised drug trials in their epidemiological context. Lancet 1990;335(8693):827–838.

50. Cutler J, Psaty B, MacMahon S, et al. Public health issues in hypertension. In: Laragh J, Brenner, B, ed. Hypertension: Pathologhysiology, Diagnosis and Management. Raven Press, New York, 1995.

51. Hebert PR, Fiebach NH, Eberlein KA, Taylor JO, Hennekens CH. The community-based randomized trials of pharmacologic treatment of mild-to-moderate hypertension. Am J Epidemiol 1988;127(3):581–590.

52. Hebert PR, Moser M, Mayer J, Glynn RJ, Hennekens CH. Recent evidence on drug therapy of mild to moderate hypertension and decreased risk of coronary heart disease. Arch Intern Med 1993;153(5):578–581.

53. Pasternak RC, Grundy SM, Levy D, Thompson PD. 27th Bethesda Conference: matching the intensity of risk factor management with the hazard for coronary disease events. Task Force 3. Spectrum of risk factors for coronary heart disease. J Am Coll Cardiol 1996;27(5):978–990.

54. Hennekens CH, Dyken ML, Fuster V. Aspirin as a therapeutic agent in cardiovascular disease: a statement for healthcare professionals from the American Heart Association. Circulation 1997;96(8):2751–2753.

55. Summary of the second report of the National Cholesterol Education Program (NCEP) Expert Panel on Detection, Evaluation, and Treatment of High Blood Cholesterol in Adults (Adult Treatment Panel II). JAMA 1993;269(23):3015–3023.

56. de Lorgeril M, Salen P, Martin J-L, et al. Mediterranean diet, traditional risk factors, and the rate of cardiovascular complications after myocardial infarction: final report of the Lyon Diet Heart Study. Circulation 1999;99(6): 779–785.

57. Esposito, K, Marfella R, Ciotola M, et al. Effect of a mediterranean-style diet on endothelial dysfunction and markers of vascular inflammation in the metabolic syndrome: a randomized trial. JAMA 2004;292(12):1440–1446.

58. Garber AJ. Vascular disease and lipids in diabetes. Med Clin North Am 1998;82(4):931–948.

59. Aronson D, Rayfield, E. Diabetes. In: Topol EJ, ed. Textbook of Cardiovascular Medicine. Lippincott-Raven, Philadelphia, PA, 1998, pp. 171–194.

60. Haffner SM, Lehto S, Ronnemaa T, Pyorala K, Laakso M. Mortality from coronary heart disease in subjects with type 2 diabetes and in nondiabetic subjects with and without prior myocardial infarction. N Engl J Med 1998;339(4):229–234.

61. Standards of Medical Care in Diabetes. Diabetes Care 2005;28(suppl 1):S4–S36.

62. Meigs JB, Singer DE, Sullivan LM, et al. Metabolic control and prevalent cardiovascular disease in non-insulin-dependent diabetes mellitus (NIDDM): The NIDDM Patient Outcome Research Team. Am J Med 1997;102(1):38–47.

63. Powell KE, Thompson PD, Caspersen CJ, Kendrick JS. Physical activity and the incidence of coronary heart disease. Annu Rev Public Health 1987;8:253–287.

64. Blair SN, Kampert JB, Kohl HW III, et al. Influences of cardiorespiratory fitness and other precursors on cardiovascular disease and all-cause mortality in men and women. JAMA 1996;276(3):205–210.

65. Blair SN, Kohl HW III, Barlow CE, Paffenbarger RS Jr, Gibbons LW, Macera CA. Changes in physical fitness and all-cause mortality. A prospective study of healthy and unhealthy men. JAMA 1995;273(14):1093–1098.

66. Erikssen G, Liestol K, Bjornholt J, Thaulow E, Sandvik L, Erikssen J. Changes in physical fitness and changes in mortality. Lancet 1998;352(9130):759–762.

67. Wannamethee SG, Shaper AG, Walker M. Changes in physical activity, mortality, and incidence of coronary heart disease in older men. Lancet 1998;351(9116):1603–1608.

68. Physical activity and cardiovascular health. NIH Consensus Development Panel on Physical Activity and Cardiovascular Health. JAMA 1996;276(3):241–246.

69. Niebauer J, Hambrecht R, Velich T, et al. Attenuated progression of coronary artery disease after 6 years of multifactorial risk intervention: role of physical exercise. Circulation 1997;96(8):2534–2541.

70. Carnethon MR, Gidding SS, Nehgme R, Sidney S, Jacobs DR Jr, Liu K. Cardiorespiratory fitness in young adulthood and the development of cardiovascular disease risk factors. JAMA 2003;290(23):3092–3100.

71. Goto C, Higashi Y, Kimura M, et al. Effect of different intensities of exercise on endothelium-dependent vasodilation in humans: role of endothelium-dependent nitric oxide and oxidative stress. Circulation 2003;108(5):530–535.

72. Watkins LL, Sherwood A, Feinglos M, et al. Effects of exercise and weight loss on cardiac risk factors associated with syndrome X. Arch Intern Med 2003;163(16):1889–1895.

73. Knowler WC, Barrett-Connor E, Fowler SE, et al. Reduction in the incidence of type 2 diabetes with lifestyle intervention or metformin. N Engl J Med 2002;346(6):393–403.

74. Eckel RH. Obesity and heart disease: a statement for healthcare professionals from the Nutrition Committee, American Heart Association. Circulation 1997;96(9):3248–3250.

75. Schwartz MW, Brunzell JD. Regulation of body adiposity and the problem of obesity. Arterioscler Thromb Vasc Biol 1997;17(2):233–238.

76. Kannel WB, D'Agostino RB, Cobb JL. Effect of weight on cardiovascular disease. Am J Clin Nutr 1996;63(3 Suppl):419S–422S.

77. Rosenbaum M, Leibel RL, Hirsch J. Obesity. N Engl J Med 1997;337(6):396–407.

78. Stone NJ. Diet, nutritional issues, and obesity. In: Topol EJ, ed. Textbook of Cardiovascular Medicine. Lippincott-Raven, Philadelphia, PA, 1998, pp. 31–58.

79. Visser M, Bouter LM, McQuillan GM, Wener MH, Harris TB. Elevated C-reactive protein levels in overweight and obese adults. JAMA 1999;282(22):2131–2135.

80. Helmer DC, Ragland DR, Syme SL. Hostility and coronary artery disease. Am J Epidemiol 1991;133(2):112–122.

81. Barefoot JC, Schroll M. Symptoms of depression, acute myocardial infarction, and total mortality in a community sample. Circulation 1996;93(11):1976–1980.

82. Frasure-Smith N, Lesperance F, Talajic M. Depression following myocardial infarction. Impact on 6-month survival. JAMA 1993;270(15):1819–1825.

83. Frasure-Smith N, Lesperance F, Talajic M. Depression and 18-month prognosis after myocardial infarction. Circulation 1995;91(4):999–1005.

84. Everson SA, Kaplan GA, Goldberg DE, Salonen R, Salonen JT. Hopelessness and 4-year progression of carotid atherosclerosis. The Kuopio Ischemic Heart Disease Risk Factor Study. Arterioscler Thromb Vasc Biol 1997;17(8):1490–1495.

85. Kubzansky LD, Kawachi I, Spiro A III, Weiss ST, Vokonas PS, Sparrow D. Is worrying bad for your heart? A prospective study of worry and coronary heart disease in the Normative Aging Study. Circulation 1997;95(4):818–824.

86. Olsen O. Impact of social network on cardiovascular mortality in middle aged Danish men. J Epidemiol Community Health 1993;47(3):176–180.

87. Berkman LF, Leo-Summers L, Horwitz RI. Emotional support and survival after myocardial infarction. A prospective, population-based study of the elderly. Ann Intern Med 1992;117(12):1003–1009.

88. Wassertheil-Smoller S, Shumaker S, Ockene J, et al. Depression and cardiovascular sequelae in postmenopausal women. The Women's Health Initiative (WHI). Arch Intern Med 2004;164(3):289–298.

89. Theorell T. The psycho-social environment, stress, and coronary heart disase. In: Marmot P, ed. Coronary Heart Disease Epidemiology: From Aetiology to Public Health, M.a.E. Oxford University Press, New York, 1992, pp. 256–273.

90. Empana JP, Sykes DH, Luc G, et al. Contributions of depressive mood and circulating inflammatory markers to coronary heart disease in healthy European men: the Prospective Epidemiological Study of Myocardial Infarction (PRIME). Circulation 2005;111(18):2299–2305.

91. Smith T, Leon A. Coronary Heart Disease: A Behavioral Perspective. Smith T, Leon, A, ed. Research Press, Champaign, IL, 1992.

92. van Dixhoorn J, Duivenvoorden HJ, Staal JA, Pool J, Verhage F. Cardiac events after myocardial infarction: possible effect of relaxation therapy. Eur Heart J 1987;8(11):1210–1214.

93. Falk E, Shah PK, Fuster V. Coronary plaque disruption. Circulation 1995;92(3):657–671.

94. Lee RT, Libby P. The unstable atheroma. Arterioscler Thromb Vasc Biol 1997;17(10):1859–1867.

95. Levine GN, Keaney JF Jr, Vita JA. Cholesterol reduction in cardiovascular disease. Clinical benefits and possible mechanisms. N Engl J Med 1995;332(8):512–521.

96. Superko HR, Krauss RM. Coronary artery disease regression. Convincing evidence for the benefit of aggressive lipoprotein management. Circulation 1994;90(2):1056–1069.

97. Treasure CB, Klein JL, Weintraub WS, et al. Beneficial effects of cholesterol-lowering therapy on the coronary endothelium in patients with coronary artery disease. N Engl J Med 1995;332(8):481–487.

98. Anderson TJ, Meredith IT, Yeung AC, Frei B, Selwyn AP, Ganz P. The effect of cholesterol-lowering and antioxidant therapy on endothelium-dependent coronary vasomotion. N Engl J Med 1995;332(8):488–493.

99. Brown BG, Zhao XQ, Sacco DE, Albers JJ. Lipid lowering and plaque regression. New insights into prevention of plaque disruption and clinical events in coronary disease. Circulation 1993;87(6):1781–1791.

100. Forrester JS, Shah PK. Lipid lowering versus revascularization: an idea whose time (for testing) has come. Circulation 1997;96(4):1360–1362.

101. Pearson TA. The epidemiologic basis for population-wide cholesterol reduction in the primary prevention of coronary artery disease. Am J Cardiol 2004;94(9A):4F–8F.

102. Unal B, Critchley JA, Capewell S. Modelling the decline in coronary heart disease deaths in England and Wales, 1981–2000: comparing contributions from primary prevention and secondary prevention. BMJ, 2005;331:614.

103. Recommendations of the Second Joint Task Force of European and Other Societies on Coronary Prevention. Prevention of coronary heart disease in clinical practice. Eur Heart J 1998;19:1434–1503.

104. 27th Bethesda Conference. Matching the Intensity of Risk Factor Management with the Hazard for Coronary Disease Events. September 14–15, 1995. J Am Coll Cardiol 1996;27(5):957–1047.

105. The seventh report of the Joint National Committee on prevention, detection, evaluation, and treatment of high blood pressure. JAMA 2003;289:2560–2571.

106. Report of the Expert Committee on the Diagnosis and Classification of Diabetes Mellitus. Diabetes Care 1997;20(7):1183–1197.

107. Greenland P, Grundy S, Pasternak RC, Lenfant C. Problems on the pathway from risk assessment to risk reduction. Circulation 1998;97(18):1761–1762.

108. Pearson TA, Peters TD. The treatment gap in coronary artery disease and heart failure: community standards and the post-discharge patient. Am J Cardiol 1997;80(8B):45H–52H.

109. Giles WH, Anda RF, Jones DH, Serdula MK, Merritt RK, DeStefano F. Recent trends in the identification and treatment of high blood cholesterol by physicians. Progress and missed opportunities. JAMA 1993;269(9):1133–1138.

110. Miller M, Konkel K, Fitzpatrick D, Burgan R, Vogel RA. Divergent reporting of coronary risk factors before coronary artery bypass surgery. Am J Cardiol 1995;75(10):736–737.

111. Low incidence of assessment and modification of risk factors in acute care patients at high risk for cardiovascular events, particularly among females and the elderly. The Clinical Quality Improvement Network (CQIN) Investigators. Am J Cardiol 1995;76(8):570–573.

112. Frame PS, Kowulich BA, Llewellyn AM. Improving physician compliance with a health maintenance protocol. J Fam Pract 1984;19(3):341–344.

113. Frolkis JP, Zyzanski SJ, Schwartz JM, Suhan PS. Physician noncompliance with the 1993 National Cholesterol Education Program (NCEP-ATPII) guidelines. Circulation 1998;98(9):851–855.

114. Cohen MV, Byrne MJ, Levine B, Gutowski T, Adelson R. Low rate of treatment of hypercholesterolemia by cardiologists in patients with suspected and proven coronary artery disease. Circulation 1991;83(4):1294–1304.

115. Campbell NC, Thain J, Deans HG, Ritchie LD, Rawles JM, Squair JL. Secondary prevention in coronary heart disease: baseline survey of provision in general practice. BMJ 1998;316(7142):1430–1434.

116. McCormick D, Gurwitz JH, Lessard D, Yarzebski J, Gore JM, Goldberg RJ. Use of aspirin, beta-blockers, and lipid-lowering medications before recurrent acute myocardial infarction: missed opportunities for prevention? Arch Intern Med 1999;159(6):561–567.

117. Schrott HG, Bittner V, Vittinghoff E, Herrington DM, Hulley S.et al. Adherence to National Cholesterol Education Program Treatment goals in postmenopausal women with heart disease. The Heart and Estrogen/Progestin Replacement Study (HERS). The HERS Research Group. JAMA 1997;277(16): 1281–1286.

118. Marcelino JJ, Feingold KR. Inadequate treatment with HMG-CoA reductase inhibitors by health care providers. Am J Med 1996;100(6):605–610.

119. Hoerger TJ, Bala MV, Bray JW, Wilcosky TC, LaRosa J. Treatment patterns and distribution of low-density lipoprotein cholesterol levels in treatment-eligible United States adults. Am J Cardiol 1998;82(1):61–65.

120. Ellerbeck EF, Jencks SF, Radford MJ, et al. Quality of care for Medicare patients with acute myocardial infarction. A four-state pilot study from the Cooperative Cardiovascular Project. JAMA 1995;273(19): 1509–1514.

121. Berlowitz DR, Ash AS, Hickey EC, et al. Inadequate management of blood pressure in a hypertensive population. N Engl J Med 1998;339(27):1957–1963.

122. Lloyd-Jones DM, Evans JC, Levy D. Hypertension in adults across the age spectrum: current outcomes and control in the community. JAMA 2005;294(4):466–472.

123. Hill, MN, Levine DM, Whelton PK. Awareness, use, and impact of the 1984 Joint National Committee consensus report on high blood pressure. Am J Public Health, 1988. 78(9):1190–1194.

124. Pearson TA, McBride PE, Miller NH, Smith SC. 27th Bethesda Conference: matching the intensity of risk factor management with the hazard for coronary disease events. Task Force 8. Organization of preventive cardiology service. J Am Coll Cardiol 1996;27(5):1039–1047.

125. Pommerenke FA, Weed DL. Physician compliance: improving skills in preventive medicine practices. Am Fam Physician 1991;43(2):560–568.

126. Lomas J, Anderson GM, Domnick-Pierre K, Vayda E, Enkin MW, Hannah WJ. Do practice guidelines guide practice? The effect of a consensus statement on the practice of physicians. N Engl J Med 1989;321(19):1306–1311.

127. Fix KN, Oberman A. Barriers to following National Cholesterol Educational Program guidelines. An appraisal of poor physician compliance. Arch Intern Med 1992;152(12):2385–2387.

128. McBride PE, Pacala JT, Dean J, Plane MB. Primary care residents and the management of hypercholesterolemia. Am J Prev Med 1990;6(2):71–76.

129. Heidenreich PA. Understanding and modifying physician behavior for prevention and management of cardiovascular disease. J Gen Intern Med 2003;18(12):1060–1061.

130. Tierney WM, Overhage JM, Murray MD, et al. Effects of computerized guidelines for managing heart disease in primary care. J Gen Intern Med 2003;18(12):967–976.

131. Ornstein S, Jenkins RG, Nietert PJ, et al. A multimethod quality improvement intervention to improve preventive cardiovascular care: a cluster randomized trial. Ann Intern Med 2004;141(7):523–532.

132. Derose SF, Dudl JR, Benson VM, Contreras R, Nakahiro RK, Ziel FH. Point-of-Service reminders for prescribing cardiovascular medications. Am J Manag Care 2005;11(5):298–304.

133. Schultz JS, O'Donnell JC, McDonough KL, Sasane R, Meyer J. Determinants of compliance with statin therapy and low-density lipoprotein cholesterol goal attainment in a managed care population. Am J Manag Care 2005;11(5):306–312.

134. Hill MN, Miller NH. Compliance enhancement. A call for multidisciplinary team approaches. Circulation 1996;93(1):4–6.

135. Sikand G, Kashyap ML, Yang I. Medical nutrition therapy lowers serum cholesterol and saves medication costs in men with hypercholesterolemia. J Am Diet Assoc 1998;98(8):889–894; quiz 895–896.

136. Shaffer J, Wexler LF. Reducing low-density lipoprotein cholesterol levels in an ambulatory care system. Results of a multidisciplinary collaborative practice lipid clinic compared with traditional physician-based care. Arch Intern Med 1995;155(21):2330–2335.

137. Haskell WL, Alderman EL, Fair JM, et al. Effects of intensive multiple risk factor reduction on coronary atherosclerosis and clinical cardiac events in men and women with coronary artery disease. The Stanford Coronary Risk Intervention Project (SCRIP). Circulation 1994;89(3):975–990.

138. Harris DE, Record NB, Gipson GW, Pearson TA. Lipid lowering in a multidisciplinary clinic compared with primary physician management. Am J Cardiol 1998;81(7):929–933.

139. Schectman G, Wolff N, Byrd JC, Hiatt JG, Hartz A. Physician extenders for cost-effective management of hypercholesterolemia. J Gen Intern Med 1996;11(5):277–286.

140. Schultz JF, Sheps SG. Management of patients with hypertension: a hypertension clinic model. Mayo Clin Proc 1994;69(10):997–999.

141. Reichgott MJ, Pearson S, Hill MN. The nurse practitioner's role in complex patient management: hypertension. J Natl Med Assoc 1983;75(12):1197–1204.

142. Weinberger M, Kirkman MS, Samsa GP, et al. A nurse-coordinated intervention for primary care patients with non-insulin-dependent diabetes mellitus: impact on glycemic control and health-related quality of life. J Gen Intern Med 1995;10(2):59–66.

143. Taylor CB, Houston-Miller N, Killen JD, DeBusk RF. Smoking cessation after acute myocardial infarction: effects of a nurse-managed intervention. Ann Intern Med 1990;113(2):118–123.

144. Taylor CB, Miller NH, Herman S, et al. A nurse-managed smoking cessation program for hospitalized smokers. Am J Public Health 1996;86(11):1557–1560.

145. Miller NH, Smith PM, DeBusk RF, Sobel DS, Taylor CB. Smoking cessation in hospitalized patients. Results of a randomized trial. Arch Intern Med 1997;157(4):409–415.

146. Lasater M. The effect of a nurse-managed CHF clinic on patient readmission and length of stay. Home Healthc Nurse 1996;14(5):351–356.

147. Blair TP, Bryant FJ, Bocuzzi S. Treating hyperlipidemia. J Cardiovasc Nurs 1988;5:55–57.

148. Bruce SL, Grove SK. The effect of a coronary artery risk evaluation program on serum lipid values and cardiovascular risk levels. Appl Nurs Res 1994;7(2):67–74.

149. Cofer LA. Aggressive cholesterol management: role of the lipid nurse specialist. Heart Lung 1997;26(5):337–344.

150. DeBusk RF, Miller NH, Superko HR. A case-management system for coronary risk factor modification after acute myocardial infarction. Ann Intern Med 1994;120(9):721–729.

151. Gerber J. Implementing quality assurance programs in multigroup practices for treating hypercholesterolemia in patients with coronary artery disease. Am J Cardiol 1997;80(8B):57H–61H.

152. Dunn PJ, Ryan MJ Jr, Hiebert M. Strategic and cost effective role for preventive cardiology. J Cardiovasc Manag 1998;9(6):13–20.

153. Dunn PJ, Superko HR, Halbrook M, Wilson S, Hiebert M. Setting up a preventive cardiology program in the real world. J Cardiovasc Manag 1998;9(2):16–21.

154. Tsuyuki RT, Johnson JA, Teo KK, et al. A randomized trial of the effect of community pharmacist intervention on cholesterol risk management: the Study of Cardiovascular Risk Intervention by Pharmacists (SCRIP). Arch Intern Med 2002;162:1149–1155.

155. Fonarow GC, Gawlinski A, Moughrabi S, et al. Improved treatment of coronary heart disease by implementation of a Cardiac Hospitalization Atherosclerosis Management Program (CHAMP). Am J Cardiol 2001;86:819–822.

INDEX

V

von Willebrand factor (vWF), function, 21
vWF, *see* von Willebrand factor

W

Weight control, *see* Obesity
Women, coronary artery disease,
  epidemiology, 217–219
  prevention,
    antioxidant therapy, 228, 229
    diet and weight loss, 227, 228
    exercise, 228
    hormone replacement therapy, 229–231
    lipid modification,
      primary prevention, 224, 225
      secondary prevention, 225–227

overview, 224
smoking cessation, 229
psychosocial aspects, 223
risk factors,
  diabetes mellitus, 220
  dyslipidemia, 219, 220
  hypertension, 220, 221
  menopause, 223, 224, 244
  obesity, 221, 222
  sedentary lifestyle, 222, 223
  smoking, 222

Z

Zyban®, *see* Bupropion